PSYCHOLOGY LIBRARY EDITIONS:
SOCIAL PSYCHOLOGY

Volume 1

THE SOCIAL PSYCHOLOGY OF THE CHILD WITH EPILEPSY

THE SOCIAL PSYCHOLOGY OF THE CHILD WITH EPILEPSY

CHRISTOPHER BAGLEY

Psychology Press
Taylor & Francis Group
LONDON AND NEW YORK

First published in 1971

This edition first published in 2015
by Psychology Press
27 Church Road, Hove BN3 2FA

and by Psychology Press
711 Third Avenue, New York, NY 10017

Psychology Press is an imprint of the Taylor & Francis Group, an informa business

British Library Cataloguing in Publication Data
A catalogue record for this book is available from the British Library

ISBN: 978-1-138-83092-9 (Set)
ISBN: 978-1-315-69455-9 (Set) (ebk)
ISBN: 978-1-138-84209-0 (Volume 1) (hbk)
ISBN: 978-1-138-84214-4 (Volume 1) (pbk)
ISBN: 978-1-315-73183-4 (Volume 1) (ebk)

Publisher's Note
The publisher has gone to great lengths to ensure the quality of this reprint but points out that some imperfections in the original copies may be apparent.

Disclaimer
The publisher has made every effort to trace copyright holders and would welcome correspondence from those they have been unable to trace.

The Social Psychology of the Child with Epilepsy

Christopher Bagley

London Routledge & Kegan Paul

First published 1971
by Routledge and Kegan Paul Ltd
Broadway House, 68-74 Carter Lane
London EC4V 5EL
Made and printed in Great Britain
by C. Tinling & Co. Ltd
London and Prescot

ISBN 0 7100 6941 3

Contents

Part three: Results and hypotheses

List of Tables

Foreword

Chronic handicaps, like diabetes, high blood pressure, are taking up an increasingly large proportion of the time and energy of many physicians, especially general practitioners. The special psychological and social problems of such patients are only now beginning to be widely studied. Such investigations involve techniques different from traditional medicine, and they require co-operative or team efforts by physicians, psychologists and others to get significant results.

Mr Bagley has chosen a topic that is especially difficult because the chief organ of adaptation to society—the central nervous system—is itself often functionally interfered with or frankly damaged by the conditions that also produce epileptic attacks. The disentangling of the numerous factors thus calls for considerable sophistication of approach. Mr Bagley has given a comprehensive critical review of past studies and his own investigation is a model of what should be done. This work is likely to be the standard reference for years—until in fact we know much more about the fundamental brain disturbances that are associated with epilepsy.

Desmond Pond,
Professor of Psychiatry,
The London Hospital

Preface

This work was begun when I was a research assistant to Dr Eliot Slater at the Institute of Neurology, University of London. The work was continued at the University of Essex, and completed at Sussex University. The bulk of the empirical analysis presented here was contained in an M.A. thesis of the University of Essex.

I am grateful to all those who have offered advice, encouragement and support during the research. In particular I am indebted to Peter Townsend, Margot Jeffreys, Michael Rutter, Carmi Schooler and William Watson. My wife compiled the index. Final responsibility for this study is, of course, my own. The study was made possible by a generous personal grant from the Nuffield Foundation.

Christopher Bagley,
Centre for Social Research,
University of Sussex

Part one
The problem, the sample and the study

1 The problem: a sociological perspective

The orientation of the present study is scientific: that is, its aim at the outset is to delineate an area of reality by means of an objective study. To what extent the inquiry has been successful the reader himself must decide. Although the study has been formally undertaken as a piece of sociological research, many of the terms and concepts employed are those more familiar to psychiatry and neurology than to sociology. This should not be taken to indicate any kind of partiality for one discipline or another. Indeed, one of the aims of the study has been to incorporate the study of social, psychological and biological variables in the same population, to see to what extent these various factors interact with one another in influencing behaviour in the population studied. To this extent the perspective of the study is socio-psychological.

The problems with which the study will deal are as follows:

1 To what extent have previous studies of epilepsy been carried out in an objective or scientific way, and to what extent have they provided definitive answers about the behaviour and intellect of the epileptic child?

2 To what extent are epileptic children psychiatrically disturbed, and what particular kinds of behaviour do they display?

3 To what extent are the psychiatric disorders endemically related to epilepsy?

4 To what extent are the psychiatric disorders related to brain damage which also causes epilepsy, rather than to epilepsy itself?

5 To what extent are the psychiatric disorders associated with factors within the child (e.g. previous personality) not related either to epilepsy, brain damage or other factors?

6 To what extent are the psychiatric disorders associated with social factors, such as a disturbed social environment, or disturbed relations with parents?

7 To what extent do these factors, if they exist, interact with one another to produce different kinds or degree of psychiatric disorder?
8 To what extent do intelligence quotients and intellectual attainments on standardized tests by the epileptic child differ from those of the normal population?
9 To what extent is the IQ and intellectual attainment associated (*a*) with kind and degree of psychiatric disorder; (*b*) type of epilepsy; (*c*) type of brain injury; (*d*) other factors, such as social environment?

Since one of the aims of the study is to provide clinicians with additional information about epileptic children that will be useful in the treatment of psychiatric disorder, the language and concepts used in finding answers to these problems will be primarily in terms familiar to those used by physicians.

In sociological language, the study is concerned with evaluating the quality of role behaviour in epileptic children and their parents, and the identification of the constraints on deviant role behaviour in the children. An implicit sociological purpose of the study is to provide some basis for attempting a systematic integration of the disciplines of sociology, psychology and human biology. As Runciman (1963) has pointed out, integration theory is still a major problem for social science:

> A significant advance has still to be made in the social sciences in the large, uncertain and difficult area where psychological factors interact or overlap with social. When our subject matter is people, their collective behaviour has to be explained by reference to factors both inside and outside of them . . . we need not only to understand the social forces acting on them (institutions, parties, economic conditions and so on) but also the psychological predispositions operating more, as it were, from within (oedipal jealousy, sibling rivalry, or even genetic predisposition). The problem which therefore confronts the social scientist is that of trying to formulate in a particular area of behaviour some general propositions about the conditions under which a proportional influence should be assigned to each type of variable.

The solution to the problem of integration theory implicit in the present study is to abstract a population of individuals from the larger social matrix and to study intensively the various factors—social, psychological and biological—which have bearing on the behaviour or social problem in question, and to study the *interaction* of these factors. The literature and problems of studying interaction are considered later in this study.

This type of approach has been advocated by some writers faced with complex clinical problems, although few systematic attempts seem to have been made to undertake such a study, which involves many complexities of organization and analysis. A model of such a study, using animal subjects, has been presented by Whimbey and Denenberg (1966), and the integrated approach has been advocated by Birch (1965), writing about brain-damaged children:

> To approach the problems meaningfully requires the pooled resources, skills, and techniques of, at the very least, such disciplines as neurology, psychology, physiology, psychiatry, education, epidemiology, sociology, pediatrics, and obstetrics. Working together, these disciplines can approach the questions of etiology, pathology, pathogenesis, and developmental interaction which emerge in any serious consideration of children with brain injury.

The present study, which uses measurements of psychiatrists, neurologists, social workers, psychologists, radiographers and electroencephalographers, is an attempt to use the kind of approach advocated by Birch and his colleagues.

2 The sample and the areas of investigation

As Pond (1952) has pointed out, any sample of epileptics derived from hospital or clinic sources will reflect the bias in selection of the hospital or clinic. A particular difficulty of many previous studies has been that their material has been selected at the outset on psychiatric grounds, so that the picture given of the behaviour of patients is by no means representative of epileptics as a whole. Ideally, a sample of epileptics in the general population should be gained. This procedure has many administrative and technical difficulties, and still may not locate those epileptics who, because of prejudice against their illness, take steps to conceal the fact that they have epilepsy. Gudmundsson's study (1966) of epileptics in Iceland is a good example of a general population study, in a country with a small and geographically discrete population where the organization of medical services made the inquiry possible.

The present study is of a sample of children seen in the neurological department of a teaching hospital. Only a very few of the children were referred to the hospital for psychiatric reasons. The sample may be expected to contain a higher proportion of children with neurological abnormalities than occur in epileptics as a whole.[1]

A record was made of all children aged 16 and under attending the hospital over a period of three years. In those cases in which a diagnosis of epilepsy uncomplicated by other physical abnormality (e.g. blindness, hemiplegia, etc.) was made by the neurologist, permission was sought from him to include the child in a research project studying the psychiatric aspects of epilepsy in children. When this permission was obtained, a letter was sent to the parents asking their co-operation in the research project.

[1] Cf. Pond (1952): 'Children referred to the Maudsley Hospital nearly always show some behaviour disorder, but lack gross neurological signs and symptoms.'

During this period 183 cases of epilepsy, uncomplicated by other physical abnormality, were diagnosed. Those children aged 15 and 16 who were working were not asked to take part in the study because of the time off work that this would involve. However, children of 15 and 16 who were still at school or had not yet found employment were included. Children aged 3 and under were not included. In a small number of cases the neurologist would not allow the child and his parents to be studied by the Psychiatric Department, and a number of parents declined to co-operate in the study. When the parent gave the difficulty of attending because of the time of appointment, a fresh appointment was given, so that a number of parents attended with their children on the second or third appointment. But a number of parents steadfastly refused to attend the hospital, while others gave no reason. Two parents specifically said that they thought that investigations would make the child's existing anxiety worse.

The final numbers studied, and the distribution of cases not seen are:

Neurologist would not give permission	9
Parents declined to attend	18
Child working, and not asked	24
Child aged 3 or under	3
Parents had moved	3
Parents attended hospital with child, but then declined to co-operate	8
Final number intensively investigated	118
Total number of epileptic children	183

Of the 144 parents asked to attend for investigation, 82 per cent or 118, finally did so.

The median age of the 118 children finally available for study was 14.0 years. Seventy-nine of the children were aged between 12 and 16. This bias towards the upper age groups in childhood epilepsy is an artefact of the referral policy of the hospital. Generally, though not always, epileptic children in the catchment area aged under 12 were seen at a pediatric hospital.

A further bias in the material is that the children are more likely than those referred to a psychiatric hospital to contain cases which are atypical, from a neurological point of view, or in whom the epilepsy proved intractable to the treatment given by the general practitioner. Very few of the children were referred to the hospital on psychiatric grounds. The sample may thus be expected to contain fewer children with psychiatric abnormalities than children at a psychiatric hospital, unless there is some connection of behaviour disorder with neurological abnormality in epilepsy, or with epilepsy which is resistant to treatment.

The occupation of the supporting parent was classified according to the Registrar General's Classification of Occupations (1961), and compared with the frequency expected, as indicated by the Registrar General's Tables for London for the 1961 Census. The results are given in Table 1.

Table 1 Social class distribution in 118 epileptic children

Social class	*Number of children*	%	*Frequency expected*	%
I and II	31	26·3	21	17·8
III	68	57·6	63	53·4
IV and V	19	16·1	34	28·8

Class I, professional and managerial: II, intermediate business and professional; III, clerical, and skilled workers; IV, semi-skilled; V, unskilled.
Overall distribution: $\chi^2 = 6{\cdot}27$, 2 d.f., P less than 0·05, greater than 0·02.

It will be seen that there is a bias in the series for children to come from parents in upper social classes, with a dearth of children coming from the lower social classes.

This bias might have been due to the selection procedure. For example, selecting only those children aged 15 or 16 who are still at school, or not working, and rejecting those who are working, might mean that the older children thus selected over-represent the upper social classes. This hypothesis was tested by comparing the social class distribution of children aged 15 and 16 with the rest of the children in the series. The results are given in Table 2.

Table 2 Social class of epileptic children by age

Social class	*Children under 15*	%	*Children aged 15 and 16*	%	*Total number*
I and II	27	28·4	4	17·4	31
III	55	57·9	13	56·5	68
IV and V	13	13·6	6	26·1	19
Totals	95	—	23	—	118

$\chi^2 = 2{\cdot}04$, 2 d.f., P less than 0·5, greater than 0·3.

There is in fact a non-significant trend for children aged 15 and 16 to be over-represented amongst the *lower* social classes. An examination of these older children shows that they were predominantly those who had not yet found work, rather than those still at school.

A possible source of the bias towards the upper social classes lies in the fact that those parents who declined to co-operate in the study might be more heavily weighted to the working classes. Of the eight parents who attended the hospital, but from whom it was not possible to obtain a full range of information, in five the social class is known: one from social class II; two from social class III; one from social class IV; and one from social class V.

The medical notes of the remaining 18 cases in which the parents declined to attend were consulted. These did not give any clue as to psychiatric condition or social class, except to indicate that the majority of these parents lived in the prosperous suburbs of north-west London. However, this fact in itself is not an indicator of social class. In two of these 18 cases, the stated reason for not attending was the belief that an extensive investigation would increase the child's anxiety about his epilepsy. In two further cases parents gave as the reason for not attending the fact that their child was studying for examinations.

The medical notes of the eight cases in which the neurologist would not give permission for a psychiatric investigation indicated that pathological factors were probably present in all of the seven sets of parents involved (two of these cases were sisters). In this latter case, the neurologist described the mother of these two girls as 'an extremely tense and excitable person given to fits of depression and despair'. In a further case, the mother's anxiety was said to accentuate the boy's fear of his attacks. In another case 'the mother was very agitated and had known someone who was epileptic and eventually committed suicide'. An 11-year-old boy was said to be in 'a morose and depressed state'. The neurologist considered that in this case the boy's father should not be told that his son had epilepsy. In another case the parents of the child were both deaf and dumb; the child also had an epileptic sibling.

It is clear from an examination of the medical notes that the neurologist thought that an extensive psychiatric investigation of the parents would tend to make worse the attitude of the child, or his parents, or both, towards epilepsy. It thus seems that these excluded cases mean that the present study will slightly underestimate the extent of parental anxiety, and possibly of behaviour disorder or anxiety in the child.

With regard to the social class bias in the series, the following conclusions can be drawn:

a This bias is not an artefact of selecting only those aged 15 and 16 who were not working.
b It is technically possible that the 18 cases who declined to co-operate could have created this bias; however, various impressionistic pieces of evidence tend to suggest these parents may not be predominantly working class.
A further bias in the series is that the cases excluded because of non-co-operation by parents, or at the request of the neurologist, may contain a high proportion of children with behaviour disorders.

In summary, the biases in the present material are as follows:

1 The cases studied can be expected to contain a higher proportion of cases with neurological abnormalities and of cases with uncontrolled epilepsy.

2 Cases in which epilepsy is associated with another clinically identifiable neurological condition (e.g. hemiplegia) have been excluded. In this respect, low intelligence has not been treated as a neurological entity, so that cases in which epilepsy and low intelligence are both apparent have been included.

3 The series is biased towards children aged between 12 and 14. Children under this age tended to be seen elsewhere, and only that proportion (23/47) of those aged 15 and 16 who were not working were seen. Children aged three and under were excluded.

4 The material is biased towards the upper social classes. This means either that epilepsy occurs with greater frequency in the children of parents in these classes (which seems unlikely) or that this bias is an artefact of referral policy, or of biases in selection.[1]

The investigation of the children and their parents

On attending the hospital, the child was examined by a child psychiatrist, who carried out a psychiatric examination and obtained a number of anthropometric measurements. During this time the parent or parents were subjected to a lengthy and systematic interview by a psychiatric social worker. The child then saw the clinical psychologist for testing, and attended the X-ray department for bone-age photography of hand and wrist. The parents were also interviewed by the psychiatrist, who completed a standard psychiatric schedule for the child's development and home background. Sometimes this rather lengthy procedure had to be spread over two sessions. With the parents' permission, a questionnaire was sent to the child's school. Where the child had been delivered in hospital, information about this was sought from the hospital involved.

[1] The variable of social class will be discussed further in a later section.

The organization of the present study

In later chapters an analysis relating to the behaviour and environment of the children, the attitudes of their parents, the manifestations and frequency of their fits, the existence of brain damage, the type of epilepsy, the intelligence and attainment and physical and developmental data will be made.

In the chapters which immediately follow a review of studies about psychiatric and social aspects of epilepsy in adolescents and children has been undertaken, in order to provide a background for the later chapters.

A note on the analysis of data

Much of the data analysed in this study has a qualitative basis, so that the assumption of normal distribution cannot usually be made. For this reason, the most powerful of significance tests, the '*t*-test' ('power' being the ability to reject the null hypothesis when it is, in fact, false) is used only occasionally.

The majority of tests used in this study are non-parametric statistical tests, which do not require that the data shall be distributed normally. Two non-parametric tests are used in this study—the χ^2 test, which is useful for data in nominal categories (i.e. categories that cannot be ranked) and the Kolmogorov-Smirnov one-tailed test. This test, described by Siegel (1956, pp. 127–36) is one of the most powerful of the non-parametric tests, and can be used for data which can be ranked.

Fisher's exact test is used for nominal data where N is less than 20; occasionally the median test is used (Siegel, 1956, pp. 111–16), in which the data for two variables are divided into four cells, according to the variation of the cases in question about the median for the whole series, and the result tested by χ^2.

Parametric versus non-parametric statistics

Since the analysis of data was undertaken, largely by hand and using non-parametric statistical tests, a debate has emerged in the literature about the usefulness of making assumptions about the normal distribution and equal interval distribution of measures (i.e. assuming that in a 1, 2, 3 measurement that 2 is twice as great as 1, and 3 is three times as great as 1). For example, in the present study we have used the numbers 0, 1, 2 and 3 to indicate the degree to which a symptom, such as 'stealing', is present; the numerical categories related to the verbal categories of 'never', 'some sign', 'definite sign', 'marked'. Now, we cannot assume that the number 1 ('some sign') is twice as great as the number 0 ('never'). The numbers are merely a convenient shorthand for the verbal categories. They do, however, indicate a definite rank order. We can assume, both numerically and verbally, that 3 is greater than 2, that 2 is greater than 1, and that 1 is greater than 0. This assumption of ranking is most important, since many of the non-parametric tests in this study make such an assumption.

The debate on the use of parametric statistics with non-parametric data was initiated by Labovitz (1967). He argued that (1) non-parametric statistics are relatively insensitive; (2) the error resulting from assigning numbers to ordinal data, and treating these numbers as if they met parametric assumptions, is very small; (3) parametric statistical tests have high power-efficiency (i.e. have a high probability of rejecting the null hypothesis when it is in fact false, and vice versa). Labovitz provides some examples to support this argument.

Champion (1968) countered Labovitz's argument with the suggestion that

> While we strive to be as 'scientific' as possible in our analyses of social phenomena, we do ourselves a great disservice when we allow ourselves to treat data as something which they are not. . . . How can we hope to be scientists when we knowingly violate assumptions regarding statistical usage?

In reply to Champion in the same issue of *Social Forces*, Labovitz again placed emphasis on the argument of the utility of parametric measures, and cited another instance where parametric measures had produced a result that was similar to that obtained from the use of the statistically pure non-parametric technique. Since means and standard deviations can be calculated with parametric statistics, this opens the way to further complex analyses which statistics based on ordinal and ranked measures cannot undertake.

Cohen (1968) has produced further arguments in favour of the use of parametric techniques with various kinds of 'soft' data.

In the present study we have maintained the purist assumptions urged by Siegel and Champion. However, we have also undertaken a parametric analysis (product moment correlations and factor analysis) of the data, and the results of this last exercise are given in Ch. 28. These results are extremely interesting, and firmly support the non-parametric analyses. They also offer fresh information on the possible existence of significant sub-groups within the main trends identified in the non-parametric analysis. But we cannot say for certain how important these results are, because the analysis necessarily ignored the non-parametric and the largely 'soft' nature of the data.

Part two
Studies of epilepsy

3 Epilepsy: definitions, incidence, causes and treatment

The review of literature

Throughout this study the epileptic child is treated phenomenologically as a *child*, as an *epileptic* child, and as a child who has often suffered *brain damage*. For this reason, a number of studies of behaviour in children will be considered, as well as studies of the behaviour of brain-damaged children, on the grounds that these studies may have relevance for the investigation of the epileptic child.

The literature on the subject during the past twenty years has been considered in a little detail. The literature on the subject before 1947 is much less frequent, and is considered only in summary form. The year 1947 heralds the period described by Guerrant and his colleagues (1962) as 'The Period of Psychomotor Peculiarity' in the study of epilepsy. Guerrant *et al.* describe three other periods in the history of the psychiatric study of epilepsy: 'The Period of Epileptic Deterioration (up to 1900)', 'The Period of the Epileptic Character (1900–30)', and 'The Period of Normality (1930–47)'.

Although this study is concerned with epileptic children and adolescents, many of the studies which are principally concerned with epileptic adults are of relevance to it, since (*a*) in the majority of epileptics the illness has its onset before the age of 14, and in a very large majority of cases the illness appears in the first two decades of life (Gudmundsson, 1966); (*b*) the period of middle and late adolescence overlaps with the age group which studies of epilepsy in adults often consider; (*c*) medical attitudes about epilepsy may tend to apply to the condition at all age levels.

A punched card bibliographic system has been used to collate studies in this area. The areas to which a paper refers, an abstract of the contents, and the source of the paper have been recorded on 124-holed punched cards. These cards have been arranged in the following systems: Epilepsy in Children; Epilepsy in Adults; Child

Psychiatry; Epilepsy and Psychosis; Anti convulsants. The maintenance of these card systems has been undertaken as an exercise in itself, so that the card systems contain much more literature than is included in the present review. The literature on epilepsy and psychosis, and on anti convulsants, has been considered in separate studies (Craske *et al.*, 1970; Davison and Bagley, 1969), although the conclusions of the review of literature on epilepsy and psychosis are drawn upon in a later chapter.

The definition, classification and general problem of epilepsy

'Epilepsy', said Banay (1961)

> is one of the persistent enigmas of medicine. Its wide-ranging symptomatology, which is a manifestation rather than an entity of disease, continues to engage the labours of investigation. In spite of advancing knowledge of the epileptic phenomena and brain pathology, as well as psychochemical action in the brain, the accumulated findings tend to consist largely of description rather than definition. After some twenty-four centuries of what the ancients called 'the sacred disease' and Hippocrates recorded as 'falling sickness', conclusive elucidation of this pathology lingers on as an item on the agenda of biological sciences for future disposal.

The neurologist Lord Brain defined epilepsy (1951) as ' . . . a paroxysmal and transitory disturbance of the function of the brain which develops suddenly, ceases spontaneously, and exhibits a conspicuous tendency to recur'.

In common terms, epilepsy is marked by sudden attacks, in which the patient loses concentration or consciousness for a long or short period, and may display violent movements of parts of the body (e.g. arms and legs). These attacks occur with little or no warning, and may occur during any activity of the patient.

Mayer-Gross, Slater and Roth (1955), in a standard textbook of psychiatry, give an overview of the general problem:

> Epileptic seizures are a common event in many forms of psychiatric illness. They are frequent and sometimes diagnostically significant in certain organic cerebral diseases . . . they also may complicate symptomatic psychoses and chemical intoxications and constitute an important item in the practice of child psychiatry. . . . The disturbance [of epilepsy] may be very localized and be shown, for instance, in the twitching of a single muscle group or in a single sensory experience in one of the special senses. In such cases there is often no general alteration of consciousness; these cases of focal

> epilepsy are the subject matter of neurology rather than psychiatry. Disturbance of brain function may, however, be general; and may then be of any degree. At one extreme there is total loss of consciousness, which may last from a fraction of a second to many minutes; at the other extreme there may be only a slight impairment in the power of attention, or a minor mood change. (p. 365)

These authors continue (p. 366):

> The essential quality of an epileptic manifestation is the occurrence of *spontaneous neuronic excitation* at some focus. . . . This local discharge may spread and ultimately produce excitation of the subcortical centres concerned in the production of the *generalized electrical disturbances of the brain.* . . . The nature of the appearance and spread of an epileptic discharge in the central nervous system appears to be intimately related to changes of a chemical and electrical nature at the cell membranes. . . . It is characteristic of epilepsy that the spread of electrical activation occurs otherwise than along the neuronic pathways involved in physiological responses, so that the events which follow have a disorderly and catastrophic character.

The significance of this description of the underlying neurological process of epilepsy may be clarified by a comparison with the normal pattern of activity of neurons (i.e. nerve cells, of which there are between 15 and 20 million in the nervous system). This account is taken from Bowsher's *Introduction to Neuroanatomy* (1961).

Attached to the nerve cell are a variable number of branching processes called 'dendrites'. The area over which the dendrites of a single nerve cell extend is called the dendritic field of that cell. In addition to the dendrites, each cell possesses a single process called the 'axon' or 'nerve fibre'. This may vary in length from less than a millimetre to over a yard. The axon may remain within the C.N.S. (central nervous system) or pass out into a peripheral nerve:

> The nerve cell and all its processes is called the neurone, and each neurone is a self-contained and independent unit. The neurone doctrine teaches that the nervous impulse is generated within the nerve cell, travels away from the cell body along the axon and its branches until it reaches the terminal button . . . this button terminal is in contact with the body of another nerve cell, a junction called the synapse. Here the nervous impulse jumps the [potential] synaptic gap to attain the cell body or centripetally-conducting dendrite of a second neurone, in which a new nervous impulse may or may not be set up . . .

Epilepsy, as described above, involved the spontaneous pathological production of a nervous impulse. This may lead to a chaotic discharge of nervous impulses between neurons, leading in turn, through the production of generalized electrical disturbances, to disco-ordination of consciousness and motor activity.

This account of the neuro-physiology of epilepsy is inevitably simplified and obscures much of the complicated process involved, but it may serve to provide a background to the rest of the study, which is principally concerned with the 'external' and, more particularly, the behavioural aspects of epilepsy.

There has been dispute and debate in recent years on the classification of types of epilepsy. Earlier writers (e.g. Page, 1947) divided epilepsy into *grand mal* (major fits); *petit mal* (minor absences); psychomotor (with some psychic features); and Jacksonian epilepsy (motor automatisms arising from a highly localized focus). This ui d of classification is still used by many writers in the clinical field. Beard (1963), for example, used a rather similar classification: *grand mal* without aura (i.e. without subjective feelings or sensations preceding the attack); *petit mal*; focal epilepsy originating in the temporal lobe; focal epilepsy originating in other sites on the brain. 'Focal' in this sense means having a localized origin, in a limited area of the brain. The psychomotor attacks usually have their origin in a temporal lobe focus, although they can originate from a focus elsewhere (Livingston, 1954). *Grand mal* attacks are characterized by total loss of consciousness and muscular spasms of arms and legs. *Petit mal* is characterized by a very short spell of unconsciousness, without motor involvement. Psychomotor seizures involve various combinations of aura and motor automatisms. They are discussed more fully in the chapter on temporal lobe epilepsy.

Whitty (1956) has laid stress on the diagnostic distinction between epilepsy which is symptomatic of some underlying cause (e.g. organic brain injury and disease) and that which is idiopathic, or cryptogenic. In this latter type no organic cause can be established, although a family history of epilepsy may be present, suggesting the possible genetic transmission of the disease.

The role of genetics in transmitting epilepsy is not clear, although a heavier incidence of epilepsy in the relatives of epileptics than in the normal population has consistently been shown. The evidence on this point is summarized by Lennox and Lennox (1960), who show that even in symptomatic epilepsy, in which a precipitating organic factor for the disease can be shown, a hereditary factor for epilepsy is sometimes present. They suggest that the actual emergence of epilepsy is due to 'a conspiracy of causes'. The study by Rodin and Gonzalez (1966) has confirmed that psychomotor epilepsy, which by definition involves an organic, focal disturbance that is acquired through an injury to the brain, has a strong hereditary component. Ounsted *et al.* (1966), who reported a similar finding, suggest that what may happen is that patients with hereditary epilepsy who suffer major fits early in life, or a series of major fits without recovery of consciousness in between the fits (*status epilepticus*) *acquire* damage to the temporal lobe, so that their later epilepsy is of the psychomotor type.

Masland (1960) reviewed the various classificatory schemes for epilepsy, and proposes a scheme dividing epilepsy into three major types, taking into account the anatomical location, the aetiology, the symptoms and the degree of disturbance of motor function of the epilepsy:

	Anatomy	*Aetiology*	*Symptom*
I. Centrencephalic	Brain as a whole	Unknown or ? genetic	(*a*) GM, (*b*) PM
II. Focal	Focal	Varied	Varied partial seizures
III. Unlocalized	*a* Known cause *b* Unknown cause	Varied	GM

GM=*grand mal*; PM=*petit mal.*

Gastaut (1964) proposed an international classification of epileptic seizures which bears some similarities to Masland's in that it proposes a major classificatory division between general and partial seizures. The partial seizures in this classification are divided into localized partial seizures and unilateral seizures, expressed predominantly on one side of the body. This latter type occurs 'almost exclusively in very young children'.

A further kind of classification is by a detailed analysis of the motor manifestations of the seizure, such as that made by Merritt (1959). Other writers classify epilepsy by the manifestations of the electrical activity of the brain, which have predictive value for the type of seizure. Vislie *et al.* (1958) classify epilepsy by five EEG (electroencephalographic) types: (1) within normal limits; (2) some abnormal features, but not predictive of epilepsy or localizing for brain damage; (3) a markedly abnormal EEG predictive of epilepsy, without focal or localizing features; (4) EEG focal in the temporal lobes; (5) EEG focal elsewhere. ('Predictive' indicates that any individual with this kind of EEG is likely also to have epilepsy.)

The usefulness of the EEG in studying epilepsy is discussed in detail in a later chapter.

The incidence of epilepsy

Brewis *et al.* (1966), who reviewed reports of the incidence of epilepsy, reported that accurate estimates of incidence were scarce because of the disagreement on how long an individual should be free of seizures, or how many seizures he should have, before the classification of epilepsy should be made. A further problem is that of legal discrimination and social prejudice, which makes the patient tend to conceal his illness, if he can. Brewis and his colleagues, studying the incidence of neurological disease in an English city (Carlisle) defined epilepsy as the occurrence of more than one epileptic-like attack, excluding febrile convulsions (associated with high temperature, and occurring before the age of 2), however long ago that attack occurred. By this definition, the lifetime incidence of epilepsy was found to be 0·55 per cent. Gudmundsson (1966) reviewed English, American, and Scandinavian studies of incidence, and reported rates varying from 0·3 per cent to 0·9 per cent.

In the large majority of epileptics the illness has its onset during the first two decades of life (Gudmundsson, 1966). Because of this, the incidence of epilepsy in children is greater than that in the population as a whole. Lennox and Lennox (1960) give an estimate of about 1 per cent for the incidence of childhood epilepsy. Epilepsy having an onset in later life is often accompanied by an underlying brain pathology, such as cerebral tumour (Pond and Bidwell, 1960).

Causes of epilepsy

As has been indicated above, epilepsy involves a malfunction of the normal activity of the brain. The studies of heredity in epileptic patients suggest that heredity can be a contributory or possibly a sole cause of epilepsy,[1] though often in combination with physiological or emotional stress. Illness or injury of the brain (e.g. birth injury, or encephalitis) can cause or precipitate epilepsy. The evidence on these points is summarized by the WHO (1957) and Lennox and Lennox (1960). Gudmundsson (1966), in an epidemiological study of 987 epileptics in the general population of Iceland, showed that early brain trauma was associated with a significantly earlier onset of epilepsy than in patients with an unknown cause; and the brain damage cases were significantly more likely to be male than female. Many studies, like Gudmundsson's, have shown a higher incidence of epilepsy in males than in females. This subject will be discussed later in this study, and some hypotheses tested.

[1] Recent work on this subject (Gastaut *et al.*, 1969) suggests that what is genetic is not epilepsy itself, but a 'convulsive predisposition' which acts in conjunction with other factors to produce epilepsy as such.

Treatment of epilepsy

Epilepsy is treated mainly (Lennox and Lennox, 1960) by drugs, of which many kinds exist. The chemical composition of these anticonvulsants is diverse, but Reynolds (1967) has suggested that a common effect of anticonvulsants, which may account for their success in controlling epilepsy, is the ability to suppress the body's levels of folic acid and/or vitamin B_{12}. In America the ketogenic diet is sometimes used for the treatment of epilepsy. This consists of a diet simulating the metabolic activity of the body during the early stages of fasting. The success of this kind of diet of controlling fits may have a metabolic link with the activity of anticonvulsants. The third treatment of epilepsy is by surgery, in those cases where a focal injury or scar of the brain is thought to be the cause of the epilepsy.

There is some evidence, summarized by the Lennoxes, that both emotional and physiological stress can precipitate convulsions, and for this reason physicians often advise the patient to seek an environment which will minimize this kind of stress. This kind of advice, however, may in the long run be dysfunctional (Szasz, 1966) if it leads to the permanent 'colonization' of the patient.

4 The electroencephalograph

Studies appearing after 1947 make frequent references to the results of electroencephalography of epileptic patients, a feature largely absent in the pre-1947 studies. This chapter is intended to place the encephalograph in critical perspective.

Electroencephalography (EEG)—the measurement of electrical activity within the brain—was pioneered in Germany in the late 1920s. Sensitive 'leads' are attached to the scalp, in the frontal, central, parietal, temporal, occipital and mastoid process areas, on each side of the head. When the patient is at rest, or asleep, abnormal rhythms may appear. These rhythms may also be induced by 'over-breathing', or photic stimulation.

The electrical activity from each lead is recorded on a graph, and is in the form of 'swoops', which appear on the graph as variations of a wavy line. The height of the swoops (or 'oscillating potentials', as Glaser (1963) calls them) is determined by the voltage of the underlying activity. Each swoop occurs with a varying frequency per second, and various combinations of frequencies and voltage types are seen.

Livingston (1954), in a textbook on the diagnosis of convulsive disorders in children, defines six types of abnormality seen in EEG records: (*a*) abnormally slow activity, seen in epilepsy, brain tumour, hypoglycaemia, migraine, possibly some types of behaviour disorder, cerebral oedema, and with increased intracranial pressure. The younger the child, the more difficult it is to judge, because of the greater possible variability in the EEG, whether or not a record is abnormal. (*b*) Abnormally fast activity (over 14 cycles per second). Sharp bursts of high voltage, fast waves usually indicate a convulsive type of activity, especially that associated with major epileptic attacks. (*c*) Amplitude asymmetry—a rather rare abnormality, and not often associated with neurological abnormality in children, though it can be associated with a one-sided cerebral disturbance. (*d*) Spikes and sharp waves are seen quite often in the interseizure records of children with major epilepsy. This record is quite common, too, in psychomotor epilepsy.[1] (*e*) Spike-and-wave forms are seen in epilepsy, and rarely elsewhere. The most typical spike-and-wave form is that occurring three times a second—a neat symmetrical pattern, from all leads, and associated with *petit mal* epilepsy. (*f*) Focal abnormalities, indicating that abnormal electrical activity (abnormally slow or fast waves, spikes, and spike and wave forms) originates in a particular area of the brain.

The judgment as to what kind of record the EEG record represents is made by the electroencephalographer. This judgment is made on the basis of the electroencephalographer's experience and powers of judgment. Usually, the recordist has other clinical details about the patient to hand, and will make a judgment about the plausibility of a particular diagnosis in the light of this and other information about the patient.

Blum (1954) has criticized the reliability of electroencephalographic judgments. He took the EEGs of 10 adult patients routinely referred for the investigation of possible pathology of the central nervous system, and asked five electroencephalographers to read the records, without having knowledge about any other clinical attributes of the patients. In only 4 of the 10 records was there complete agreement on indicators of organic pathology: in 3 in 10 records there was complete agreement for cerebral localization; and in only 1 in 10 complete agreement for both cerebral localization and organic pathology.

Hill (1956) suggests that in psychiatry the EEG cannot provide any 'grand answers' about mental functioning, but must be used to answer specific and perhaps limited questions about the cerebral functioning of particular patients. The same author (1958) suggests that the EEG should be used (1) for the location of a neuronal area in which epilepsy originates—that is, to establish the presence or absence of focal epilepsy—and (2) to decide what the nature of the pathological process underlying epilepsy is. These two uses are termed 'topographic' and 'aetiological'. The EEG only has a limited role in answering the second question. Hill stresses that the use of the EEG to decide whether symptoms are epileptic or psychogenic in origin is an abuse of the electroencephalographic technique, and provides only the most inconclusive evidence.

Pond (1957) has expressed a similar point of view, suggesting that

[1] Epilepsy having a focal origin, usually in the temporal lobe, and affecting the sensory motor system. The attack may therefore be accompanied by 'feelings of familiarity, strangeness or depersonalization and . . . complex visual and auditory hallucinations . . . ' (Mayer-Gross *et al.*, 1955, p.379).

the hypothesis that conditions such as temper tantrums are 'epileptic equivalents' merely confuses the task of trying to elucidate the behaviour disorders associated with epilepsy. The EEG cannot, he urges, provide reasonable evidence that behaviour manifested at some time in the past was an equivalent to epilepsy. The hypothesis that *during* the disturbed behaviour the patient was undergoing an equivalent of an epileptic attack is completely untenable. The only EEG evidence that can be considered is that taken during the disturbed behaviour itself, and evidence of this kind is extremely rare. Even this does not prove that behaviour was an epileptic equivalent.

Aird (1959) suggests that the role of the EEG in diagnosing epilepsy is itself limited, and should be used as a clinical tool for elucidating those neurophysiological mechanisms which vary greatly with each epileptic. Beard, however, (1963), suggested that the EEG was a bettei diagnostic indicator of epilepsy than clinical factors. Nuffield (1961), in a study of 236 epileptic children, found that the EEG diagnosis had greater predictive quality than diagnosis based on fit pattern, in terms of the scatter of behavioural scores. This led him to suggest that the EEG was the most reliable categorizer of epilepsy.

B. Tizard (1962), reviewing the methodology of studies of personality in epilepsy criticized the EEG studies on the grounds that

> . . . . no study shows an adequate appreciation of the problems of bias and reliability in the judgments made. Precautions are not reported to prevent contamination of EEG interpretation by clinical data and the reliability of the EEG and clinical diagnoses is not assessed.

The validity of studies of epilepsy, she suggested, wuuld be increased if the individual making the assessment of the EEG had no knowledge of the patient's psychiatric status, or of other clinical data which might bias his judgment.

Bingel (1967) found that the first 200 records judged by an encephalographer are liable to error. The incidence of errors is reduced with experience—but errors can still occur.

It is clear, from these studies, that the electroencephalograph can be a useful tool for classifying epilepsy, but the interpretation of factors associated with the EEG must proceed with extreme care: the reliability of the EEG must be considered in each study, and statements about cause based on the associations of the EEG should be avoided. The chain of reasoning: A has epilepsy, and an *x*-type EEG; B has disturbed behaviour, but no epilepsy. He has, however, an x-type EEG and therefore his disturbed behaviour is an epileptic equivalent—is without logical validity.

Further discussion on the use of EEG records in studying epilepsy will be made in the sections on 'Temporal Lobe Epilepsy' and 'Epileptic Equivalents', pp. 53–70 and 71–7.

5 Psychiatric aspects of epilepsy since 1947

The pre-1947 studies

The scientific studies of epilepsy before 1947—if we can grace them with the name 'scientific'—gave epilepsy a bad press. The methods they used left much to be desired. Epilepsy itself was poorly and over-inclusively defined in many studies, as were the supposedly resulting behaviour and personality traits. The source of the population studied was not often specified. The actual incidence of the alleged behaviour in epileptics was rarely presented in any statistical form. A common feature of such studies was to associate epilepsy with a wide range of adverse traits, the evidence being either the authors' impressions of unspecified epileptic populations or the accretion of previous opinions. The fallacies of inferring 'this or these epileptics are antisocial; therefore all epileptics are antisocial' and 'this behaviour followed epilepsy, and was therefore caused by it', are common.

The kinds of study to which we are referring (e.g. Clark, 1917; Wiersma, 1923; Baker and Traphagen, 1936; Fenichel, 1945) suggested that epileptics, both children and adults, presented a very wide range of abnormal and anti-social behaviour, including crime. These traits were related to an epileptic constitution of a biological kind. Another kind of study, with equally poor methology, was based on psychoanalytical formulations. But the conclusions were rather similar to those of the physicians who laid so much stress on an inherent, anti-social 'epileptic personality'. These psychoanalytical studies asserted that the epileptic possesses primitive and aggressive drives whose repression causes epileptic fits.

A small number of studies, especially after 1930, came to the conclusion that the 'epileptic constitution' was basically normal, and that behaviour disorders seen in epilepsy were the result of adverse reactions of people in the epileptic's environment. A special proponent of this view was Bridge (1934), who, like earlier writers, relied on the case history method: but in a more comprehensive study (1949) Bridge put his theories to a systematic test.

Studies of psychiatric aspects of epilepsy since 1947

Jensen (1947), describing a series of 22 epileptic children, stressed the importance of emotional factors in precipitating fits. In 4 of the cases a parent also had epilepsy, and 3 of the mothers experienced pregnancy and birth difficulties. Ten of the children came from broken homes, while in another 10 there was discernible tension in the home. Intensive sibling rivalry existed in 11 of the patients. Jensen stresses the interaction of a number of factors—genetic, neurological and psychological, which act together in precipitating fits.

Carter (1947) studied children's expressed attitudes toward their epilepsy, a field in which very little woik has been done. He categorized the responses of 165 children to their epilepsy into eight groups:

1 The child reports the epilepsy in matter-of-fact way as if the fact of occurrence of 'turns' had no particular emotional significance for him.

2 The child is very worried and concerned about the epilepsy, reflecting gross anxiety in his parents. His attitude is one of hopelessness, and he fears he may die during an attack.

3 The child confines his expressed attitudes to the aura which precede the attack.

4 Many children were concerned with the etiology of their condition. Some of their utterances were repetitious of adults' wisdom, but others reflected spontaneous preoccupation.

5 Some of the children expressed anxiety about the effect of their condition upon others.

6 Many of the children voiced the complaint that their condition, and more particularly the overprotective attitude of others (both parents and school) toward their condition, prevented them from living a normal life. An 8-year-old girl said, 'I don't have anyone to play with me. I'm not allowed to run or anything in case I have another one [attack].'

7 Several children expressed resentment over the fact that they had been accused of 'putting on the spells' or of making themselves have spells.

8 Some children expressed complete or partial ignorance of their condition.

Carter concluded:

> The epileptic child should be regarded as something more than a convulsion with a positive electroencephalogram who makes a response of some type to the latest medication. He should be

> viewed as an individual who is struggling with an important problem. He should be given opportunities to express his attitudes towards that problem, and these attitudes should be taken into consideration by his physician in dealing with him, his parents and his environment.

Davidoff (1947) categorized children in colonies for epileptics into five types:

1 The uncomplicated epileptic.

2 The mildly handicapped, e.g. with physical or mild emotional problems.

3 The emotional child—with neurotic or personality disorder.

4 The anti-social, aggressive child.

5 The defective child, of very low intelligence.

Excluding the last category, this classification is rather similar to that suggested by Turner in 1927. The problem of the classification of behaviour, in children and in epileptic children, will be discussed in detail later in this book.

Bradley (1947) presented an impressionistic review of the four major types of problem encountered in a series of 200 epileptic children:

1 Because of the danger of fits, the child has often been excluded from the activity of other children.

2 He is very apt to have certain personality characteristics which appear directly linked to his convulsive tendencies. Particularly noticeable among these are variability in mood, hypermotility, impulsiveness, short wandering attention-span, vacillations in ability to recall material which has previously been learned everything else being equal, more difficult in arithmetic than in other school subjects. These traits have been observed in children with electroencephalographic tracings characteristic of convulsive disorders even when seizures themselves have not occurred, which suggests that they are symptoms of the same type of disturbance which produce convulsions. They are much more constant than the secondary symptoms about to be mentioned.

3 Any child who has repeated seizures, and over-solicitous or over-protective care, with exclusion from the company of other children, will inevitably develop distorted emotional attitudes toward life. 'It is helpful to think of these attitudes as symptoms which are secondary to the convulsive disorder itself and the personality characteristic more directly linked to it as mentioned in (2).'

4 As with most children's problems, parents and family naturally tend to adopt attitudes or actions which, because of the dramatic nature of a convulsive disorder, vary from the objective, constructive

outlook of parents which is considered most helpful to the growing child.

The model for studying the epileptic child which Bradley implicitly presents has two major components—the 'innate' effects of epilepsy or brain damage upon the child's behaviour, and the effects on behaviour which environmental and interpersonal factors may elicit. A number of subsequent writers, particularly those dealing with brain damage in children, have developed similar models. Valuable as this kind of exercise is, many important details are lacking in Bradley's study. What is the incidence of these innate traits, and external stresses, in the population of epileptic children? How did Bradley measure them? What validity is to be attached to his impressions and to his reports of EEG findings in the absence of specified methods of study? How, if at all, do these factors interact with one another, and how is this interaction to be measured?

Altable (1947) studied Rorschach responses in 30 epileptic children and saw the following 'characteristic pictures': (*a*) deficient intellectual control over the affective, emotional and instinctive spheres; (*b*) anxiety; (*c*) aggressiveness; (*d*) an extraverted reaction; (*e*) tendency towards opposition; (*f*) poor mental efficiency; (*g*) slight bradypsychia (mental slowness). Since there is no comparison with controls, the usefulness of the study must be held in doubt. Studies indicated below, which have used matched controls, have indicated that there is no characteristic epileptic Rorschach response.

Lisansky (1948) compared 10 epileptics with 10 diabetics of similar age and education and similar age of onset and duration of the respective illnesses. IQs were similar and in the normal range. The epileptic displayed more 'neurotic signs' on the Rorschach test than the diabetics. Lisansky found that the more maladjusted epileptics had a more recent onset of epilepsy, and suggested that there was an initial neurotic response to the illness which disappeared as the patient grew accustomed to his condition. The findings of this study must be tempered by the fact that the numbers were too small for adequate significance testing to be made.

Bridge (1949) studied in detail 742 cases of epilepsy in children attending the Johns Hopkins Hospital, Baltimore, between 1927 and 1940. He classified the behaviour of these children into severe (the child seriously jeopardized by personality problems from carrying on normal life in home, school, or community), 9 per cent, mild (some degree of difficulty in home or school, but managing to get along tolerably), 37 per cent, and normal, 54 per cent.

Bridge suggests that:

> At one extreme were the highly intelligent, well-adjusted children, with excellent insight into their situations and able to

> co-operate in the programme of the clinic in a responsible way. At the other extreme were the insecure, antisocial individuals, sometimes underdeveloped intellectually, who required custodial care for the protection of the community in which they lived.

Unfortunately, Bridge does not make it clear whether his estimate of intelligence is based on standardized IQ testing, and no statistical material is presented in support of this conclusion.

Of the 65 (9 per cent of total) children described as having a 'severe' personality disorder, 40 suffered from insecurity (fears, shyness, sensitiveness to criticism, dependency); 27 presented 'spoiled child' reactions to lax discipline, and inconsistency and indulgence on the part of parents; 26 showed antagonism and resentment to the parents; 12 showed temper tantrums; 10 were unmanageable and destructive; 9 were prone to fighting; 8 had anxiety concerning seizures; 7 displayed sexual delinquency; and 5 were otherwise delinquent. How these traits overlap in the 65 children Bridge does not say; nor does he give any indication of the methods of measurement used in assessing these traits and assigning children to the 'severe', 'mild', and 'normal' groups.

Bridge suggests that there is a neurological underlay of epilepsy characterized by irritability and short attention-span. The child interacts badly with his environment, which in turn shows him intolerance, leading to demanding behaviour and temper tantrums. The environment, in turn, begins to think of the child as endemically bad, and the parents see the child as a troublemaker— '. . . as time goes on, the child's way of reacting becomes set into a pattern, and elements of what is called "the epileptic personality" appear.'

The child can develop three alternative kinds of reaction: withdrawal, with fears, anxiety and depression; aggression, showing antagonism against all the apparent agents of frustration; or the child seeks success where he can, with relatively normal adjustment.

A follow-up of 411 of the 742 children when they were in their late teens, by a social worker using unspecified methods, suggested that 18 per cent then had a severe handicap of personality maladjustment, and 40 per cent had a mild disability. Bridge suggests that because of the interaction of factors producing maladjustment in epilepsy, the passage of time is likely to see the maladjustment become worse. However, he stresses that the epileptic personality is not a clearly defined clinical entity, and is by no means a universal accompaniment of epilepsy.

Bridge attempted to measure environment stresses upon the epileptic child, on a 5 point scale ranging from 0 (no stress) to 4 (maximal stress). The 'sources of strain' in 60 cases are listed: unsatisfactory habit training in 40 cases: broken home in 26 cases:

psychosis or psychoneurosis in parent in 22 cases: unsatisfactory home setting in 21 cases: family incompetence or irresponsibility in 14 cases: misunderstanding of epilepsy in 11 cases: family and marital discord in 10 cases: puritanical and perfectionist attitudes in 9 cases: promiscuity in 7 cases: alcoholism in 6 cases: and school problems in 2 cases. No information is given as to what judgments went into making the estimate of 'unsatisfactory home setting' and 'family incompetence and irresponsibility', both of which must depend heavily on the value perceptions of the observer. The most frequent variable is 'unsatisfactory habit training', but Bridge does not say how the dangers of making a tautologous judgment were faced. No information is given as to what kinds of stress relate to which kinds of disturbed behaviour.

Correlation coefficients are presented for the relationship between brain injury; heredity for epilepsy; physiological factors which precipitate fits (e.g. disturbed fluid regulation, hypoglycaemia, frequent fatigue); and the amount of personality problems. Bridge's results are as follows:

	Environment	*Personality*	*Physiology*	*Brain injury*
Heredity	+0·076	−0·004	+0·083*	−0·121*
Brain injury	−0·133*	−0·102*	−0·242*	
Physiology	+0·226*	+0·292*		
Personality problems	+0·673*			

* = a statistically significant result.

It is seen that there is a very strong and positive correlation between personality problems and environmental difficulties. The negative relation between heredity and brain injury is to be expected, but the negative association of brain damage and personality disturbance is interesting, since an opposite conclusion has been drawn by other writers.

Bridge discusses the neurological aspects of the epilepsy in the 742 cases in some detail (e.g. kind of fit manifested), but does not relate this to the other information he presents. He does not analyse, either, the intellectual factors which he apparently attaches much importance to.

We must conclude of Bridge's study that, although it shows the possibility of more sophisticated studies of epilepsy, and the results, in so far as they are reliable, are extremely interesting, it indicates some crucial problems in the area of measurement and analysis: measurement which depends on the evaluative judgment of the investigator must be carefully controlled, and the methods specified. The interrelation of a large number of variables provides tempting possibilities for cross-analysis. Bridge goes part of the way towards this with his correlation matrix for a limited number of variables, but he makes no proposals for testing his interesting theory of interaction in the production of epileptic behaviour disorder.

M. Eysenck (1950) compared the results of the performance of 38 epileptic patients (adults and adolescents) to normal means on a number of tests designed to measure emotional instability and neuroticism (Crown's word ranking test; the Maudsley personality inventory; and the Rorschach ranking test). On all three tests the average score of the epileptics was about one standard deviation below that of normal, clearly indicating that these epileptics have neurotic personality. No correlation could be found between the length of the illness and the degree of neuroticism—'a result which would seem to negative the theory that neuroticism in the epileptic is merely a reaction to his illness'. Eysenck showed that the more neurotic subjects had lower abstract intelligence scores and poorer vocabulary and conceptual quotient scores (a possible indication of intellectual deterioration). These results, she concludes, imply that the neuroticism has organic aetiology.

One possible intervening variable which Eysenck does not mention is fit frequency, which could cause organic impairment, and also evoke a neurotic reaction in the patient. Since this and other intervening variables (e.g. kind of fit, environmental situation) are not considered, it must be concluded that Eysenck's material by no means proves that neuroticism in epileptics is directly related to organic pathology.

Price (1950) studied 50 epileptic children in the public schools in Ohio, and reported that 28, or 56 per cent, were subject to malbehaviour, mental impairment, or symptoms arising from brain injury, such as overactivity:

> Intrafamily discord was described as the primary cause of school disturbance in six different instances, or 12 per cent. In some cases, frequency of attacks, mental retardation and malbehaviour are of much less importance to the school authorities than mother dependency, anxiety, and fear of attacks.

Price suggested that hereditary epilepsy was likely to be benign behaviourally compared with epilepsy due to brain damage, an opposite conclusion to that of Bridge. He suggested that a disturbed attitude to epilepsy in the child's relatives in combination with epilepsy from brain damage was more likely to cause behaviour disorder than in combination with epilepsy that was not due to brain damage.

Bradley (1951) reported, without giving details of data collection or the population studied, that there were five behaviour traits which characterized the epileptic child, and did not appear in this combination in any other illness:

1 Erratic variability in mood or behaviour.
2 Hypermotility.
3 Irritability.
4 Short and vacillating attention span.
5 A rather selective difficulty in mathematics as a school subject.

Although the author states that these traits do not appear in all epileptic children, he gives no estimate of incidence.

Kaye (1951) studied maladjustment in 17 children with *petit mal* epilepsy. Using methods of intensive investigation of family and social history, he suggested that the maladjustment in these children was due to impairment of parent-child relationships. The disturbed attitude of the parents existed in a number of cases even before the onset of epilepsy, and was thought to be causal for the maladjustment in the child. The effect of the seizures on personality was minimal.

Zimmerman *et al.* (1951) carried out a detailed study of 100 epileptic children aged 3 to 16. Epilepsy of symptomatic origin was said to display more 'personality deviation' on the Rorschach test than the other cases. These symptomatic cases also had the lowest intelligence. The highest intelligence, and the least personality disorder, was found in the *petit mal* cases.

Pond (1952) studied 150 epileptic children seen at the Maudsley Hospital, London. He stressed that no hospital has an unbiased sample of epilepsy—the Maudsley Hospital tended to get cases in which behaviour disorder, rather than neurological features, were paramount. Pond does not give statistical accounts of incidence of the features he describes, but gives a series of clinical impressions from the material. He comments:

> All the usual factors which may produce disturbances in children, such as rejecting or overprotective parents, sibling rivalry, can be seen in the epileptic child . . . this special disability causes disturbed interpersonal relationships, and arouses great anxiety in parents, and rejection or overprotection. A severe behaviour disorder can arise because of parents' attitude to epilepsy.

Pond suggests that the *petit mal* children tend to be slightly built, have fair hair and blue eyes, over protective, anxious mothers, and often display symptoms of the neurotic type. The brain-injured child, by contrast, tends to be violently aggressive, explosive, irritable, unpredictable, has a short span of attention, with poor concentration. EEGs tend to show a focus in the temporal region. The children tend to be stocky, and there is often a bad family history of psychopathy and a socially unsatisfactory background. These factors, Pond suggests, are almost as important as the brain injury itself in producing behaviour disorder. He notes that brain-damaged children without behaviour disorder will tend to be referred to a neurological hospital.

Commenting on the epileptic personality, Pond indicates that there is not one, but several personality types found in association with epileptic fits: these types are the product of many constitutional and environmental factors.

Deutsch (1953) compared 30 patients with symptomatic epilepsy (i.e. because of organic illness or injury of the brain) with 30 patients with idiopathic epilepsy (no identifiable organic cause) and 30 normal control subjects. The Rozenzweig picture test, a projection test of personality responses to 'frustration' situations, failed to show any differences between the three groups.

Henderson (1953) reported the results of an investigation of epilepsy in schoolchildren in England and Wales, by means of a 6 per cent stratified sample carried out by the Ministry of Health. This survey revealed 430 schoolchildren with epilepsy. Of the 430 children, Henderson investigated 365 in detail, and suggested that 44 (12 per cent) were emotionally disturbed or badly behaved. Thirty-seven of these children had major seizures, and nearly half of them were feeble-minded. Henderson noted that these behaviour disorder cases had a much lower intelligence than the remainder of the epileptic children. A number of the parents of the disturbed children were said to be emotionally immature, or over-protective, but no figures of incidence for the two groups, normal and abnormal, were given. Henderson concluded:

> If this sample was representative, the bulk of epileptic children outside institutions are no more difficult than normal children. Those who are emotionally disturbed, are, however, exceedingly troublesome.

Hill (1953), in a review of the psychiatric problems of epilepsy, suggested that 30 per cent of behaviour disorder cases were of well below average intelligence; in the remainder, social or domestic stresses were responsible for the child's difficulties. This view is based on Maudsley Hospital material, which had been previously referred to by Pond (1952).

Fuster *et al.* (1954) studied sleep terrors in 228 epileptic children, compared with 139 non-epileptics. Of the 228 epileptics (who were specially referred because of psychological problems), 52 (22·9 per cent) had sleep terrors. Of these, 49 had an EEG centred in the parieto-temporo-occipital region. In the 139 non-epileptics, 13 (9·4 per cent) had sleep terrors, and in 8 of these cases an EEG showed a localization in the parieto-temporo-occipital region. Electroencephalography during the sleep terrors confirmed the authors' view that the terrors, in both epileptics and non-epileptics, have an organic origin. The higher incidence in epilepsy was most likely due to the fact that epilepsy itself is a disease of organic origin.

This is an important study, since it seems to suggest, by careful investigation, that at least one manifestation of disturbed behaviour in epilepsy can have a direct origin in disturbances in an area of the brain.

Pond and Bidwell (1954) discussed the problems of management of behaviour disorders in epileptic children in '50 highly selected cases'. The authors did not say whether these cases overlap with the 150 cases examined by Pond in his 1952 paper. In addition to the two groups, *petit mal* plus nervousness and temporal lobe epilepsy plus aggression, described in 1952, the authors distinguished a third group of 'mentally defective epileptics'. These fall into two kinds: those with minor attacks and tantrums and behaviour disorder in between the fits, and those with multiple epileptogenic foci, but an unclear pattern of seizures, and behaviour characterized by slowness, 'stickiness' and mutism. This appears to be a physiological result of the seizures, operating on an unknown basis. Commenting on the intelligence of the temporal lobe group, the authors say that they 'usually have a low average intelligence, but a genius for annoying people'.

The authors make a number of comments on the behaviour and attitudes of the parents of the epileptic children, but without indicating their methods of investigation or giving details of incidence. The characteristic parent of the *petit mal* child is said to show 'an astonishing contempt for their weakly, passive youngsters'. These parents are essentially middle class in outlook, even when poor. There is a subtle rejection of these children by their parents, and the family stresses can be so severe that the child's removal to a colony is necessitated. This description of the parents of the *petit mal* child seems to differ from Pond's description (1952) of these parents as 'over protective'.

One important point that Pond and Bidwell do not discuss is the problem of numbers of the *petit mal* population. More recent studies (Currier *et al.*, 1963; Lees and Liversedge, 1962), have shown that carefully defined classic *petit mal* (both with and without 3 per second spike-and-wave EEG) does not occur in more than 10 per cent of epileptic children, and in less than 3 per cent of epileptic adults. This means that a very large total population of epileptic children is necessary before adequate numbers of *petit mal* cases are obtained for study. Pond (1952) presumably was making generalizations (e.g. having blue eyes and fair hair) from a population of 15 or less, which does not appear to be a large enough number for reliable generalizations to be made. Pond and Bidwell do not specify the total number of epileptics in their 1952 study, nor do they specify the numbers of *petit mal* cases.

On the parental background of the temporal lobe children, Pond and Bidwell suggest that a frequent characteristic is for the home to be broken, and the care of the child transferred to institution or foster-home. Where the home is intact,

> the unconscious hostility of one parent for another sometimes finds its expression in the rejection of a child who might resemble, in fact as in fantasy, unpleasant character traits of the mother, or his or her whole family. Or if abortion has been tried, the divine disease seems divine punishment for wrong-doing. . . .

In view of the lack of information about the methods used to arrive at these conclusions, the confidence with which they are presented is a little surprising.

Navratil and Strotzka, in a carefully conducted study carried out in Vienna (1954), studied the responses to the Minnesota Multiphasic Personality Inventory of 100 mothers of epileptic children, and 100 mothers of normal children. After examining the statistical differences between the two sets of responses, they concluded that the epileptic mothers resembled Kanner's 'compensatory overprotection' type of mother who was over-solicitous and over-controlling towards her child.

Delay *et al.* (1955) reviewed what studies existed on Rorschach testing, with appropriate normal controls, of epileptic children. They concluded that these studies showed no characteristic personality pattern in epileptics.

Halstead (1957) studied 68 epileptic children in Birmingham, 28 attending normal school, 28 attending residential school, and 12 attending a school for the physically handicapped. Twenty children were said to be 'badly behaved'—aggressive, violent, bad-tempered, insolent, spiteful, destructive, sadistic, in need of constant supervision. A further 15 were said to be 'negatively behaved'—sullen, solitary, low-spirited, easily led, timid, unstable, over-sensitive, moody, immature, dependent. The remaining 33 children were said to be 'polite, happy, lovable, pleasant, and popular'. Apparently there were no intermediate groups on these behavioural dimensions. Halstead does not specify the methods of investigation of behavioural abnormalities in these children.

Associations with 'bad behaviour' (the aggressive group) are given as: low intelligence; male sex; brain injury; grossly abnormal EEG; *petit mal* seizures; frequent seizures; late development; longer duration of epilepsy. These associations, the author stresses, are trends rather than significant associations, since the numbers studied were small. The finding that *petit mal* epilepsy is associated with aggressive behaviour is the reverse of Pond's earlier impression. As with Pond's study, the number of *petit mal* cases is not specified. (There is a possibility that Halstead may have followed the pattern of some earlier writers in confusing *petit mal* with minor (e.g. temporal lobe) epilepsy, which would account for this disparity.)

Associations with 'negative behaviour' (the neurotic group) are: normal intelligence; *grand mal* seizures; being first-born; attendance at normal schools; female sex; shorter duration of epilepsy.

Shaw and Cruickshank (1957) compared the Rorschach responses of 25 epileptic children, and 25 age and IQ matched controls. No differences in response were observed, a finding similar to that of Delay *et al.* in their review (1955).

A fresh sample of Maudsley Hospital epileptic children was studied by Grunberg and Pond (1957). These were studied by more intensive and clearly defined methods than in the previous Maudsley studies.

The authors considered 53 epileptic children with conduct disorders (i.e. with behaviour of the aggressive type), 53 epileptic children without behaviour disorder, and 35 non-epileptic children with conduct disorder. Epileptic children with neuroticism or anxious behaviour were not considered. The ages of the children ranged from 5 to 16, and their IQs from 65 to 130. The groups of children were 'homogeneous, but not exactly matched'.

Firstly, the two groups of 53 epileptic children were compared. With regard to organic and genetic factors, the only significant difference found was that more of the children with conduct disorder had psychopathic individuals in their family than the normal epileptics. With regard to environment, in all five areas studied the epileptics with conduct disorder had a significantly higher incidence than normal epileptics of: maternal attitude disturbed; paternal attitude disturbed; sibling rivalry; marital disharmony; upsets in environment. What the disturbed maternal and paternal attitudes actually were the authors do not say; nor do they specify the 'upsets in the environment'.

Secondly, 35 epileptic children with conduct disorder were compared, for the same areas, with 35 non-epileptic children with conduct disorder. The only difference which appeared was that the epileptic children had a significantly higher incidence of epilepsy in near relatives.

The most marked factor in the disturbed cases, both epileptic and non-epileptic, was the disturbance of maternal attitude, which occurred in over 60 per cent of cases. The clinical and social data were gathered by a variety of physicians investigating the children, and the authors do not discuss the problem of heterogeneous criteria to which the physicians may have referred in making judgments about such factors as disturbed maternal attitude.

The authors conclude:

> . . . conduct disorders in epileptic children cannot be properly investigated or treated save by the methods of child psychiatry, which alone can make a full study of the emotional development of the child and its relation to the social milieu.

It will be noted that Grunberg and Pond make no analysis of the neurological kinds of epilepsy associated with the behaviour disorder they describe.

Cazzullo (1959) presents a model for studying the behaviour of the epileptic: the inputs of this model are the pre-morbid personality of the individual; his status as an epileptic; and the neurological substrate of his illness, such as the causation of aggressive behaviour by temporal lobe damage. These factors interact with one another, suggests the author.

Psychiatric aspects of epilepsy were reviewed by Pond (1957) in a paper intended for those in general practice.

He concluded:

> The characteristics of the neurotic reaction depend less on the epileptic phenomena and more on the factors of previous personality, family relationships, etc., that mould the form of neurotic disorders without epilepsy. Further research may of course find further sub-groups within this undifferentiated whole.

However, Pond stresses that organic factors may cause psychiatric abnormality in epilepsy. The two principal types are the hyperkinetic pictures in childhood and the paranoid hallucinatory psychoses seen in adults.

The conclusion of a seminar of 16 international experts on juvenile epilepsy were published by the World Health Organization in 1957. On the psychological disturbances of epilepsy, they concluded: 'Every clinician knows that many epileptic children show disturbances of behaviour and intelligence, but there is no agreement as to their frequency and causes.'

Hill (1959) suggested that 15 per cent of epileptics suffered from personality disorder. He said that these patients were likely to have brain damage incurred early in life and temporal lobe epilepsy. No details of the patient population from which these generalizations were made were given. It will be noticed that Hill's view is in direct contrast with Bridge's finding (1949) that personality disorder in epilepsy is negatively associated with brain damage.

Lennox and Lennox (1960) reported their investigation, over many years, of 1,270 epileptic patients. Fifty per cent of the patients were said to be normal, 25 per cent were 'irritable, quick-tempered, highly strung', 16 per cent were 'depressed and sluggish', 13 per cent were 'over active', 12 per cent were 'unstable', and 10 per cent were 'seclusive'. It is not stated in what proportion these latter symptoms overlap with one another. The authors indicate that the most abnormal pictures are associated with essential (metabolic) epilepsy, rather than with that due to brain damage (agreeing with Bridge), but provide no supporting evidence.

The Lennoxes surveyed the school population of Boston, (92,000) and found an incidence of 1 case in 643, an incidence much lower than that found in other studies. They concluded that this was because parents tended to conceal the fact that their child had epilepsy because of the attached social stigma. In the clinical experience of these authors, the removal of social and family stresses, and the control of fits by drugs, resulted in a normal behavioural adjustment on the part of the patient, even in cases where over-active behaviour results from underlying brain damage.

Pond and Bidwell (1960) and Pond, Bidwell and Stein (1960) surveyed epilepsy in children and adults in fourteen general practices in southern England, in an attempt to escape the bias of hospital studies. They found that about a quarter of the 100 epileptic children thus located suffered from some kind of psychological handicap.

Williams (1963) suggested that the psychological aspects of epilepsy could be divided into five areas:

1 The effect of associated physical brain damage on bodily structure, bodily function, intellectual capacity and personality and behaviour.

2 The effect of fits themselves upon the person's behaviour and thought as well as upon his life pattern (for example, the child feeling resentful because of the restriction of his activities by parents).

3 The results of medical or surgical treatment reflected in alteration of intellect or behaviour (for example, the effect of bromide, a common anticonvulsant in past years).

4 The development of neurosis because of the subject's disturbed life pattern, whether or not he is brain-damaged.

5 The influence of intercurrent and apparently unrelated neuroses upon the epilepsy itself, e.g. tension and fatigue states which precipitate fits.

Nuffield (1961) set out to examine the behaviour characteristics of different diagnostic groups of epileptic children attending the

Maudsley Hospital. He examined 332 epileptic children, 59·6 per cent of whom had behaviour disorder. Nuffield suggested that the incidence of behaviour disorder in an unselected sample of epileptic children might be as low as 10 per cent.

The behaviour disorders were divided into 'aggressive' or 'neurotic' according to the classification of Kanner. A behaviour score on each of these dimensions was obtained from a check list of behavioural traits thought to be associated with aggression and neuroticism in children. This classification was an *a priori* one, based on previous theoretical work in child psychiatry, and it was not known how closely the classification accorded with the actual distribution or clustering of behavioural symptoms in epileptic children.

Boys were found to be more aggressive than girls, and girls more neurotic than boys. There was no significant relation between intelligence and type of behaviour. Associations between an EEG classification and the behaviour scores were studied, after the 'unpure' EEG cases and those with IQ below 50 were eliminated, leaving a final number of 233 cases.

Significance testing of this result showed that:

a The 40 temporal lobe children were significantly more aggressive than the remainder of the children.

b The 3 per second spike-and-wave children ($n = 28$) were significantly more neurotic than controls.

c The irregular spike-and-wave children ($n = 44$) were intermediate between these two groups, having both moderate aggressive and neurotic scores.

A 'striking incidental finding' was that the temporal lobe cases had very low neurotic scores. Children with normal EEG ($n = 29$) had low scores on both kinds of behaviour disorder. The three remaining groups (parietal/central/occipital/frontal, $n = 30$; diffuse spikes, $n = 32$; and non-specific abnormality, $n = 33$), occupied non-significant intermediate positions.

Nuffield then attempted to relate environmental factors to the diagnostic groups, dividing the environment into 'good', 'fair' and 'bad'. No significant difference appeared for any group, a finding which Nuffield found surprising, in view of the work of Pond and his colleagues at the same hospital showing environment to be an important factor in epileptic behaviour disorder. However, 'environment' as Nuffield uses it seems to be a very broad, over-inclusive concept. A much more detailed breakdown and evaluation of different environment mental factors would seem necessary before confidence could be placed on a negative finding. It should be noted that neither Nuffield nor Bridge distinguishes between general disorder in the environment (poverty, overcrowding, breaks in environment, lack of play space, etc.) and direct disturbance of interaction between the child and emotionally significant individuals, such as parents, in their general measures of 'environment'.

Pond (1961) studied a series of brain-damaged children without epilepsy at the Maudsley Hospital, and suggested that the brain-damaged child closely resembles the epileptic child with regard to behavioural symptoms and their relation to environment; however, the brain-damaged children manifest a lower mean IQ than the epileptics. Pond suggests that a suitable framework for studying both the epileptic and brain-damaged child (often an overlapping population) is the interaction between the before-injury (or onset of fits) personality of the child and the after-injury treatment and environment.

Keating (1962) reviewed some post-war studies on epilepsy and behaviour in children, and reported that they produced 'controversial and contradictory' results.

B. Tizard (1962) reviewed some of the studies on epileptic personality, and concluded:

> No study shows an adequate appreciation of the problems of bias and reliability in the judgments made. Precautions are not reported to prevent contamination of EEG interpretation by clinical data, and the reliability of the EEG and clinical diagnoses are not assessed . . . the position is worse in respect of the assessment of the presence or type of psychiatric disturbance. This is left undefined in all studies and is never made without knowledge of clinical status. Nor is the reliability of the judgments assessed.

The only study that Tizard exempts from this criticism is that of Nuffield (1961). Tizard suggests that future studies must examine the relationship of a broad range of carefully defined variables, including the presence or influence of brain lesions.

Geist (1962) summarized 'years of intensive research and work with epileptic patients' in a book which asserted that the cause of idiopathic epilepsy was a need to release pressing material in the unconscious. The mechanism by which this release takes place is physiological, in the form of an epileptic fit. Geist's evidence for this proposition is based on psychoanalysis of epileptic patients, and his view is reminiscent of that of earlier writers, such as Clark (1917).

Juul-Jensen (1962) reported the findings of an epidemiological study of 1,020 epileptics in the general population of Denmark, aged 16 and over. He found that the social prognosis (in terms of adaption to work and society) was poorest in those patients in whom epilepsy began in childhood or early youth. Temporal lobe epileptics had the most difficulty in social adjustment. This difficulty was encountered in 60 per cent of the 221 temporal cases, and in 35 per cent of the remainder.

Guerrant *et al.* (1962) studied psychiatric illness in matched groups of 32 adults with temporal lobe epilepsy, 26 with idiopathic *grand mal* epilepsy, and 26 without epilepsy, but with chronic medical illness. In all three groups they found a 90 per cent incidence of functional emotional disorder, although the two epileptic groups had a higher incidence of personality disorder and a lower incidence of neurotic disorder than the chronic illness group. The authors conclude that epilepsy does not seem to present a picture of 'organic' mental illness; rather, the psychiatric pictures seen are a reaction to having a chronic illness, and are not peculiar to epilepsy. In view of the careful methods employed in the study, these findings are particularly important.

Dutra (1963), in a Brazilian study, categorized the epileptic child's behaviour as (*a*) a neurotic reaction to having the illness, with its disturbing effect on others; and (*b*) sudden discharges of behaviour, e.g. aggression or temper, which have an organic basis.

Tureen and Woolsey (1964) arrived at a rather similar conclusion, but suggested that there was no *specific* organic brain syndrome in epilepsy, contrary to Bradley's earlier view. The behavioural disorders were, rather, 'responses of the patient to being an epileptic and his frequently inadequate struggle with an environment hostile to his illness'. No details of cases, material and methods of study are given in these two studies.

Winston and Chilman (1964) discussed social, psychological and educational aspects of epilepsy in a review article intended for American social service workers. They conclude:

> There are almost no research findings available regarding personality characteristics with epilepsy. In carrying out such research, difficulties exist both in obtaining adequate samples and control groups and in establishing reliable and valid measures of personality.

They observe that irritability, hyperactivity, hostility, depression, anxiety and low self-esteem have been associated with epilepsy, but

> Further research is needed before any precise statements can be made on how common such symptoms are among persons with epilepsy and to what extent such symptoms can be ascribed to life experiences, response to medication, or basic physical disabilities.

Unfortunately, the authors do not give references in their study. Their statement, 'There are no research findings available on the subject of family and marital relations of persons with epilepsy', is puzzling, since there are a number of research reports on the family relationships of epileptic children, and of the marital patterns and adjustment of the adult epileptic.

Rodin *et al.* (1964) coded a wide range of data (neurological, psychological and psychiatric) relating to 57 adult epileptics hospitalized for uncontrolled seizures or 'unacceptable social behaviour'. The data were analysed by correlation coefficients and factor analysis. The fact that there was a small but significant correlation between psychomotor epilepsy and epilepsy with psychosis leads the authors to suggest:

> Factor 3 tends to confirm this relationship [between psychosis and psychomotor fits] but the factor loading of the variable history of psychomotor automatisms is quite small. This probably explains why some investigators [Small *et al.*, 1962] reported that no difference between psychomotor epileptics and patients with other seizure types can be demonstrated as far as mental symptomatology is concerned. The reason for the small factor loading lies probably in the fact that only a portion of psychomotor epileptics show a psychotic picture. If one examines, however, a number of psychotic epileptic patients and makes the presence of psychosis the classifying criterion, as has recently been demonstrated by Slater *et al.*, then the majority of these patients suffer from psychomotoı epilepsy.

A further interesting correlation of epilepsy with psychosis is that of history of difficulty at birth ($r = 0{\cdot}46$), which supports the suggestion of Slater *et al.* (1963) that a brain injury may be causal for both the epilepsy and the psychosis. Rodin *et al.* used the term 'psychomotor automatisms' as equivalent to the term 'temporal lobe symptoms'. However, as Gibbs and Gibbs (1963) demonstrated, psychomotor symptoms coincide with temporal lobe location of epilepsy in 80 per cent of cases only, the other 20 per cent of psychomotor attacks having a focal location elsewhere in the brain.

Wilson and Harris (1966) compared the psychiatric pictures in 83 American children with frontal, central (*petit mal*) and temporal lobe epilepsy. Of the 39 temporal lobe children, 29 were normal, 9 were hyperkinetic and 1 was hypokinetic. Of the 11 frontal cases, 9 were normal and 2 hyperkinetic. Of the 33 central cases, 24 were normal, 8 were hyperkinetic, and 1 was hypokinetic. There were no significant findings on the incidence of neurotic or aggressive pictures. This study suggests an incidence of behaviour disorder in an out-patient population of 25 per cent. Commenting on the higher incidence found in studies of adults (e.g. Guerrant *et al.* cited above), the authors suggest that this may be due to a reaction to epilepsy as a chronic disease. The similarity of the psychiatric pictures and the incidence in the different types of epileptic population do not implicate organic factors in the aetiology of behaviour disorder in epileptics.

Rutter *et al.* (1966) have studied the incidence of severe reading retardation, epilepsy, neurological disorder and maladjustment in children aged 9 to 12 in the school population of the Isle of Wight, the total number of such children being 2,299. Using multiple screening procedures for school health records, school performance, interviews with parents, and other sources, 62 children with epilepsy and neurological disorder were found. Thirty of the children (1 in 100 of the total population at risk) had epilepsy. The authors report that in the 30 children with epilepsy there was the expected incidence of disorders associated with brain damage, such as child psychosis and hyperkinesis (over active, distractable behaviour), but there was a much higher rate of maladjustment than in the children without epilepsy (of whom 5·7 per cent, according to psychiatrists' judgment and teachers' ratings, were maladjusted). The authors do not give the incidence of maladjustment in the epileptic children, but say:

> That the disorders were mostly similar in type [to those in non-epileptics] suggests that the increase in maladjustment was not due in any direct way to the effects of brain damage. The nature of the association will be considered in more detail on another occasion.

The further reports of this study are awaited with much interest.

Gudmundsson (1966) studied the entire epileptic population of Iceland, a small country with a non-migratory population, in which contact with all medical practitioners was possible. He suggested that 'a survey of the literature of the last decades will reveal how markedly the views of the authors diverge on the kind and incidence of mental abnormality', a suggestion which is borne out by the present review. Gudmundsson estimated, by standard psychiatric interview, that 52 per cent of the epileptics showed mental changes to a greater or lesser degree. Sixty-one of these patients were psychotic, the remainder having neurotic or personality disorders.

A relationship, significant at the 1 per cent level, was found between early brain injury (especially at birth) and the psychiatric pictures in the adult epileptics. The younger the onset of the epilepsy, the more likely it was that the patient would be psychiatrically abnormal. There was also a significant relationship between early brain damage and low intelligence. Psychiatric disorder was also associated with a lack of control of the fits, and minor fits (most likely to be connected with brain damage) which were the most difficult to control. Gudmundsson suggests two possibilities for the causation of the psychiatric disorder: the socio-psychological stress of continuing uncontrolled fits; and in underlying brain injury. His final view is that:

The conclusions of this investigation suggest that it is not possible to attribute the mental changes to any one cause, but that they are the result of various factors. An important factor is brain damage, though certain inherited defects are also involved, besides socio-psychological influences.

It will be noted that Gudmundsson's finding on the association of brain damage and psychiatric disturbance is the opposite to that of Bridge (1949) on epileptic children.

Conclusions

1 The methodology of many studies is open to criticism. Some writers give their clinical impressions without specifying the number of patients studied, how these patients were studied, or what the methods of study and analysis were. Often, where comparison with a control group would be appropriate, this has not been done. The difficult problems of categorizing behaviour and individuals into behavioural groups, and measuring the behaviour and attitudes of parents are rarely discussed. Intervening variables which might have accounted for the behaviour observed, but which were not measured, are not often considered.

A particularly difficult problem in the study of epilepsy is the problem of gaining a population for study that is representative of the population of epileptics as a whole. Psychiatric clinic or hospital sources will obviously contain an excess of psychiatric pictures; it might be more useful to avoid this bias by taking a sample from a neurological hospital, although this sample would be likely to contain an excess of patients with neurological abnormalities. General population studies are difficult to undertake, and meet the problem of the concealment of epilepsy.

2 The estimates of the prevalence of personality disorder in epilepsy, and the kinds of behaviour observed, are given in the following tables:

Table 3 The incidence and type of personality disorder in epilepsy

Study	*Incidence of personality disorder*	*Categorization of the disorder*	*Source and type of population*
Davidoff 1947		*a* Neurosis *b* Aggression *c* Mental defect	Children in epileptic colonies
Bradley 1947		*a* Overactivity, impulsiveness	Clinic children

Table 3—*continued*

Study	*Incidence of personality disorder*	*Categorization of the disorder*	*Source and type of population*
Bradley 1947		*b* Neurotic overlay to *a*	
Deutsch and Wiener 1948		*a* Antisocial *b* Neurotic *c* Prepsychotic *d* Organic *e* Mental defect	Clinic children
Bridge 1949	46%	*a* Anxiety, depression *b* Aggression	Pediatric hospital
Pond 1952		*a* Neurosis *b* Aggression	Psychiatric hospital children
Henderson 1953	12%		Random sample of English normal school population
Pond and Bidwell 1954		*a* Neurosis *b* Aggression *c* Mental defect	Psychiatric hospital children
Halstead 1957	51%	*a* Neurosis *b* Aggression	Children at normal and special schools
Hill 1959	15%		Unstated—? all epileptics
Lennox and Lennox 1960	50%	*a* Irritable, quick-tempered *b* Depressed *c* Unstable *d* Over active	Epilepsy clinic—all ages
Pond, Bidwell and Stein 1960	25%		Children in general practice survey
Nuffield 1961	59·6%	*a* Neurosis *b* Aggression	Psychiatric hospital children
Dutra 1963		*a* Neurosis *b* Aggression	
Rutter *et al.* 1966	Much higher than 5·7% personality disorder in non-epileptics		All children in normal school, aged 9–12, in Isle of Wight
Gudmundsson 1966	52%	*a* Neurosis *b* Psychosis *c* Intellectual deterioration	All epileptics in Iceland

The various incidences of personality disorder in epilepsy given by these studies obviously reflect the different populations studies, the different definitions of personality disorder, and the different methods used for measuring this disorder. There seems to be general agreement, however, that personality disorders are much more common than in the general population.

There is also fairly general agreement as to the main types of personality disorder seen in epileptic children. These are (*a*) a neurotic picture, marked by anxiety, depression, fears, inhibition, etc.; (*b*) aggression with temper tantrums and anti-social behaviour; (c) over-active or hyperkinetic behaviour; (*d*) mental defect. However, little indication is given of exactly what precise traits of behaviour distinguish children in categories (*a*) and (*b*).

3 The research since 1947 has produced a variety of findings by a variety of methods of research. The findings often seem to conflict with one another. In summary, the findings are:

Brain damage

There is an innate, brain damage pattern of mood variability, hyperactivity, impulsiveness, short attention-span and learning difficulties, especially in mathematics.

A neurotic picture, being a reaction to environmental difficulties, may overlay the brain damage picture.

Brain damage and abnormal personality are positively correlated.

Brain damage and abnormal personality disorder are inversely correlated.

Epileptic children with brain damage are likely to have a temporal lobe focus.

Hyperactivity in epileptic children is associated with brain damage in the temporal lobe.

Personality disorder in epilepsy is a reaction to a chronic disease; there is no organic picture of personality disorder.

Hyperactive children with temporal lobe damage tend to be stockily built and have a poor family history.

Brain damage causes sleep-terrors and fear attacks.

Temporal lobe cases have lower intelligence.

Temporal lobe cases are particularly likely to have personality disorder.

Essential epilepsy, rather than organic (brain damage) epilepsy is likely to be associated with personality disorder. When social and interpersonal stresses are removed, the brain-damaged epileptic tends to be normal.

Children and adults with temporal lobe epilepsy have no more personality disorder than other epileptics, with similar duration and onset of the illness.

Brain damage cases have an earlier onset of epilepsy.

Intelligence[1]

Behaviour disorder and low intelligence are associated.

Low intelligence is associated with aggressive behaviour disorder.

Neurosis is associated with normal intelligence.

There is no relationship between behaviour and intelligence.

Petit mal cases have the highest intelligence and the most neurotic pictures.

Temporal lobe cases have the lowest intelligence and are most likely to display aggressive, anti-social behaviour.

Temporal lobe cases have normal intelligence.

Fits

The longer the duration of the fits, the less marked are the disorders of personality.

The longer the duration of the fits, the more marked are the disorders of personality.

Personality disorder is a reaction to a chronic disease, so the longer the duration of fits, the more personality disorder.

Personality disorder in epilepsy bears no relation to the duration of fits.

The earlier the onset of fits, the more the personality disorder.

Temporal lobe fits are the most resistant to control, and are associated with the most personality disorder.

Fits associated with brain damage have an earlier onset, and are associated with personality disorder.

Uncontrolled fits are associated with a deterioration of intelligence.

Psychological stress can precipitate fits.

The control of fits by surgery is associated with the cessation of personality disorder.

The control of fits by anticonvulsants is sometimes associated with the onset of personality disorder.

Aggressive behaviour disorder is associated with an earlier onset of seizures, and a more frequent onset of seizures.

Environment

The disturbances of the environment of the epileptic child with

[1] The literature on intelligence and epilepsy is reviewed more fully in a later section.

personality disorder is similar to that of the non-epileptic child with personality disorder.

Disturbances in the environment are the cause of aggressive behaviour.

Mental illness in the relatives of the epileptic, acting as an environmental hazard for the child, causes aggressive personality disorder.

Disturbed environment and family relationships, which are more common in the families of epileptics than in the normal population, mean that often the behaviour disorder has its onset before the onset of epilepsy.

Poor environment, together with an early onset of epilepsy, often of the temporal lobe type, is associated with personality disorder.

There is no significant relationship between disturbed environment and personality disorder; the personality disorder, however, correlates with clinical categories of epilepsy.

Parents

Anxiety in the parents of epileptics is associated with personality disorder in their children.

Parents of epileptic children often reject or over-protect them, with the adverse results encountered in other fields of child psychiatry.

Mothers of epileptic children are over-compensatory and over-solicitous.

Adverse parental behaviour is associated with aggressive behaviour in epileptic children.

Adverse parental behaviour is associated with anxious behaviour in epileptic children.

Sex

Males tend to be aggressive: females tend to be neurotic.

Males tend more often than females to appear in epileptic populations. (This finding is discussed more fully in a later section.)

Personality

The behaviour pictures seen in epilepsy are a compound of the premorbid personality of the child, the factor of epilepsy and associated variables.

Body build

This may be a correlate of personality, and may be associated with particular kinds of behaviour disorder: stocky, athletic children tend to be aggressive; lean children tend to be anxious. (These findings are discussed more fully in a later section.)

Petit mal

Children with *petit mal* are slender, with fair hair and blue eyes, have over-protective, anxious mothers, and tend to be neurotic.

Petit mal children tend to be more aggressive than other kinds of epileptic children.

Petit mal children tend to be more intelligent than other epileptic children.

Interaction

Personality disorder in epilepsy is the result of the complex interaction of the personality existing before the onset of epilepsy, the effect of the epilepsy itself, brain damage underlying the epilepsy, the parental reactions, the environmental reactions to the epileptic child, and perhaps the effect of anti-convulsants.

Some of the findings summarized above seem to be directly contradictory to one another. The possible reasons for this are the different definitions and methods of study used, and the fact that different populations may have been described. Other findings may be complementary: for example, the finding of the association of behaviour disorder with brain damage *might* be explained by the fact that in these cases the fits tend to occur earlier and be more difficult to control, rather than as a direct result of the influence of brain damage on behaviour.

The most promising hypothesis seems to be the interaction one. It is, however, extremely difficult to test, and no suggestions as to how it might be undertaken have appeared in the literature on epilepsy. If there are, say, six hypothetical constraints on personality (previous personality-body build; effect of epilepsy; effect of brain damage; effect of environment; effect of parental reactions; effect of drugs) and these are ranked 1 or 2 according to their seriousness, in combination with a ranking of personality disorder 1 or 2, there would be 128 possible combinations of personality disorder and its hypothetical correlates. Considered in this light, it may not be surprising that previous research has sometimes produced conflicting findings. Only when a large number of variables are measured, and the interactions of each variable with each other variable assessed, can any firm generalizations be made about the background of personality disorder in epilepsy.

6 Epilepsy and psychosis

The literature since 1900 to the present day on the relationship between epilepsy and psychosis resembling schizophrenia in adolescents and adults has been reviewed by the present writer, in conjunction with Dr K. Davison, as part of a larger review of the literature on the relationship of organic brain disease and schizophrenia (Davison and Bagley, 1970).

The conclusion of this review on epilepsy and psychosis is:

1 An inter-ictal psychosis resembling schizophrenia occurs more often in epileptic patients than chance expectation.

2 The epilepsy is usually secondary to a cerebral lesion, particularly in the temporal lobe and the psychosis is aetiologically related to the lesion rather than the fits.

3 The psychosis is genetically distinct from 'true' schizophrenia, but claims that distinction can be made on personality, psychopathological or prognostic differences are insecurely based.

4 There probably exists a separate group of episodic epileptic psychoses which are psychologically similar but related to changes in medication and to the suppression of EEG epileptiform activity.

A common pattern in these cases of schizophrenia is for the epilepsy to begin in childhood or adolescence, and for the schizophrenia to have an onset some years later. The modal interval between epilepsy and schizophrenia is 12–14 years (Slater *et al.*, 1963). The appearance of 'schizophrenia' during childhood and early adolescence is extremely rare (Pond, 1952), and takes the special forms described by Creak *et al.* (1961). This psychosis in children seems to have a relationship, possibly aetiological, to early brain damage (Rimland, 1964). Childhood schizophrenia seems to have an association with epilepsy that is much higher than chance incidence, and the occurrence of epilepsy is probably related to the underlying brain damage which causes both conditions.

Bender (1961) reported 51 cases of childhood schizophrenia associated with convulsive states. Ten children were autistic from an early age. All of these cases developed convulsions, as well as a chronic psychotic state. Eight children displayed over activity, tics, stuttering, temper tantrums and marked mood swings, and explosive laughter and speech obscenities. Three of the cases were diagnosed as Gilles de la Tourette syndrome. The prognosis was poor. All had major, minor or psychomotor fits. Thirteen children with early schizophrenia developed fits during adolescence. One boy was reported to have committed 'the rape murder of a small girl' shortly before the onset of his first temporal lobe attack. In 9 children there was a hereditary history of schizophrenia (unlike all the other cases). The epilepsy in all these cases seemed related to early brain damage. In a further 11 children, isolated convulsions occurred during the schizophrenia.

Creak (1963) reviewed 100 cases of childhood psychosis, and found that 12 of them were also epileptic. In 7 of these cases the fits occurred some time after the onset of psychosis.

The conclusion, from the fairly scanty literature on the association of psychosis and epilepsy in children, is that although more epileptic children than would be expected by chance develop psychosis when they are adults, the association of epilepsy and childhood schizophrenia is extremely rare.[1] However, childhood schizophrenia itself is an extremely rare condition. The association of epilepsy with childhood schizophrenia seems to be greater than chance expectation. This may be due to an underlying brain damage which causes both epilepsy and psychosis.

[1] This conclusion is supported by recent work on the natural history of childhood psychosis by Dr M. Rutter and his colleagues at the Maudsley Hospital, London.

7 Temporal lobe epilepsy and psychiatric disorder

Interest in temporal lobe epilepsy as a clinical entity has developed rapidly since 1950, following advances in electroencephalographic methods and equipment (Gibbs and Gibbs, 1952). Most of the earlier studies ignored temporal lobe epilepsy (e.g. Bridge, 1949) for the reason that accurate diagnostic facilities for its identification were not available. A literature, mainly on neurophysiological aspects, has rapidly built up, and there have been a number of studies suggesting relationships between temporal lobe epilepsy and psychiatric abnormality. The review of literature on epilepsy and psychosis has been indicated above. The conclusion of this review was that 'the epilepsy is usually secondary to a cerebral lesion, particularly in the temporal lobe and the psychosis is aetiologically related to the lesion rather than the fits.'

The literature reviewed below is concerned with non-psychotic disturbances.

Merritt (1959) in his *Textbook of Neurology* states that the term 'psychomotor attacks' was previously used to describe practically all forms of epilepsy which did not conform to the classical description of *grand mal*, focal or *petit mal* seizures. Psychomotor attacks involve a brief loss of consciousness, superficially similar to that which occurs in *petit mal*. However, the attack is longer, lasting from 30 to 120 seconds, and is accompanied by muscular movements. The range of these movements is great—'twisting or writhing of the extremities or trunk, smacking lips, incoherent speech, involuntary acts, resistance to aid. The clouding of consciousness is deeper, and involves complete amnesia.' The EEG shows a focus in the anterior portion of one or both temporal lobes, with slow, high voltage, square-topped waves, at the rate of two to four a second.

Gibbs and Gibbs (1963) have shown that psychomotor attacks have an origin in the temporal lobes (from EEG evidence) in some

80 per cent of cases. In the other 20 per cent the psychomotor attacks can be located focally in other areas, such as the frontal lobes. Major attacks may also have an origin in a temporal lobe focus.

Falconer, a pioneer in surgery of the temporal lobe, has outlined the functions of the temporal lobe, with special regard to affective behaviour in epileptic seizures (1965). Falconer points out that the temporal lobes have an extremely complex function, since they comprise the cortical representation of the greater part of the autonomic nervous system, including smell and taste sensibility, as well as providing a mechanism of memory storage through which present experiences can be collated with the past. In the superior portion of the superior temporal gyri on each side are the areas concerned with the cortical representation of hearing and of equilibration, while in the posterior part of the dominant temporal lobe are the areas concerned with speech.

Anatomically speaking, the temporal lobe can be divided into two portions: one an older part consisting of mesial temporal lobe structures which have close reciprocal connections with certain midline grey masses, including the hypothalamus and the brain-stem; and a more recent acquisition (from an evolutionary point of view), the temporal neocortex, which has close connections with the older part, but which probably has different although related functions. Falconer suggests that the older part is among other things directly concerned with the control of the emotions, while the newer part is an interpretative area and analyses incoming stimuli in the light of past experiences and leads to an appropriate response.

Williams (1966) observes that the temporal lobe integrates the perception of stimuli with the 'feelings arising within the person, including the emotions and moods, . . . to achieve the sense of being'. Patients with temporal lobe epilepsy may therefore, shortly before or during an attack, experience sensory illusions or hallucinations or disturbances of emotion or mood. 'They may also experience disintegration of the self with feelings of depersonalization or derealization which result from disturbances of the integrative function of the lobe.'

Serafetinides (1965) reviews animal evidence which indicates that both fear and aggression originate in areas of the temporal lobe. The reduction of aggression in humans after temporal lobectomy suggests that the temporal lobes may be responsible for aggression in humans. The author also cites his earlier research, which show that aggression was only reduced by temporal lobectomy if fits were also controlled by this operation. This finding, however, offers no direct proof of the association of temporal lobe epilepsy with aggression, since the intervening variables, such as the effect of fits on social adjustment and consequent behaviour, must be effectively discounted before a primary association between epilepsy and aggression can be established. This point is developed more fully in the section on epileptic equivalents.

The strongest conclusion about the influence of temporal lobe dysfunction on behaviour during an attack is that this behaviour may become disco-ordinated, and emotions disturbed. These emotions may be fear or aggression. Given that a psychomotor attack lasts at the most for three minutes, and the subject loses the ability to co-ordinate activity, it seems implausible that crimes of violence should result during a psychomotor attack. However, as will emerge from the following reviews on temporal lobe epilepsy, and epileptic equivalents, medical writers often express the opinion that this may be possible.

The finding that lesions of the temporal lobe may cause both epilepsy and psychosis does not logically relate the epilepsy to the disturbed behaviour. The overwhelming evidence, which Davison and Bagley have reviewed (1970), is that in psychosis where there is organic brain disease the brain damage is causal for both epilepsy and disturbed behaviour. There is strong evidence, in fact, from the EEG and from clinical observations that epilepsy and disturbed behaviour have an inverse relation to one another. Landolt (1958) suggests that the epileptic EEG is therapeutic for disturbances of behaviour. In this respect, it is important to note that the successful treatment of psychiatric disorder by means of induced convulsions followed the observation of the antagonism of epileptic attacks and psychiatric abnormality.

Although a history of brain damage is more frequent in temporal lobe epilepsy than in *petit mal* and *grand mal* (Wada and Lennox, 1955) genetic factors probably have a fairly significant role in the onset of temporal lobe epilepsy. Lennox and Lennox (1960) found that the incidence of epilepsy in near relatives of temporal lobe cases was five times that in the normal population, and they postulate a 'conspiracy of causes'—genetic, acquired brain damage, infection, physiological or emotional stress—which may act together in various combinations in precipitating epilepsy. Rodin and Gonzalez (1966) compared the encephalograph records of 80 epileptic patients with those of their near relatives, and employed the same procedure with 30 normal controls. This study showed that nearly half of the family members of those with psychomotor epilepsy had abnormal EEGs, in marked contrast to the non-epileptic controls. Like the Lennoxes, these authors suggest that the actual emergence of epilepsy is the result of a combination of factors.

Hill (1958) estimated that between a quarter and one third of all cases of epilepsy are of the temporal lobe type. Because of the age of onset, temporal lobe epilepsy tends to occur later than in other forms of epilepsy, so that the incidence of younger children may be less than 25 per cent (Robertiello, 1953). Glaser and Dixon (1956) reported that 30 per cent of a series of epileptic children had psychomotor epilepsy, a type which coincides with temporal lobe location in the majority of cases.

The literature reviewed in the following pages on the psychiatric disorders apparently associated with temporal lobe epilepsy will be confined to non-psychotic cases, since the literature on psychosis and epilepsy has been discussed above.

It is rare to find a discussion of psychiatric aspects of temporal lobe epilepsy before 1949, and Bridge (1949), in his study of 742 epileptic children, made no mention of the concept in his analysis of personality disturbance.

Rey, Pond and Evans (1949) studied 59 temporal lobe cases referred to the Maudsley Hospital as psychiatric problems. Forty of these cases were said to show the traits: inability to keep a job or friends, or adapt to an environment, or face responsibility, irritability, egocentricity, unfriendliness to a marked degree; the remaining 19 cases displayed these traits to a lesser degree. Case histories were given for a number of children in this series, and the authors suggested that 44 of these patients showed 'aggression of an overt type, and to a pathological degree'. They were also said to display anxiety differing from the 'normal' psychoneurotic type, being of a 'lower' level of experience, expressed in body as well as in mind. The authors do not elucidate this rather obscure concept.

It was reported that in 32 of the 59 cases a family history of neurosis, psychopathy, psychosis and alcoholism was found. The authors do not attempt to relate these factors to the aetiology of the behaviour disorder, but instead hypothesize that the behaviour disorder may be due to a delayed maturation of the central nervous system. No supporting evidence is given for this hypothesis.

Pond (1952), in a study critically reviewed earlier, divided epileptic children into three types: the *petit mal* child, with neurotic syptoms; the brain-injury child with focal abnormalities in the temporal lobe, with violently aggressive, irritable, unpredictable behaviour, and often with a family history of psychopathy and socially unsatisfactory backgrounds; and the group of mentally defective epileptic children, with severe brain injury. The psychomotor (temporal lobe) cases appeared to have a 'nightmare' aspect in their waking lives, which Pond suggested might explain their greater psychological disturbance than that seen in the other types of epilepsy. Frank psychotic episodes in these children were extremely rare.

Pond does not make it clear whether these are meant to be exhaustive categories of epileptic children, although there presumably exists the psychiatrically normal epileptic child who is not referred to the Maudsley Hospital.

Hill (1952), writing of his clinical impressions with Maudsley Hospital patients, suggested that about 50 per cent of temporal lobe epileptics had severe personality disorder, characterized by irritability, impulsiveness, bad temper, anti-social behaviour, over-sensitive suspiciousness, egocentricity, perseveration and religiosity. Transient hysterical, depressive and anxiety states were also common. These characteristics, said Hill, made up what earlier writers referred to as 'the epileptic personality'. This personality, he suggests, exists only in temporal lobe cases; these individuals 'are a burden to themselves, their families, and their employers'. Hill does not make clear how selective his material was of temporal lobe epileptics as a whole, nor how the diverse psychiatric symptoms were measured, and related to one another.

Robertiello (1953), reporting his clinical experience with children with temporal lobe epilepsy, suggested a dominant psychiatric picture of a child who was over-controlled, quiet and shy. Occasionally, when this rigid control system failed, the child would be subject to gross rages. For the large majority of the time, the temporal lobe child did not display markedly disturbed behaviour. This picture of the temporal lobe child differs from that of the Maudsley Hospital workers'; it may be that Robertiello is reporting on a less psychiatrically selected population.

Falconer and Pond (1953) reported two cases of children with severe personality disorder and temporal lobe epilepsy. The first case was of a two-year-old girl in whom 'dreamy state' attacks had an inverse relationship to temper tantrums. Surgical removal of a temporal lobe lesion was followed by the cessation of both fits and behaviour disorder. The second case was of a 14-year-old girl with highly disturbed behaviour who was liable to be 'wilful, insolent and vulgar and at times expose herself . . . a group of attacks such as she always frequently experienced just before menstruation always caused her to be subdued and manageable for a few days . . .'. This inverse relation between fits and disturbed behaviour has been reported in a number of studies of epilepsy.

Surgical removal of part of the right anterior temporal lobe caused a remission of the epileptic attacks. The general practitioner, teachers and social worker involved with the girl 'all testified that she was now a normal girl, well-behaved, getting on well at school, and completely free of any suggestion of epilepsy'. This is an interesting case, since the spectacular cessation of disturbed behaviour does suggest a possible organic basis for both the epilepsy and the behaviour. However, there are other possible influences on behaviour. The fits themselves were controlled, and the behaviour may have ceased because the resulting disturbed interaction with environment also ceased. The effect of hospitalization, having one's head shaved and part of one's brain removed may well have a profound effect on the patient's feeling and self-perception, quite apart from any organic effect. Another variable is the fact that physicians, surgeons, parents and teachers have a strong emotional expectation of the results of brain surgery. For parents and teachers brain surgery for an adolescent must seem a physically dangerous and spectacular event, and may well affect both the quality and kind of interactions with the patient.

The remission of the disturbed behaviour cannot be definitively said to be due to the removal of a part of the brain directly causing the disturbed behaviour, since so many other possible causal factors were not investigated.

Fuster *et al.* (1954), in a study referred to above, showed that night terrors, in which the child sits up, screams and is intensely anguished, fighting and struggling and crying for help, is related in epilepsy to an EEG located in the parieto-temporo-occipital region. It was rare for epileptics without this kind of localization to have night terrors. This careful study does provide some support for the view that anxiety in temporal lobe epilepsy may have an organic origin. Penfield and Flanigan (1950) observed fear as a prominent symptom during the temporal lobe epileptic attack. Macrae (1954) also reported isolated fear as a temporal lobe aura in seven cases, with meningiomas in the medial aspect of the temporal lobe. There is evidence, said Macrae, for the physiological control of the emotions in this area. The suggestion that extreme anxiety, both during an attack, and perhaps at other times, is associated with temporal lobe dysfunction, seems on much firmer ground than the attempts (below) to implicate diverse anti-social traits, such as fetishism, as a concomitant of epilepsy.

Williams (1956) studied 100 patients who felt an emotional experience as *part of* an epileptic attack. The ictal[1] emotions observed were fear; depression; pleasure; displeasure; and possibly anger. One of Williams's case histories is of interest, since it apparently demonstrates the existence of fear as an inter-ictal phenomenon (i.e. occurring in between fits, as well as in association with them):

> A 7 year old epileptic boy experienced very frequent attacks of pure fear. . . . If this boy were about the waıd he would impulsively rush to the nearest nurse, or failing a nurse, a male patient, clasp them round the legs and bury his face in them . . . he later became an aggressive delinquent and at the age of 14

[1] 'Ictal' indicates an event occurring *during* an epileptic attack; 'inter-ictal' in between attacks.

had an extensive right temporal lobotomy . . . with cessation of the fear attacks.

The experimental work, reviewed by Liberson (1955), on the stimulation of the rhinencephalon in animals and man, supports the view that the temporal lobes are involved in the control of emotions. Further supportive work is cited in the review by Adey (1959).

Ounsted (1955) studied a consecutive, unselected sample of 70 over-active epileptic children. The EEGs of these children showed either a general spike-and-wave manifestation (but not *petit mal*) or a focal temporal lobe electrical discharge. Ounsted does not discuss the incidence of hyperkinesis (extreme over-activity) in the total population of children with temporal lobe epilepsy.

These hyperkinetic children were frequently known to have suffered brain damage. The children were extremely difficult to manage, since they would rarely rest, and were constantly seeking new situations to interest them, and were often aggressively impatient of environment frustrations to their over-activity. Distractability and short attention-span was revealed in IQ sub-tests. Ingram (1956) described 25 over-active, brain-damaged children, 13 of whom had epilepsy. The behavioural and intellectual pictures were similar to those described by Ounsted. In Ingram's 13 epileptic children, however, the EEG, while frequently showing gross abnormalities, was as likely to implicate other foci as it was to implicate a focus in the temporal lobe.

There appear to be certain similarities between these children and the aggressive temporal lobe children described by Pond (1952). The hyperkinetic syndrome will be discussed in detail in a later section.

Glaser and Dixon (1956) studied psychiatric symptoms in 25 children with psychomotor epilepsy (a major correlate of a temporal lobe focus). These children represented 30 per cent of the children with epilepsy at the authors' pediatric hospital. Nineteen of the 25 children were psychiatrically disturbed, and displayed a common picture of excitability, irritability, 'nervousness', hyperactivity, aggression, temper tantrums, and depression.

The WHO study group on epilepsy (1957) suggested that

> So striking are the associations between severe temporal lobe behaviour disorders and disturbed family background that one is tempted to postulate a genetic or familial factor to account for it. Such an idea is, of course, but a revival of the 'epileptic constitution', but in a new form that may be heuristically more useful.'

This is a puzzling statement, since although a number of reliable studies have shown an increased incidence of disturbed behaviour in the families of epileptics, especially in the families of those in whom hereditary transmission of epilepsy is likely, there do not appear to be any reliable studies of the incidence of mental disorder and disturbed behaviour in the families of specified populations of temporal lobe epileptics. Although Rey, Pond and Evans (1949), for example, found a poor family history in 32 of the 59 disturbed temporal lobe epileptics, it is not specified in this study what proportion of all temporal lobe epileptics were in fact thought to be disturbed: nor whether an adverse family history was found in other kinds of disturbed epileptic.

Peterman (1958) studied behaviour in 65 children with temporal lobe epilepsy. Forty-six of these displayed 14 and 6 cycles per second positive spikes on the EEG. A wide variety of psychiatric pictures were seen, with no picture predominant. Peterman comments:

> A study of epilepsy in children leads inevitably to the view that there is an important constitutional element which interacts with the social situation to produce symptoms. Factors within the child himself can be many and complex: the character of the epileptic process, the presence or absence of acquired brain damage, intellectual capacities, body build, etc.

In 22 of the 65 cases Peterman found a history of epilepsy in close relatives. Although many writers use the diagnosis of temporal lobe epilepsy to assume implicitly an accompanying diagnosis of brain damage, the fact that a history of brain damage could be shown in only 25 cases, and the incidence of familial epilepsy was much higher than that expected in a normal population, leads the author to suggest that there is a group of 'idiopathic' temporal lobe cases. (But see Ounsted *et al.*, 1966, *infra.*)

Davis (1959), reporting on an unspecified population of children with explosive or episodic behaviour disorder, suggested that a common finding was an abnormal EEG in the temporal lobe area. On these grounds he termed the behaviour disorders 'epileptic equivalents'.

Gibbs and Stamps (1958) suggested that 'hypermobility, excitement, and agitation are sometimes encountered in patients with epilepsy, particularly in children with temporal lobe foci'. No details of case material were given.

The Lennoxes (1960), in their textbook on epilepsy, tend to associate temporal lobe epilepsy with disturbed inter-ictal behaviour on an organic basis:

> Abnormalities of personality and behaviour in both adults and children [with psychomotor epilepsy] occupy an area of wide

> uncertainty and debate. Some of the persons in this area clearly are epileptics: others just as clearly are not . . . many chronic epileptics, especially those with severe psychomotor seizures in addition to discrete attacks, have periods of moodiness, negativity, bad temper, increased irritability, or even destructiveness, awareness and consciousness being maintained. At such times the EEG is likely to display more than the person's usual abnormality; hence these unpleasant periods, though not sufficiently discrete to be termed an attack, are like the smoke that surrounds a fire. Abnormal or anti social acts assume many forms. A child will mutilate with a knife or scissors, set fire, steal without purpose, run away, display temper tantrums or fits of screaming, or crying and breath-holding spells followed by unconsciousness.

No account is given of the number of cases in which the authors may have verified these views by EEG recording during disturbed behaviour. However, they recommend four types of investigation which may, they suggest, connect disturbed behaviour with epilepsy (*a*) Did the behaviour come up abruptly, with no warning or abnormal frustration? Did it end just as quickly? Was the mind blank afterwards? (*b*) Is there epilepsy in relatives? Did the subject have febrile convulsions (i.e during infancy)? (*c*) Is there an abnormal EEG, especially one having seizure discharges? (*d*) Do anticonvulsants improve behaviour?

This is controversial advice. Hill (1958) and Pond (1957) have both argued strongly that the EEG cannot legitimately be used to prove that an individual who has an epileptic EEG at the time he is tested, committed some act in the past under the influence of the cortical irritations of epilepsy 'like the smoke that surrounds a fire'. None of the investigations which the Lennoxes suggest can prove or disprove that disturbed behaviour in an individual has an organic underlay. A much more careful kind of inquiry which shows epileptic discharges *during* the disturbed behaviour is required. In addition, the investigation must be carried out by systematic methods with a clearly defined population.

Parsons and Kemp (1960) studied responses to the Minnesota Multiphasic Personality Inventory of 15 psychomotor epileptics, and 15 subjects of similar age and duration of fits, and 15 matched controls. The results showed that personality responses in both kinds of epilepsy were not significantly different from those of normal subjects.

Nuffield's paper (1961) compared 40 children with temporal lobe epilepsy, and compared the mean aggression and neuroticism scores of this group with those of 6 other diagnostic groups. This comparison showed that the temporal lobe group had significantly higher aggressive scores, and significantly lower neuroticism scores than all of the other groups. Correlations between fit pattern (as opposed to the EEG localization of epilepsy) confirmed this result for psychomotor epilepsy. Nuffield was unable to show that the temporal lobe cases had a significantly worse environment than the other types of epilepsy. However, since Nuffield evaluated 'environment' as a single variable, without any apparent sub-categories, this last finding may be open to error.

However, the association of behaviour and neurophysiology revealed by Nuffield's study is of great importance, in view of the careful methods he used. One possible biasing factor must be considered—the pre-selection of the clinical material by general practitioners naming referrals to the Maudsley Hospital. As Pond (1952) pointed out, the Maudsley Hospital treats a highly selected psychiatric population, and epilepsy in which neurological rather than psychiatric features are prominent tend to be referred elsewhere. It is possible that general practitioners would refer to the Maudsley Hospital children with psychomotor epilepsy (i.e. epilepsy with temporal lobe aurae) and with markedly aggressive behaviour, since the hospital has experience of treating this type of child, as exemplified in the writings of Pond and Hill. Considered in this light, Nuffield's findings might refer to a specially selected population, and not to children with temporal lobe epilepsy in general. Stevens (1966) criticizing studies on the psychiatric implications of psychomotor epilepsy has suggested that:

> A . . . serious criticism of the majority of published reports which document the high incidence of psychopathology in patients with psychomotor or temporal lobe epilepsy is the failure of all but a few studies to select relatively unbiased groups of patients for evaluation and to employ suitable controls.

Guerrant *et al.* (1962), in a study outlined above, found a high incidence of emotional disorder and maladaptation in sexual and personal relations in all the three groups investigated—psychomotor epileptics, idiopathic *grand mal*, and non-epileptic chronic illness not involving the central nervous system. No significant psychiatric differences could be found between the three groups, which were matched for sex, age and duration of illness. The ratings of psychiatric status were carried out by a team of six, making judgments about the patients in a variety of areas. The careful methods and controls used in this study make the findings extremely important. The authors' hypothesis is that the psychiatric disturbance is a reaction to having a chronic illness, the implication being that the psychiatric disorder increases the longer the patient's illness is uncontrolled. The finding of Wilson and Harris (1966) that the incidence of psychiatric problems in 83 young children with epilepsy was very low is in keeping with this hypothesis, since the epilepsy in this group was of recent onset. The children with temporal lobe epilepsy in this study showed no difference in incidence of disturbance from the two other groups, frontal focal, and *petit mal*. It must be noted, however, that Lisansky (1948), who compared Rorschach responses in epileptics and a matched group of diabetics found that the more recent the onset of the illness, the more neurotic signs the epileptics displayed. Lisansky suggested that the longer the period of epilepsy, the more the patient would be likely to adjust to his condition. It is possible that an explanation for the difference between the findings of Lisansky and Guerrant *et al* might lie in the different methods used to establish disturbance of personality.

Small *et al.* (1962) tested the hypothesis that temporal lobe epileptics would display more psychopathology than patients with other kinds of epilepsy. Twenty-five patients with temporal lobe epilepsy were compared with 25 matched controls with minor fits of the centrencephalic type (i.e. *petit mal*). The diagnoses were made by a neurologist, and the psychiatric evaluation carried out by a psychiatrist and a psychologist without knowledge of this diagnosis. Ratings were made for impulsivity, anxiety, hysteria, rigidity, schizoid traits, passivity and aggression. No significant differences were shown between the two groups, thus rejecting the hypothesis of increased psychopathology in the temporal lobe cases. This study by Small and his colleagues is carefully designed and executed, and is in contrast to some contemporary studies.

Bennett (1962) reported that an EEG study of 100 children with severe behaviour with aggression and violence showed a focus of 6 to 14 per second spiking in the areas of the temporal lobe, suggesting the possibility of 'hidden epilepsy'. Bennett generalizes from his clinical experience of epileptic patients, without giving details of incidence, measurement techniques and comparison with a control group:

> Undoubtedly epilepsy goes unrecognized in a large number of cases because patients have mental symptoms only. Such cases may not all be of the psychomotor type. Unrecognized epilepsy may show feelings of hostility and surges of hatred without overt seizures. Or the patients may have difficulty in adjusting to life situations or social relations. . . . Anxiety reaction in the form of terrifying dreams, nightmares, peculiar fears, queer head sensations, with apprehension and panic without adequate psychogenesis may be a manifestation of epilepsy. . . .

> Behaviour disorders in both adults and children may be of epileptic origin . . . a child may commit anti social acts without purpose—set fires, steal, run away, display temper tantrums or have fits of screaming, crying or breath-holding to the point of unconsciousness.

The question must be asked: How does Bennett know that behaviour disorder represents disguised epilepsy if the patient never displays epilepsy? His chain of reasoning seems to be: This individual displays behaviour disorder. He has an EEG similar to that displayed by some epileptics. Therefore he is an epileptic and the epilepsy has caused the behaviour disorder. (Bennett does not in fact say whether an EEG was taken in the cases cited in the quotation above.) This chain of reasoning is fallacious, and cannot provide any logical proof for Bennett's assumptions. The only possible grounds for hypothesizing an epileptic equivalent seem to be where a patient displays an EEG pattern *during* disturbed behaviour similar to that which he displays during an epileptic attack. The only behaviour which has been subjected to this kind of test are the night terrors, fears, and anxiety attacks discussed above.

Bennett repeats his assertions about temporal lobe epilepsy in a further paper (1965), making the same generalization with the same kind of evidence, and he asserts that 'Many horrible crimes are attributable to epilepsy'.

Pond (1963) suggested that the temporal lobe epileptic may display a withdrawal of interest and motivation as a basic personality pattern. Pond admitted that this view was reminiscent of some of the older writers on the epileptic personality. No case histories or methods of investigation are provided in support of this view, although animal evidence is cited that motivation falls as a result of rhinencephalic lesions (i.e. those associated with temporal lobe epilepsy). Pond suggests that the hyperkinetic child, although over-active in childhood, becomes apathetic after adolescence.

Juul-Jensen (1964) found that 60 per cent of the temporal lobe epileptics he studied (221 cases) had difficulties in social adjustment, compared with 35 per cent of the remaining 694 cases of other types of epilepsy. He suggested that an intervening variable in this association was the failure of anticonvulsants to check temporal lobe epilepsy, in comparison with other types of epilepsy, since when the temporal lobe group was compared with a group matched for severity and frequency of attacks, no differences in the incidence of social adjustment could be found.

Whitmore (1964), generalizing from material available from school medical officers, estimated that 1 in 3 children with temporal lobe epilepsy had behaviour disorder, and they tended to display the symptoms of tensions, lack of toleration, quickness to quarrel, aggressiveness, moodiness and temper tantrums.

Krych and his seven co-workers (1964) studied in great detail clinical and other factors in fourteen Polish children with temporal lobe epilepsy. The cases were compared according to the presence or absence of behaviour disorder. The only neurological feature associated with behaviour disorder was the existence of EEG lateralization in the dominant hemisphere. They concluded: 'The occurrence of character disorders clearly correlates with unfavourable environmental conditions. Disturbed family situation and a rejecting attitude towards the child seem to be of a particular detrimental influence.' The small number of cases involved did not permit significance testing of the different incidence of the extra-clinical factors.

Serafetinides (1965) studied 100 temporal lobe epileptics at the Maudsley Hospital in whom a well-localized epileptogenic lesion allowed a unilaterial operation on the temporal lobe. These patients were specially referred to the Maudsley Hospital because of their psychiatric characteristics, and the most common picture of disturbed behaviour was that of aggression, 36 of the 100 patients displaying aggression. The aggressive group were more likely to be male, and to have an earlier onset of fits.

A number of social factors were studied (normal home, broken home, family strife, unhappy childhood, step-parents, illegitimacy, mental illness in parents). In contrast to the study of Krych *et al.* (1965), no excess of environmental pathology could be found in the aggressive cases: in fact, there was a trend in the opposite direction: 11 per cent of the non-aggressive cases came from a broken home, and none of the aggressive cases; 20·5 per cent of the non-aggressive cases had a maladjusted father, compared with 5·5 per cent of the aggressive cases. The findings were in accord with Krych's study for the factor of lateralization, in that in most of the aggressive cases the focus was on the dominant side of the brain (i.e. the left side for most subjects, who are righthanded). The success of the surgical removal of the epileptogenic area of the temporal lobe in reducing the aggressive behaviour leads Serafitinides to suggest that this behaviour is organic in origin. The majority of the patients in this study were aged 19 or less, the modal age being 3 to 9 years.

Small *et al.* (1966) compared fifty subjects with temporal lobe epilepsy with fifty matched controls having other types of epilepsy. The incidence of the 'sociopathic' personality sometimes attributed to the temporal lobe epileptic (e.g. Hill, 1952) was found to be the same in both the temporal lobe cases and the controls.

Stevens (1966) studied 100 consecutive adult patients referred to an epilepsy clinic. Fifty-four of the cases had psychomotor epilepsy with a temporal lobe location. Stevens concluded that the increased risk of psychiatric hospitalization of this group, compared with the other types of epilepsy, could be adequately explained by the coincidence of temporal lobe epilepsy with an age cohort particularly susceptible to mental illness. Controlling the age factor indicated that there was no difference in psychiatric abnormality between temporal lobe and other types of epilepsy.

Ounsted *et al.* (1966) studied 'biological factors in temporal lobe epilepsy' in a series of 100 children, selected from a much larger population of epileptic children in Oxford because of the unequivocal electrical evidence of temporal lobe epilepsy. The children were studied for a period of 10 years. Thirty-five had clear evidence of an 'aetiological organic cerebral insult', with 7 more cases having a suspicion of brain injury at birth. In the organic insult group, the incidence of epilepsy in siblings was 2 per cent; in a group having no insult, but *status epilepticus*, the sibling risk was 30 per cent; in the group with neither insult nor *status*, the sibling risk was 9·3 per cent. These differences were highly significant. The authors suggest that early *status*, caused by a genetic predisposition to epilepsy, causes damage to Ammon's horn. Sclerosis follows, and an epileptogenic lesion arises. The early onset of epilepsy in the *status* group supports this view.

The IQ of the cerebral insult group ($N = 35$) and the *status* group ($N=32$) was significantly lower than that of the remaining children, with neither insult nor *status* ($N=28$). The earlier the insult or the *status*, the greater the intellectual loss.

Hyperkinesis, as described by Ounsted (1955), was present in 26 of the 100 children. Hyperkinesis was significantly associated with cerebral insult, *status*, low intelligence and male sex, and early onset of epilepsy. Only 3 of the hyperkinetic children did not have a history of cerebral insult or *status*. This fact, and the fact that hyperkinesis occurs in children with brain damage but without epilepsy, suggests (the authors conclude) that brain damage rather than epilepsy is the significant aetiological factor in these cases.

Thirty-six of the children were found to display 'catastrophic rage'—that is, outbursts of extreme rage and anger apparently out of proportion to the stimuli which provoked this behaviour. This rage had the effect of making schooling and social relationships for the child particularly difficult. The significant associations with these rage outbursts were a history of cerebral insult or *status*. However, although hyperkinesis and rage were often associated, they also occurred independently. Only in girls was catastrophic rage associated with low IQ and early onset of epilepsy, an enigmatic finding. Children who had never had *grand mal* fits were free from rages.

The home of the epileptic child was considered to be 'disordered' if one or more of the following five factors was present: (1) gross poverty; (2) death of mother at an early age; (3) grossly aggressive father; (4) psychosis in one or both parents; (5) gross chronic neurotic illness in one or both parents. There was a significant association between a 'disordered' home and the existence of catastrophic rage in the epileptic child. The data suggest the possibility that hyperkinesis has an organic origin, but rage can occur in those hyperkinetic cases which have a poor environment. The finding that has been made by other writers, of a notably high incidence of psychopathy or disturbed behaviour in the parents of the children, again occurred in this study. It will be noted that the authors merge diverse factors, such as poverty, with other factors with which they have only a loose conceptual relation, such as aggression of the child's father.

The careful observation of the children over a ten-year period indicated that only in 15 was there no personality abnormality. The pictures observed were: hyperkinesis plus rage; hyperkinesis plus a milder aggression; neurotic reactions, usually of a mixed form; general psychological problems arising for the first time at adolescence; and, in middle and late 'teens, schizophrenia and severe aggressive psychopathy.

One interesting case report is of a 7-year-old boy who developed hyperkinesis *after* the successful control of fits. This case is reminiscent of those cases in which disturbed behaviour shows an inverse relationship to the occurrence of fits.

This carefully conducted study, in which the population and methods of study were carefully specified, is in contrast to the many poorly conducted studies of temporal lobe epilepsy reported in earlier literature. The study has the merit that it does not overgeneralize about cause, leaving 'residual areas' open to further investigation. The obvious areas suggested are a fuller investigation of the neurotic pictures, and a more detailed investigation of environment and interaction between parents and children.

Aird *et al.* (1967) studied the antecedents of temporal lobe epilepsy in 193 patients. They found that the epilepsy had an onset earlier than was previously suspected—42 per cent of cases had an onset in the first decade and 75 per cent in the first two decades. Comparison with normal controls showed that the temporal lobe group had a significantly higher percentage of anoxia, more abnormalities of development, behaviour problems of childhood, and unusual nocturnal phenomena. The authors suggest: 'These findings suggest that serious dysfunction of the CNS had long antedated the final development of an overt form of temporal lobe epilepsy in approximately 50 per cent of the 156 patients with an onset of epilepsy after the age of 10'. The authors suggest that the same underlying dysfunction of the central nervous system creates a continuum of disturbance, ranging from abnormal behaviour to frank convulsions. However, some doubt must be cast on this conclusion, in view of the fact that the authors did not consider other possible factors which precipitate behaviour disorder, such as abnormal family environment or abnormal personality in the parents. These variables were not measured for subjects or controls. WHO (1957) has in fact indicated findings that in temporal lobe epilepsy there is often a marked picture of abnormal personality in the family members of the patient.

Conclusions

The conclusions from this review of the literature on temporal lobe epilepsy and psychiatric disorder (not including schizophrenic-like psychosis, which is reviewed elsewhere) is that there are a number of conflicting views about the kind and degrees of psychiatric disorder in temporal lobe epilepsy, and about the nature of the relationship of temporal lobe epilepsy and disturbed behaviour.

The suggestions that have been made about the behaviour of temporal lobe epileptics (children, adolescents, and some adults) are that the temporal lobe epileptic has:

Inability to keep friends.
Unadaptability.
Irresponsibility.
Unfriendliness.
Overt aggression to a pathological degree.
A deep-seated anxiety.
A family history of neurosis, psychopathy, psychosis and alcoholism.
Delayed maturation of the central nervous system.
A 'nightmare' anxiety.
Irritability.
Impulsivity.
Anti-social behaviour.
Over-sensitiveness.
Egocentricity.
Religiousness.
Transient hysterical depression and anxiety states.
Quiet, shy, over-controlled behaviour, with occasional rage outbursts when this control fails.
Psychic anxiety as *part of* the epileptic attack.
Fear in between epileptic attacks.
Fetishism; hyposexuality.

Hyperactivity, with short attention-span and low frustration tolerance, excitability and occasional depression.
An interaction of brain damage, the epileptic process, social factors, intelligence and bodybuild in producing the psychiatric picture.
Diverse psychiatric reactions, with no consistent picture.
Severe anti-social behaviour, perhaps as an epileptic equivalent.
Criminal behaviour.
Behaviour disorder which is no different from that in other epileptics, but more marked because fits are more difficult to control.
Behaviour disorder because of the reactions of environment.
Behaviour disorder because of the reaction of parents.
Aggression dominating the psychiatric picture.
No excess of environmental disturbance.
A deficit of neurotic reactions, in comparison with other epileptics.
The disappearance of aggression after surgery of the temporal lobe.
Hyperkinesis, often associated with catastrophic rage; in some cases a mixed neurotic picture is seen.
No difference in psychiatric symptoms when compared with other epileptics matched for age and duration of illness.
Hyperactivity, excitement and agitation.

These diverse and sometimes contradictory findings may be accounted for by the biases in selection of the populations studied, and the methods of study. The general picture of the temporal lobe epileptic that emerges from these studies is that of aggression, sometimes associated with anxiety, and sometimes with hyperactivity. However, this picture is by no means consistent, and some writers have seen the temporal lobe epileptic as normal, or with aggression completely dominating, or with anxiety tending to dominate. There are various accounts, too, of the causes of this behaviour. It is obvious that further study will have to attempt to provide answers to the following questions:

What kinds of psychiatric picture, and with what frequency, are seen in temporal lobe epilepsy?
How do these pictures relate to those seen in other kinds of epilepsy?
To what extent are the psychiatric disturbances caused by brain damage in the temporal lobe area?
To what extent are the psychiatric disturbances caused by difficulties in the environment of the patient?
To what extent are the psychiatric disturbances caused by reactions to epilepsy or the existence of a chronic disease?
To what extent are the psychiatric disturbances caused by the reactions and behaviour of the parents of the epileptic?

To what extent are the psychiatric disturbances associated with the pre-morbid personality of the epileptic?
To what extent do the above five factors interact with one another to produce the psychiatric pictures seen in temporal lobe epilepsy?

8 Epileptic equivalents

In the section on electroencephalography (pp. 22–5, above) it was concluded that the EEG should be used with great care, since it is liable to error in interpretation. However, as a classifiying tool it may be more useful than purely clinical data. It was suggested that arguments about 'epileptic equivalents' based on the manifestation of an epileptic-like EEG in a patient who has disturbed behaviour at other times in his life can have little logical validity.

However, a number of physicians commit themselves to the view that disturbed behaviour can be an epileptic equivalent, and the temporal lobes have been mentioned frequently as being the cerebral location of the epileptic-like discharges. A number of these reports are critically discussed in the section on temporal lobe epilepsy (ch. 7, above).

The Lennoxes (1960), have suggested additional criteria for assessing equivalents: the sudden appearance of the disturbed behaviour without adequate psychogenic cause; its rapid disappearance; a family history of epilepsy; and a favourable response to anticonvulsants, even when there are no clinical manifestations of epilepsy. The stress on a genetical causation of the supposed equivalent is in contrast to those writers who point to brain damage as causative of both epilepsy and disturbed behaviour. There is, in fact, evidence that epilepsy can be incidental to a clearly defined brain damage syndrome (e.g. hyperkinesis, reviewed in a later section, p. 86); and that in some cases there is an *inverse* relationship between an epileptic EEG and disturbed behaviour.

The observation of a systematically inverse relation between fits and disturbed behaviour has been made by many authors (Müller, 1930; Yde *et al.*, 1941; Hill 1948; Gibbs, 1951; Lavitola and Vitzioli, 1955; Landolt, 1955, 1957, 1958; Schorsch and Hedenstrom, 1957; Christian, 1957, 1962; Hachiya, 1960; Tellenbach, 1965; Fischer *et al.*, 1965).

This evidence of the inverse relation between epilepsy and behaviour disorder seems to be in direct conflict with the views that disturbed behaviour is *caused* by a sub-epileptic activity (for which the evidence seems to be doubtful). Either there are two different *kinds* of reaction to an epileptic EEG, as Brady (1964) suggests (psychomotor states + abnormal EEG, and generalized abnormal EEG + normal mental states), or there is a direct conflict of views. Glaser *et al.* (1963) report that it is possible, although unusual, for an inter-ictal mental disturbance in temporal lobe epilepsy to be accompanied by an abnormal EEG. Much more work will have to be done in this field before a definite answer about the exact nature of the inverse relation of epilepsy and mental disorder is arrived at. But the number of careful findings which do report an inverse relation between fits and psychiatric disturbance bring many of the statements about 'epileptic equivalents' into question.

Foxe (1948) has argued strongly and persuasively against the idea of the epileptic equivalent:

> The equivalence idea [in epilepsy] is as fallacious as if one were to say that, because hyper reflexia and the Babinski sign are both present in pyramidal tract disease, they are equivalents. Two symptoms must be equivalent quantitatively, qualitatively, or temporally. The so-called equivalents of epilepsy do not meet these requirements. . . . The whole theory of epileptic equivalence . . . has attained a dogmatic position. . . . This is all important from the point of view of anti social aspects of epilepsy, because it is rarely scientific fact, but scientific dogma that is responsible for the scapegoat or scapegrace use of the disease.

Foxe is saying, in effect, what we have argued above: that it is fallacious to infer cause from association. Psychological phenomena are totally different from an epileptic fit, as Foxe says, qualitatively and quantitatively, and occur at different times. The idea of the epileptic equivalent is extraordinary and unscientific, yet it gains frequent utterance by physicians.

A similar point of view to that of Foxe was expressed by the WHO Study Group on Juvenile Epilepsy (1957):

> The finding of epileptic discharges at other times in the patient's life does not prove an epileptic basis to the symptoms any more than it would prove the epileptic origin of ingrowing toe-nails if spike-and-wave were found in such patients. This logical fallacy comes out clearly in the literature on the periodic syndrome, which contains a number of reports on cases showing spike-and-wave and other specific epileptic discharges. . . .

Pasamanick (1951) used anticonvulsants to treat 21 children with behaviour disorder, and with various EEG abnormalities, on the assumption that the behaviour might be an epileptic equivalent. The results were uniformly disappointing, leading the author to call in question the notion of an epileptic equivalent.

Kennard (1953) reviewed 127 studies on the encephalogram in psychological disorder, and concluded:

> . . . in spite of repeated attempts to prove otherwise, most authors concede that the majority of patients having psychopathology have no other disorder related to organic focal pathology. This includes epilepsy, if, by the latter, is meant recurrent paroxysmal seizures resulting from cortical discharges and dependent upon a hyperexcitable focus within the central nervous system.

The only exceptions to the above conclusion were the few studies reporting a possible association between temporal lobe foci and aggression.

Ervin *et al.* (1955), who compared two groups of subjects having temporal lobe spikes on the EEG, but only one group having epilepsy, found similar patterns of disturbed behaviour (psychosis, neurosis, or instability) in both groups. They concluded that the disturbed behaviour in the forty-two subjects was related, not to epilepsy, but to temporal lobe pathology.

Schwade and Geiger (1956) studied the EEGs of 623 subjects with both normal and abnormal behaviour, including five patients committing bizarre, impulsive murders. Twenty-three patients had epileptic patterns, but none of these had behaviour disorder. Fourteen and six per second positive spiking occurred only rarely, and seemed to be associated with brain damage rather than epilepsy. It was suggested that the murderers had organic disease of the thalamus or hypothalamus, causing personality disintegration. There was no suggestion of epilepsy in these cases.

Pond (1957), reviewing studies on psychiatric aspects of epilepsy, concluded that in 'aggressive psychopathy' (a poorly defined concept, with definitions varying from study to study) EEG studies showed a lack of maturation rather than any relation to epilepsy.

Poser and Ziegler (1958) examined the EEGs of 2,209 patients taken in routine examination in a neurological hospital in the period 1956–8. A total of 136 of these EEGs (6·4 per cent) showed '14 and 6 per second positive spike-and-wave complexes' a pattern which some previous writers had seen in epilepsy of thalamic origin. Of the 136, 58, or 42 per cent, had epilepsy. Twenty per cent of cases had organic disease of the central nervous system. Case records of 55 of the patients without epilepsy were available for examination, and 21 were found to display behaviour disorder. A case history of a 10-year-old girl is given, without epilepsy, but with 14 and 6 per second spikes, who was disobedient, displayed temper tantrums and hyper-irritability, and whose behaviour improved when she was given anti-convulsants. These findings led the authors to suggest that this behaviour is an epileptic equivalent. This view is subject to the logical difficulties outlined above.

Kellaway *et al.* (1959), in a paper entitled, 'A Specific EEG Correlate of Convulsive Equivalent Disorders in Children', assumed at the outset of their study that epileptic equivalents were a well-defined category. In a study of 550 children with 14 and 6 per second positive spikes, the authors found a marked incidence of headache, abdominal pain, and behaviour disorder in children without epilepsy. These symptoms they referred to as a special syndrome of epileptic equivalence. Koegler *et al.* (1961) were critical of studies associating 14 and 6 per second positive spiking on the EEG with behaviour disorder, on the grounds that very few of the studies had used careful behavioural criteria and adequate control subjects. Livingston (1963) came to a similar conclusion.

Green (1961) studied 10 children with EEG spikes localized in the temporal or occipital lobes (a similar pattern to that seen in psychomotor seizures) and without epilepsy. Five were hyperactive with short attention span and probable intellectual deficit; 3 had normal intelligence and varied behaviour problems; and 2 had sudden, sharp headaches. Anticonvulsants were successful only with the latter 2 children.

Rodin *et al.* (1963) coded and analysed by computer, data relating to 72 children with behaviour disorder or poor academic progress. The data included medical history, neurological examination, and EEG results. EEG abnormalities were found to correlate with birth injury and with hyperactivity, but an epileptic-like EEG could not be implicated as associating with behaviour disorder. The authors concluded: ' . . . anti social behaviour is as a rule not the result of organic cerebral disturbances. . . . Tendencies towards epilepsy as revealed by paroxysmal EEG abnormalities in the waking record are not of major etiological importance in behaviour-disorder children.'

Goldensohn (1963) has pointed to the difficulty of knowing exactly what the EEG correlates of abnormal behaviour are. After showing that an epileptic attack, and its aura, can have no EEG correlate at all, he concludes:

> Are there predictable scalp EEG correlates for consciousness? It appears not. For interferences with memory? It appears not. What are the scalp EEG correlates for ictal hallucinatory and other psychic and mood experiences? Practically none. Is there a characteristic type of scalp EEG discharge during psychomotor attacks? No, not always. When

does a seizure start? When does it end? The scalp EEG frequently does not tell us.

If the EEG correlates of disturbed behaviour in epilepsy are so difficult to establish, it is obviously an even more hazardous task to establish that an EEG during disturbed behaviour is similar to that seen during epilepsy itself, a primary criterion for establishing the validity of the notion of an epileptic equivalent.

Henry (1963), reviewing 107 papers on the association of positive spike discharges in the EEG associated with behaviour abnormality (but not necessarily with epilepsy), concludes:

> As of this writing the real clinical significance of this pattern, *if there be any*, is anything but clear. There is a surfeit of possible clinical relationships, too often resulting from uncontrolled studies, but almost nothing is known of the basic neurophysiological substrate that might produce such an unorthodox discharge. And even if one chooses to ignore the cases not predicted by history and the apparent normals with such activity, there is the problem of causal vs non-causal relationship between clinical and EEG data. Some type of causal association is frankly assumed or at least implicit in most papers. Our own laboratory experience suggests that bursts of positive spiking might be regarded as a neurophysiological handicap, the importance of which varies as a function of the environment of the patient.
>
> A child subjected to the dual stress of 6 and 14/sec. positive spiking and a poor behavioural environment may well react with an unacceptable clinical response that would not be elicited if he lived in a less stressful situation.

Reading the studies of Goldensohn and Henry together, it seems that studies which posit behaviour disorder associated with abnormal spiking as an epileptic equivalent are on a weak empirical as well as logical foundation.

Maura *et al.* (1964), in a Brazilian study, reported that epilepsy in children having as its chief manifestation a paroxysmal disturbance of the autonomic nervous system affecting abdominal functions had a correlate of 14 and 6 spike activity. This kind of epilepsy apparently resembles the abdominal pain described by Kellaway *et al.* (1959) as an epileptic equivalent.

Gross and Wilson (1964) took the view that previous studies had provided evidence for the existence of behaviour disorder as an equivalent to epilepsy: 'There is a considerable body of evidence pointing to a syndrome, which the authors have termed "sub-convulsive cerebral dysrhythmia" of mild but definite organic brain disease, not having overt convulsions or neurological signs.'

The authors studied 122 children with behaviour disorder in two years. Routine electroencephalography showed 'subconvulsive cerebral dysrhythmia', and treatment with anticonvulsants seemed successful in controlling the behaviour disorder. A comparative study with a placebo was not undertaken.

Davidoff and Johnson (1964) studied 36 patients with generalized paroxysmal abnormal outbursts on the EEG. The authors could demonstrate no connection between disturbed behaviour in these patients and the occurrence of the EEG abnormalities. The EEG of the patients was studied for 90 minutes on a battery of mental and motor tests. While intellectual performance was impaired during the periods of paroxysmal discharge, abnormal behaviour was completely unconnected with these discharges.

Chen and Higgins (1966) studied the EEG patterns in 46 children having temper tantrums, truancy, theft, and sexual misbehaviour, and in whom an organic involvement was thought possible. The EEG results were divided into three major categories: paroxysmal features; incidence of Δ rhythms; and incidence of Θ rhythms. No relation could be found between EEG disturbances and disturbed behaviour. The authors concluded that the disturbed behaviour was a function of a disturbed social environment, rather than because of any organic impairment, such as an epileptic EEG.

Jonas (1967) suggested that large numbers of the population suffer from 'epileptic equivalents'. He reports that he observed 124 children during an hour's play activity at school. Five of these children received knocks on the head in various activities. These, he suggested (from other neurological work), could cause microscopic scars on the brain which could develop into abnormally firing foci. These foci, he suggests, produce tension states leading to disturbed behaviour. This kind of state is conventionally treated by tranquillizers, but since some of these (e.g. phenothiazine derivatives) have epileptogenic properties, they may actually make the behaviour disorder worse. Jonas gives a case history in which the withdrawal of tranquillization and the substitution of an anticonvulsant produced a remission of the disturbed behaviour.

This paper, which appeared in an eminent medical journal, the *International Journal of Neuropsychiatry*, is particularly interesting, since it indicates the kind of views of epilepsy, and the kind of evidence still considered as proving the existence of epileptic equivalents, which can still exist among clinicians. The study of Bennett (1965) cited above in the section on temporal lobe epilepsy, (p. 65), which asserted, on the basis of unproduced evidence, that 'many horrible crimes are attributable to epilepsy'—even where there are no clinical signs of epilepsy—is another recent comment of interest for the same reason. This study was written by an established

Californian physician, and published in the internationally regarded journal, *Diseases of the Nervous System.*

It is difficult to avoid the conclusion of Foxe (1948) in regard to these modern studies: that they are 'scientific dogma that is responsible for the scapegoat or scapegrace use of the disease'.

Conclusions

1 The logical and practical difficulties of establishing whether or not behaviour in the epileptic patient is an 'equivalent' of epilepsy seem clear.
2 Despite this, many physicians have committed themselves to the view that epileptic equivalents do exist.
3 A close examination of the evidence seems to indicate that, because of methodological difficulties in interpreting EEG results and the common absence of control subjects, there is little positive evidence of an association of abnormal discharges from the thalamus and the temporal lobe being integrally connected with disturbed behaviour.
4 This conclusion does not discount the possibility that brain damage may cause both disturbed behaviour and epilepsy. However, there is some evidence that the occurrence of an epileptic EEG is *inversely* related to disturbed behaviour.

9 Epilepsy and crime

The literature on epilepsy and crime before 1947 frequently attributed anti-social, sexual and violent crimes to the epileptic on extremely doubtful evidence. Physicians and criminologists writing under the influence of Lombroso almost seemed to regard 'the epileptic constitution' and 'the criminal constitution' as almost interchangeable concepts. The methodology of such studies was, however, extremely poor.[1]

Further papers reporting the association of crime and epilepsy have been critically reviewed above in the sections on 'Temporal Lobe Epilepsy' and 'Epileptic Equivalents' (pp. 53–70 and 71–7).

Foxe (1948), reporting his clinical experience with epileptics of all ages, suggested that they tended to be somewhat less crimogenic than the average individual.

Stafford-Clark and Taylor (1949) studied the EEG records of 64 prisoners charged with murder. Seven records showed severely unspecific abnormalities, and a further 8 showed specific epileptic discharges. Fourteen of the patients had been diagnosed previously as epileptics, while 7 others had received severe head injury without subsequent epilepsy. The authors suggested that there was a correlation between motiveless crime and a history of epilepsy.

Alström (1950), in a study of 345 adult epileptics in the general population of Sweden, found over 25 years a criminal detection rate of 7 per cent, which was not significantly higher than that for the normal population. However, the incidence of crime in the psychologically normal epileptics was 5 per cent, identical with the general population rate; but the crime rate in the psychologically abnormal epileptics was 10 per cent. None of the classical, heinous 'epileptic

[1] See, for example, the studies of Stekel, 1923 and 1933; Krafft-Ebing, 1926; Holmes, 1936; and Norwood East, 1936.

crimes' was observed, and no relation could be found between offence and seizure.

Hill and Pond (1952) studied 100 alleged murderers, in 27 of whom the plea of epileptic automatism had been entered. Nine of these latter cases had specific epileptic EEG abnormalities, 9 had no abnormal EEG, but a clear history of epilepsy in the past, while in the remaining 9 cases evidence of epilepsy was not apparent. The authors suggest:

> The evidence, therefore, for some relationship existing between murder and epilepsy in some murderers is undoubted but this is not to say that such murders are committed in an epileptic seizure or a post-epileptic automatism. In those cases we have had the opportunity to follow-up in the courts . . . we have not observed a case in which we were not in the end satisfied that the chance of an epileptic seizure preceding the murder was extremely remote.

The authors point out that in automatic states, when consciousness is clouded, the patient is rarely sufficiently co-ordinated to permit complex aggressive acts.

Hodge *et al.* (1953) studied EEGs in 100 consecutive admissions to a classifying school for delinquent boys aged 10 to 17. EEGs were outside the normal range in 84 per cent. In 5 per cent there was an EEG compatible with epilepsy. However, this did not provide clinical evidence of epilepsy itself, and the incidence of 5 per cent having an epileptic EEG is probably not much greater than that found in a normal population (Lennox and Lennox, 1960).

De River (1956) in a textbook on the sexual criminal, under the heading of 'Sadistic Bestiality', states that the proponents of this crime

> are usually vagabonds, psychopathic wanderers, such as herdsmen or schizoid tramps. These personalities practise sadistic bestiality whenever the opportunity presents itself. To this group may also be added the criminal epileptics and mental inferiors [morons], who because of lack of desire for sexual gratification with human beings, practice all forms of sexual perversion with animals and fowl.

No case histories of the 'criminal epileptics' are given, nor accounts of the incidence of this kind of behaviour among epileptics, nor an estimate of the proportion of 'criminal epileptics' in this kind of population.

Sethna (1956), in a textbook on sociological aspects of criminology, suggests that epilepsy is a cause of pyromania and theft. He quotes Lombroso with approval: 'Lombroso has told us of so many cases of epileptic assassins and rapists. . . . '.

The WHO Group (1957) report a study by Scott, specially carried out for this study group, which found 7 epileptics in 294 consecutive boys referred for psychiatric report at a London remand home (2·3 per cent). This percentage is somewhat higher than the association that would be expected by chance combination alone.

Lennox and Lennox (1960), giving their clinical experience of many years of investigating the possibility that criminal behaviour in some individuals may have been due to epilepsy, arrive at negative conclusions. Even when the EEG is positive, there are so many possible intervening variables that could account for the behaviour that a direct relation between epilepsy and crime cannot be established, they conclude.

Walker (1961), in an article entitled, 'Murder or Epilepsy?' reports the case of a man who stabbed his wife. Examination found him to be a temporal lobe epileptic. Walker suggests that the man may have killed during a post-ictal automatism. A review of literature, however, showed that such cases seemed to be very rare.

Banay (1961) reports his personal conviction that an epileptic may commit a crime of violence in a post-ictal state. Whilst he was interviewing an epileptic, the patient had an attack, and then proceeded to attempt to strangle Banay. Fortunately, the psychiatrist was able to resist the attack. The patient recovered consciousness, and confessed no knowledge of the incident. Banay cites a number of other cases of violent crimes committed by epileptics, but does not provide clear evidence linking the actual epileptic fit with the crime. However, he quotes with approval the views of Maudsley and Lombroso on the integral connection of epilepsy and violence. Banay also commits himself to the view that a number of violent criminals in whom there is no clear evidence of epilepsy are in fact epileptics, on an 'equivalence' basis.

Livingston (1963) concluded that 'There are, in my opinion, no reports in the current literature which prove that there is a higher rate of criminal action among epileptics than among other individuals'. On the supposed relationship between thalamic or temporal lobe epilepsy, associated with 14 and 6 per second wave-and-spike EEG, and having an apparently high incidence of violent crime, he suggests that much more work, using control subjects, is necessary before any firm conclusions can be drawn.

Woddis (1964) reported the findings of the examination of 91 cases over the age of 16, referred from English courts for psychiatric examination. In 10 cases there was a possibility of epilepsy. A case is reported of a youth aged 17, with a long history of epilepsy associated with behaviour disorder. Apparently the boy, in a post-ictal phase, enacted a sadistic fantasy which commonly accompanied masturbation. The result was that he murdered a small girl who was nearby.

While this case seems to show a fairly strong relationship between the post-ictal behaviour and the crime itself, the pre-existence of sadistic components in the offender's psyche, which emerged in the post-ictal confusional state, bears no necessary integral connection with the epilepsy.

Juul-Jensen (1964) studied 960 epileptics in the general population of Denmark, and found a crime rate of 9·5 per cent for men and 1·9 per cent for women. These figures were identical with those for the general population. No correlation could be found between seizures and the criminal acts. There was no preponderance of arson, sexual or violent crimes.

Gudmundsson (1966) studied the incidence of crime in 987 epileptics in the general population in Iceland. He found an incidence of criminal convictions of 8·3 per cent in males and 0·59 per cent of women, in comparison with rates for the general population of 2·5 per cent for men and 0·3 per cent for women. Gudmundsson found that the offenders were significantly over-represented in the categories of mentally abnormal epileptics. A common form of conviction was found to be that for drunkenness or 'liquor offences'.

A statement by the secretary of the British Epilepsy Association (Burden, 1966) suggested that 1 in 50 of the British prison population was suffering from epilepsy, compared with 1 in 200 of the general population. The prevalence of epilepsy in prisoners has recently been investigated by Gunn in a continuing study (1969). He made a one month census of all men received into prison in England and Wales in December 1966, and calculated that the rate of epilepsy was 8·8 per 1,000 in prisoners, compared with a rate of 5·0 per 1,000 in the general population, after making allowances for the age and sex composition of the prisoners. There was an exceptional excess of epileptics in prisoners aged 15 to 24; among these prisoners the rate was 11·4 per 1,000, compared with 6·0 per 1,000 in the general population.

Gunn compared 158 prisoners with epilepsy with 180 prisoners without epilepsy, and found significantly more epileptics than controls with affective symptoms (depression and anxiety). A similar difference was found for the expression of suicidal ideas. No less than 39 per cent of epileptic prisoners had made a previous suicidal attempt, compared with 22 per cent of the controls (p less than 0·001). Moreover, there was a significant correlation between temporal lobe epilepsy and a previous suicide attempt. The two epileptic groups with the highest amount of psychiatric symptomatology were those with temporal lobe epilepsy, and those with an 'unrateable' or atypical EEG.

Significant intercorrelations were found between epilepsy, CNS abnormality, and the amount of previous unemployment. The fact of this unemployment may have had some influence on deliquent behaviour in the epileptics. Gunn found a 'surprisingly high' level of neurological abnormalities in the control group of non-epileptics, and suggests that this might be an aıea for further research.

The authoı found a similar incidence of a disturbed early environment and other possible social factors influencing delinquency in epileptics and controls. These results suggest that social as well as some neurological factors may play an important part in influencing delinquency in this epileptic population. Gunn found no relationship between type of crime and epilepsy. Nor did he find any relationship between type and dosage of anticonvulsants and psychiatric symptoms.

Conclusions

1 Among a number of writers the idea of an integral relationship between epilepsy and some bizarre and violent crimes, which was common in earlier writers, still exists. The evidence for such an association, however, is extremely weak.

2 Statistical surveys of epilepsy among the prison population, and criminal behaviour among epileptics, suggest that a higher proportion of epileptics than would be expected by chance are found in such populations. This finding, however, has not been made consistently. There is no suggestion of violent or sexual crimes being over-represented in epileptics in prison. There are many possible social variables (the effect of prejudice, difficulties in employment, etc.) which could account for this apparent excess.

10 Drugs and personality disorder in epileptic children

The epileptic is given powerful anticonvulsants to suppress the epileptic activity of the EEG, and so control fits or reduce their frequency. What evidence is there of an effect of these drugs on the mental state and behaviour of the epileptic patient?

In an early, but meticulously designed and executed study, Somerfeld-Siskind and Siskind (1940) compared 50 previously untreated epileptics, of all ages, before and after receiving phenobarbital, with 50 epileptics not receiving an anticonvulsant. Mental testing was given to subjects and controls before and after the administration of phenobarbital. After one month, no significant intellectual changes were found in either group. However, testing after one year showed that the epileptics on phenobarbital were significantly *more* intelligent than controls, with an average gain in mental age, compared with controls, of six months. The drug was successful in controlling fits in 79 per cent of cases, leading to the suggestion that controlling the fits, quite apart from any sedative action the drug might have, increased mental clarity. Mayman and Rapaport (1948) suggested that their clinical experience pointed to the same conclusion.

Bradley (1951) pointed to the paradoxical effect of phenobarbital on hyperkinetic epileptic children. This drug, normally a sedative, had the effect of increasing their overactivity; Pond (1952) referring to epilepsy in children with brain damage and psychomotor seizures, but without referring diiectly to the hyperactive syndrome suggested that phenobarbital was contra-indicated for this kind of child, since it often increased irritability.

Ounsted (1955) suggested that amphetamines (usually a stimulant) had the effect of depressing over-active behaviour in hyperactive epileptic children. However, anticonvulsants were particularly unsuccessful in controlling fits in this type of child. Ingram (1956) confirmed the impression of previous writers that phenobarbital tended to make the symptoms of the hyperactive epileptic child worse, while amphetamine had the reverse effect.

Loveland *et al* (1957) compared 26 epileptics and 26 normal controls, matched for age, intelligence and education, by means of a battery of psychological tests and reported:

> Our test data, supported by the clinical ratings, yield negative evidence of interest to the clinician who prescribes anticonvulsant drugs, namely, the drugs administered to this group of epileptics had little if any effect on their total adjustment to their environment as measured by these tests and ratings, and to the extent that medication might have had an influence, it was as often favourable as unfavourable.

Gibbs and Stamps (1959) suggested that if too high a medication was given to the patient, this could produce drowsiness, double vision, or inco-ordination, giving the erroneous impression of feeble-mindedness. Royo and Martin (1959) studied in great detail, over time, the effect of anticonvulsants on the mental proficiency of three young epileptics. They concluded: '(1) Ill-balanced therapy can lower intellectual functioning, including visuo-perceptive and visuo- spatial structuring. (2) Proper combination of anticonvulsants can *increase* intellectual efficiency'.

Chaundry and Pond (1961) compared 28 epileptic children with deteriorating intelligence (a fall of 20 points or more in IQ in 3 years) with 28 epileptic controls in whom intelligence was not deteriorating. No significant difference between the two groups were found with respect to site and extent of brain damage; age at brain damage; age at onset of epilepsy; amount and duration of anticonvulsants; or associated emotional and behavioural problems. However, the deteriorating children had significantly more seizures, a poorer response to anticonvulsants and more generalized abnormality, and focal features on the EEG.

Wapner, *et al.* (1962) gave the Stanford-Binet IQ test to 36 children before and after the administration of phenobarbital for the control of epilepsy, compared with 36 matched controls. No significant differences in IQ were found.[1]

A review of the side effects of anticonvulsants (Craske *et al.*, 1969) has shown that the occurrence of abnormal mental states, including psychosis, is a consistent result—even though it occurs in only a small percentage of cases in each trial—of the successful control of fits by anticonvulsants. This outcome might be directly related to the toxic effect of the anticonvulsant. There is considerable evidence

[1] But cf. the effect of high doses of phenobarbitone on perceptual and motor tasks in three of four adult normal subjects (Hutt *et al.*, 1968).

(reviewed above, pp. 71–2) of an inverse relationship between an epileptic EEG and disturbed behaviour. Reynolds and his colleagues (1967) have suggested that a possible reason for this inverse relationship is the fact that many anticonvulsants induce a folic acid deficiency in patients—a deficiency previously known to be associated with mental disorder.

On *a priori* grounds, the administration of folic acid to epileptics who have a folate deficiency and disturbed behaviour should cause improvements in behaviour. Reynold's experimental work has shown this to be so. Reynolds has communicated to the writer details of a case of a 17-year-old epileptic girl with long-standing but now successfully controlled fits and a severe behaviour disorder of an aggressive kind, which made her virtually unemployable. She was found to be folate deficient. The administration of folic acid was followed in a few weeks by a complete remission of her behaviour disorder, and her general practitioner described her as 'a changed personality'. Reynolds has suggested that a folate deficiency can be particularly injurous to an immature nervous system. Further experimental results in this field are awaited with interest.

The evidence of the effect of anticonvulsants on the mental state of epileptics suggests the following conclusions: Intelligence does not seem adversely affected, and may in fact be enhanced when anticonvulsants control fits. However, it is possible that in certain cases a dose of anticonvulsants, higher than that necessary to control fits, can cause mental dullness. Phenobarbital seems to have a particular adverse effect on the behaviour of the hyperkinetic child. The mental disturbances seen in some epileptics when fits are controlled may be due to folic acid deficiency induced by anticonvulsants. In this respect, then, drugs may be an important causative factor in the personality disturbance associated with epilepsy.

11 Epilepsy, brain damage and the hyperkinetic syndrome in children

In 1941 Bradley described the hyperkinetic syndrome as being characterized by hyperactivity, short attention-span, impulsivity, explosiveness, erratic school performance, and poor social adjustment. The same author in 1951 described the 'primary, neurophysiological' behavioural characteristics of the epileptic child in rather similar terms: erratic variability in mood or behaviour; hyperactivity; irritability; short and vacillating attention-span; and a selective difficulty with mathematics at school. These two descriptions suggest the possibility that the hyperkinetic syndrome may often coincide with epilepsy. In view of the fact that brain damage is a suspected cause of both hyperkinesis and epilepsy, the view that the two conditions may coincide is not implausible.

Ounsted (1955) investigated the incidence of the hyperkinetic syndrome in an unselected sample of epileptic children at a pediatric hospital, and reported an incidence of hyperactivity of approximately 8 per cent of such children. The hyperactive children displayed common 'brain-injured features' of distractability, short attention-span, wide scatter on IQ sub-tests, mood fluctuation with euphoria as the abiding background, aggressive outbursts, diminution or absence of spontaneously affectionate behaviour, lack of shyness and lack of fear. The IQ range was from idiotic to normal. Boys (79 per cent) were much more often seen as hyperactive than girls. The behaviour of the children was said to be intolerable in home, school and hospital. The children appeared to have a predominantly mesomorphic body build, compared with mentally normal epileptic children. The response to anticonvulsants was often disappointing. The predominant EEG pattern was a temporal lobe focus or a generalized spike-and-wave formation. Cerebral insult (birth injury, meningitis, and encephalitis, or *status epilepticus*) was known to have occurred in 51 per cent of cases.

Ounsted found that in the mothers of the hyperactive children there was often 'excessive parental devotion', leading to physical and emotional exhaustion in the family, and conflict with the medical and school authorities. The child's behaviour seemed to be made worse by this excessive devotion, since placing the child in an emotionally neutral environment often had the effect of improving behaviour and reducing fits.

Ingram (1956) studied 'a characteristic form of behaviour' in 25 children with a known history of brain damage. Thirteen of these children had epilepsy. Intelligence was low, and a family history of epilepsy, mental deficiency and mental illness was often seen. The behavioural characteristics of these children are similar to those described by Ounsted. However, *lack* of affection, rather than an excess of it, was observed in the parents of the children.

Hutt and Hutt (1964) studied 16 continuous referrals to a neuropsychiatric unit. The subjects were brain-damaged hyperkinetic children, 14 of whom were epileptic. Comparison on a range of tests of attention and reactions to stimuli, with 16 matched, normal controls showed a number of significant differences. The reactions of the hyperkinetic children appeared to be similar to those of the extraverts described by Eysenck (1957), and the authors concluded: 'It may be suggested that in may ways the hyperkinetic child is the extravert *par excellence*.'

Ounsted *et al.* (1966) investigated 100 cases of children with temporal lobe epilepsy found that 26 per cent were hyperkinetic, a much higher percentage than the 8 per cent seen in epileptic children as a whole. This finding clearly implicates children with temporal lobe damage as being more susceptible to hyperkinesis, or the 'minimal brain damage syndrome', as some writers term it. In the review of temporal lobe epilepsy (*vide supra*, pp. 53–70), a number of writers associated hyperactive symptoms with this kind of epilepsy, although this finding was often difficult to evaluate because of the lack of clear specification of methods of investigation used.

Hyperkinesis and the minimal brain damage syndrome

If something like 8 per cent of epileptic children suffer from hyperkinesis, it is obviously of importance in studying epileptic children to examine the findings which have been made about the behaviour, and the influence on behaviour, of hyperkinetic children.

Birch *et al.* (1964) point out that the syndrome of epilepsy, in so far as epilepsy is connected with brain damage, overlaps with the minimal brain damage syndrome. However, the incidence of epilepsy in the hyperkinetic population is apparently unknown.

Laufer and Denhoff (1957) suggested that the hyperactive syndrome (hyperactivity, short attention-span, impulsiveness, and distractability, explosiveness, variability in mood and poor school work, was a fairly common behaviour disorder in children, but tended to disappear spontaneously by early adulthood. Since disturbed reactions on the part of parents tended to make the reactions of the child increasingly adverse, psychological guidance of parents, as well as psychotherapy for the children, often had beneficial effects. Eisenberg (1957) confirmed this behavioural picture, and stressed that factors in the social environment were extremely important for the emergence of *anti-social* behaviour.

Levy (1959) reported 100 cases of post-encephalitic disorder in children. Encephalitis may cause, through brain damage, both epilepsy and behaviour disorder. Hyperkinesis is quite often seen by itself as a post-encephalitic behaviour disorder.

Pond (1961), in a study of a series of brain-damaged children seen at the Maudsley Hospital, suggested that, with regard to adverse environment, age, and behavioural symptoms, the brain-damaged children with behaviour disorder were similar to epileptic children with behaviour disorder.

Kennedy and Ramirez (1965) quote the history of an 8-year-old child with minor Jacksonian attacks and hyperkinesis. An air encephalogram indicated left cerebral atrophy. Surgery (hemispherectomy) cured both epilepsy and the behavioural symptoms of hyperkinesis. The authors give further case histories to show that the brain of the newborn infant, because of its immature state, may suffer from extensive injury which can go unrecognized for a period of years, but may have an outcome of learning and behaviour disorder, sometimes accompanied by epilepsy. A common involvement is in the lower brain centres, which are particularly liable to be injured by encephalitis. The fact that this is a *minimal* brain damage syndrome is stressed:

> It is clear that the tools for the recognition of previous brain injury are grossly inadequate and that the cause for behavioural aberrations in many instances must go undiscovered. There is reason to believe that even if the brain of the individual in question were available for pathologic examination, the answer would not be exclusively forthcoming, because of changes in histology which occur over time.

Eisenberg (1964) points out that an aetiology of brain damage cannot be implicated in every case of hyperkinesis. The absence of a clear indication of brain damage does not, however, mean that no brain damage in fact took place: 'There is extensive epidemiological evidence that children with behaviour disorders but without other neurological manifestations have a disproportionate loading of foetal and neo-natal complications known to be associated with CNS pathology.'

Eisenberg suggests that the brain-damaged child is *more* at the mercy of an adverse environment than a normal child: for full development, he needs a *better* than average environment:

> The dependence of the brain damaged child upon his environment is nowhere more clear than in his family relations. His defect, if it is obvious at birth, may alter parental attitudes towards him. What is the impact on the development of maternal feelings of having a child who does not respond as he should, who is a source of frustration rather than pride? Parental behaviour may be so skewed as to induce in the child the very patterns of disturbance we would have recognized as psychogenic had the presence of brain damage not pre-empted our attention . . . consider what it means to the child if he finds himself rejected for something he cannot control and does not understand . . . how the child thinks about himself has a major influence on his behaviour . . . if his parents cannot provide the warm acceptance that underlies the sense of personal worth for the normal child, the inner-core of his self-concept will be one of worthlessness. His extra-familial experiences with peers and teachers often cause further self-deprecation as others display impatience with his limitations and share his companions. . . .

The brain-damaged child is subject to outbursts or rage he cannot control. He *wants*, Eisenberg suggests, a firm environment, which understands his functions, and the organic state underlying them. Permissive child-rearing makes things worse, and intensifies his guilt. The picture of the brain-damaged child, his environment, and 'rage reactions' is similar to that given by Ounsted (above, p. 87) of the hyperkinetic epileptic child.

Eisenberg notes that parents of the brain-damaged child often themselves display personality disorder. He suggests two alternative explanations: only those hyperkinetic children who have disturbed or non-understanding parents, who provoke further behaviour disorder, tend to come to clinics and hospitals for treatment; or the hyperkinetic child provokes disturbed behaviour on the part of the parent. There is a possible interaction of both causes.

Richardson (1965) has stressed the extreme importance of social environment in eliciting particular behaviour outcomes from the brain-damaged child.

Birch, Thomas and Chess (1964) studied in great detail the longitudinal development of three brain-damaged children. They argue that 'the course of behavioural development in brain-damaged children is the complex production of the interaction of a child having a given set of response tendencies with parental attitudes and practices and more general features in the environment'. This extremely important theory of interaction will be outlined in more detail below, when other theories and accounts of interaction will be considered.

Lucas *et al.* (1965) studied 72 children referred for school problems. Twenty-seven were found to be hyperactive, with poor impulse control. Statistically significant correlations were found between hyperactivity and a number of clinical abnormalities on the neurological examination, and with a history of difficulty at birth. Some of the hyperactive children were found to have 'associated neurotic problems, with acting out behaviour'. This was suggested to be a neurotic overlay to a neurological syndrome.

Burton (1965) studied 20 children who had been involved in road accidents, compared with matched controls. Hyperkinesis and birth injury were common in the children who had been in accidents, and absent in controls. Stewart *et al.* (1966) compared 37 children described as hyperactive with 36 children of similar age in normal school classes. Three of the 36 normal children themselves displayed hyperkinesis—8 per cent—which suggests that the hyperkinesis might be quite common. The finding that children involved in road accidents have a high proportion of hyperkinetics among them supports this view. Stewart and his colleagues, on the basis of their work in schools, suggest that there is on average about one hyperkinetic child in each class.

Stott (1966) argues that much disturbed behaviour in children has an origin in early brain damage. After studying 305 school truants, he suggested that there is a relationship between poor and overcrowded conditions which impair the reproductive capacity of the mother, and influence the appearance of multiple congenital impairment, of both health and behaviour, in some of her children. A special study of 33 'troublesome children' found that 5 also had neurological problems, 2 having epilepsy. The findings of Hare and Shaw (1965) offer support for Stott's work. These authors studied mental health on old and new housing estates in a London suburb. They suggested:

> The present finding of an association between nervous disturbance and a history of certain infections or of brain injury is in line with recent work suggesting that many kinds of apparently minor physical or physiological damage to the nervous system, especially at an early age, may lead to increased vulnerability to illness. The search for the origin of this vulnerable group provides opportunities for future study.

Halton (1966) has suggested that the prevalence of the minimal damage syndrome necessitates the neurological examination of all schoolchildren acting abnormally, or showing enigmatic problems with learning. Widrow (1966) suggests that the child with minimal brain damage suffers from a delayed maturation of the CNS. He suggests that about 5 per cent of the normal school population in Australia suffers from hyperkinesis of varying degree.

A variant of the minimal brain damage or hyperactive syndrome is the choreiform syndrome, which involves certain slight jerky movements of sudden occurrence and short duration which occur quite irregularly and arhythmically in different muscles. Woolf and Hurwitz (1966) reported that it was significantly more frequent in delinquents; American and Japanese studies had indicated that it occurred in about 12 per cent of children, and a ratio of 3 : 1 of boys to girls. Other associations were learning difficulties, severe emotional disorder and early brain damage.

Rutter *et al.* (1966) carried out an assessment of choreiform movements, by an observational method, in 252 children aged 9 to 11 in the normal school population of the Isle of Wight. Choreiform movements were found to be significantly associated with low intelligence, but the expected relationship with birth difficulties and with neurological and behavioural abnormalities did not appear.

The implications of the study of the minimal brain damage syndrome

The first and most obvious implication has already been pointed out —a significant number of epileptic children are brain-damaged, and suffer from this syndrome of hyperkinetic, over-active behaviour. The evidence supports the view (Birch *et al.*, 1964) that damage to the brain[1] can cause a variety of syndromes: epilepsy, mental subnormality, cerebral palsy, hyperkinesis. The damage to the brain is often slight from the point of view of detection by present methods, but the outcome of this damage is often profound. It appears possible that some unfortunate children will suffer from all four of these syndromes, others from combinations of them, and some brain-damaged children suffer no apparent ill-effects whatever. Why this should be so is unknown. A further enigmatic outcome of brain damage is childhood schizophrenia (Baer, 1961; Rimland, 1964).[2]

Secondly, the studies of brain damage in children appear to have been carried out in a more sophisticated way, in terms of scientific detachment, critical assessment of methods and material, and reasoning about cause, and the outcome of the various combinations

[1] For a validation of the concept of the 'brain damage' syndrome in children see Hertzig *et al.* (1969).

[2] Note, too, early brain damage as a possible aetiological factor in psychosis in *adult* life (Davison and Bagley, 1970).

of factors. In fact, the work on brain-damaged children may provide a model for the study of epilepsy in children, a field which has been dogged by an adverse emotional involvement with the clinical material.

Thirdly, studies of brain damage have provided some extremely important models for the study of interaction of a variety of factors in producing behaviour in children. Some further studies in this field will be reviewed in the section on interaction, p. 114–28, below.

Conclusions

1 The most important brain damage syndrome, from the point of view of adverse behaviour, is the hyperkinetic syndrome, which may result from minimal damage to the brain.

2 The damage to the brain which causes hyperkinesis may also cause epilepsy. Approximately 20 per cent of epileptic children are apparently hyperkinetic.

3 The studies of brain damage in children provide models for the study of the epileptic child.

12 Body build and personality disorder in epilepsy

Pond (1961) has suggested that behaviour disorders in epileptic children are the result of the pre-morbid personality of the child, interacting with the effect of the epilepsy itself, and the reactions of environment and parents to the child having epilepsy. It seems plausible, on an *a priori* basis, that the child's basic personality (e.g. the dimensions of extraversion-introversion, and neuroticism, described by Eysenck, 1970) will be an important factor in what kind of behaviour disorder he will show—if he displays a behaviour disorder at all—when he has epilepsy. However, this variable is extremely difficult to investigate, since it is impossible to know with any degree of accuracy what the child's personality was like before epilepsy. The only way of knowing this directly seems to be to apply personality testing to a large population, checking, in subsequent years, those who develop epilepsy. However, a very large initial sample is required.

An alternative is to follow up children who are more at risk than the general population to develop epilepsy, such as premature children or those with a history of difficult birth. Although a longitudinal study of this type is in progress (Wortis *et al.* 1964) with children who have suffered early brain damage and premature children, no findings are available for a large epileptic population. However, the findings of Thomas and his co-workers (1964) for brain-damaged children do suggest that the child has an innate, biologically determined personality from birth, which interacts with his subsequent environment and history to produce the final outcome of personality.

Body build and personality: findings in non-epileptics

There is an alternative to personality testing itself for predicting personality: the method of somatyping, or measuring body build, which has been found to have a correlation with personality. Although somatyping has a long history in psychiatry, it has been surrounded by controversy, proponents of the various schools of somatyping criticizing the methods of the others. The elements of this controversy have been reviewed by Eysenck (1959). Skottowe (1965) has pointed out that surprisingly little account is paid to somatyping by psychiatric textbooks, perhaps because of the controversy that surrounds the technique and measurement of the correlates of body build.

Despite this controversy, some positive findings have emerged from research. Epps and Parnell (1952) compared 177 girls and young women at Borstal with 123 women undergraduates of similar age, and found the delinquents to be heavier and shorter in build, with more muscle and fat. The correlative personality of the delinquents—being assertive, adventurous, energetic, and enjoying risk, also differentiated them from the undergraduates, who were more likely to be quiet, restrained, and lovers of privacy. Somewhat similar findings with delinquents were made by Glueck and Glueck (1950).

Davidson *et al.* (1957) studied the amount of fat, bone and muscle relative to height and weight, and the linearity (height over cube root of weight) in 100 healthy children within 6 months of their seventh birthday. The three traditional body types thus assembled had the following associations: ectomorphy (leanness) correlated with anxiety, high moral standards, and an 'inner world', in which the child's intelligence was not used in responses to the world, but 'internally' in a fantasy world—the description according with that of the typical introvert. The ectomorphs had more night terrors, and tended to be more suspicious and resentful. The other two body types (mesomorphy, describing high bone and muscle development; and endomorphy, describing roundness of physique and the ability to grow fat) tended to be much lower on these characteristics.

An alternative type of somatyping has been used by Eysenck and his colleagues (Rees and Eysenck, 1945; Eysenck, 1959). This has been carried out by factorial studies, which have extracted those combinations of body measurement having maximum predictive value for psychological characteristics. A comparison of other kinds of somatyping with the same data seems to show fairly conclusively the superiority of the Rees-Eysenck system, which has two factors, rather than three, as in the Sheldonian system, which was used by Davidson *et al.* The two factors were height, or length (*L*), and width or breadth (*B*). An equation of *B* and *L* gives a single index of body build, which distributes normally, and has a good correlation with the extraversion-introversion dimension.

Eysenck (1959) reanalysed the data given by Davidson and his colleagues (1957) to show that the three body types could in fact be reduced to a single dimension without loss of predictive value. Linearity, leanness, or a low amount of muscle and fat at one end of the dimension correlates with introversion, high intelligence, neurosis, social conformity, and more schizoid personality traits; and at the other end of the curve, marked muscularity in combination with the amount of fat correlates with extraversion, lower intelligence, poor school record, and low incidence of schizophrenia.

Children who are introverted tend to develop neurotic, anxious disorders, while extraverted children tend to develop aggressive behaviour disorders under stress (Eysenck, 1960). Deductively, epileptic children who are lean should tend to become neurotic or anxious after the onset of epilepsy, if accompanying stresses occur, while muscular children should tend to become aggressive. Body build does not change with epilepsy (although there is some suggestion in the literature, reviewed below, that it might be affected by early brain injury), so that it can be measured after the onset of epilepsy. On the interaction hypothesis, extreme linearity and extreme muscularity should place epileptic children especially at risk for behaviour disorder.

Body build and epilepsy

Some of the early work on body build and type of mental illness has been summarized by Kallman and Sander (1948). The work of Westphal and Kretschmer cited in this review indicated that epileptics had the lowest proportion of pyknic ('tubby') individuals, compared with schizophrenics and manic depressives. Schizophrenics had the highest proportion of asthenic ('lean') individuals, epileptics having only a moderate number, but more than manic depressives. The modal body type of the epileptics was found to be athletic ('muscular'), a type occurring less frequently in manic depression, and only rarely in schizophrenia. A high proportion of the epileptics were also found to be unclassifiable on the Kretschmer scheme, in contrast to the body types of schizophrenia and manic depression, which were much more easily classifiable.

Before any significance is attached to these findings, some qualifications should be made. Schizophrenia and manic depression are by definition mental diseases, but epilepsy is not. It is not possible to tell, from the material provided by Kallman and Sander, to what extent the body build of the epileptic individual differs from that of the normal population, if at all. The only generalization that can be made from these findings is that schizophrenics have a strong tendency to be lean or thin individuals, while manic depressives tend to display the opposite characteristics of tubbiness or fat. Epileptics seem to fall in the middle of this spectrum, having a predominance of muscular individuals. If Eysenck's 'normal curve' hypothesis for body build is correct, this kind of distribution occurs in the normal population, so that the excess of 'muscular' body types among epileptics would probably place them in the normal population so far as body build is concerned.

Janz (1940) studied aggressive, anti-social disorder in 200 epileptics, and found that the athletic and dysplastic (unclassified) types were heavily over-represented among those epileptics who displayed what he called the 'traditional epileptic personality'. Janz hypothesized that a hypophyseal lesion of some kind was responsible for the predominance of these kinds of body development in epileptics. There is a slight plausibility in this hypothesis, since hypophyseal tumours are a known cause of precocious puberty in children. However, Janz was unable to show any difference between the body types of epileptics in whom brain damage was a known aetiological factor, and epileptics in whom the cause of fits was unknown.

Rey *et al.* (1949) reported on a series of 57 cases with temporal lobe epilepsy (including a number of children). The predominant body type was found to be asthenic, or lean (33 per cent), 19 per cent of the cases having an athletic body build.

Pond (1952) found in 150 epileptic children, 'The slightly built, retiring boy with *petit mal* seizures contrasts with the stockier build of the child with major seizures and an aggressive behaviour problem'. Numbers are not given, and it is not clear whether systematic somatyping was undertaken.

Siegmund and Pache (1953) studied minor and atypical epilepsy in 70 children, and found a correlation between Kretschmer's athletic-viscosic constitution and behaviour of the aggressive type.

Ounsted (1955), describing 70 epileptic children with hyperkinesis, found a preponderance of mesomorphic or muscular body types among them: 'The large majority of children had rosy plump faces, short necks, square chests, and solid trunks with heavy muscular development in the limbs. They gave an impression of marked mesomorphy when compared with mentally normal epileptic children.' It does not appear, from this account, that systematic body measurements of the children were taken and compared with those from normal epileptic children. However, assuming the validity of the finding (of low tolerance for frustration and a tendency to act in an aggressive manner), there seem to be three theoretical possibilities: (*a*) Hyperkinesis of a mild degree occurs in a higher proportion of epileptic children than the 8 per cent having *marked* hyperkinesis described by Ounsted. The emergence of hyperkinesis, of a marked degree and in association with aggressive behaviour, depends on the coincidence of the minimal brain damage syndrome with a child having a muscular body type. (*b*) The early brain damage causing the hyperkinesis also causes accelerated muscular and body development. If, as many writers suggest, hyperkinesis is associated with organic impairment of the rhinencephalon, the involvement of the hypophysis cerebri, which is an important endocrine centre for structural development, has some anatomical plausibility. (*c*) Children with a biologically innate athletic constitution tend to be larger at birth, and therefore are more susceptible to injury to the nervous system. The evidence summarized by Montagu (1964) provides some support for this view. However, detailed evidence from obstetrics and developmental neurology is not available to provide very much support for this hypothesis. It should be noted, however, that boys have a higher birth weight than girls (Tanner, 1958), and also that boys are heavily over-represented in hyperkinetic population (Ounsted, 1955).

A recent writer on the hyperkinetic syndrome (Widrow, 1966) has suggested that hyperkinetic children were likely to be *underdeveloped*, and to suffer from maturational delays of the central nervous system. This finding seems difficult to reconcile with Ounsted's finding of an athletic constitution, unless physical overdevelopment is accompanied, in a paradoxical way, by underdevelopment of the nervous system. It is obvious that this is an important field for further work.

The literature on body build, reviewed above, suggests the following conclusions:

1 In non-epileptic children, muscularity seems associated with outgoing, extraverted, or aggressive behaviour; leanness or lack of muscularity seems associated with in-turned, introverted, anxious behaviour.

2 *A priori*, one would expect the same kind of reaction from epileptic children with lean and muscular body builds when faced with stress.

3 There does appear to be some evidence that epileptics with a muscular body build tend to behave in an aggressive way.

4 There has been a suggestion that *petit mal* is associated with leanness and an anxious type of personality.

5 Hyperkinesis is apparently associated with muscular body build, in contrast to normal behavioural pictures seen in epilepsy. Why this should be so is not clear.

13 The social environment of the epileptic

The review of liteıature above has indicated numerous studies which stress the fact that adverse factors in the environment—a rejecting peer group, anxiety or rejection by parents, and a hostile social world—may cause behavioural disturbances in the epileptic. This behaviour may serve to reinforce the adverse picture that others have of the epileptic. A number of writers have laid stress on brain damage as causative of disturbed behaviour in epilepsy. Some have suggested that the disturbed behaviour is a neurological equivalent to epilepsy, while others have suggested that there is a complex interaction of social environment, early personality, the effect of fits, and brain damage influencing behaviour in epilepsy.

The present section will consider in detail some particular problems in the social environment of the epileptic: social prejudice, the problem of finding work, and the environment created by the personality of family members. The direct interaction between parents and epileptic children will be considered in detail in a later section

Social prejudice

Levy *et al.* (1964) studied epilepsy in a population of Africans in Southern Rhodesia. In a population of 17,500, 130 epileptics were discovered. The authors reported that in children ridicule of epilepsy was common, and adults with epilepsy were likely to be social outcasts, without jobs. A similar situation has been reported by Giel (1968) in Ethiopia.

Aall-Jilek (1965) studied epilepsy in the Wapagora tribe in Tanganyika. This tribe was isolated geographically from other tribes. A very high incidence of epilepsy—1·5 per cent—was found (101 patients). The occurrence of epilepsy was surrounded by rituals which seemed to be incorporated into the social system of the tribe.

During and after an attack the epileptic was untouchable; he had to live in his own hut, apart from the village. His food was prepared separately. Epilepsy in children was attributed to sexual indulgence on the part of their parents (cf. the views of the general practitioner in early twentieth century England, cited by Russell, 1967). The epileptic was poorly nourished, and often suffered severe burns through falling into the fire and not being rescued. This treatment created a particular kind of personality in the epileptics (or perhaps there was a particular kind of ascribed role for the epileptic): 'They are shy, humble, and timid people who in mute apathy have resigned themselves to their fate, without hope or complaint. They have lost interest in keeping clean . . . '. The control of attacks by luminal had a strong effect on the personality of the epileptics, so that their behaviour and self-concept returned to normal.

An interesting point made by Aall-Jilek is that only patients who had major attacks were feared. The occurrence of minor forms did not seem to be associated with prejudice. The author suggests that there are many rituals in the tribe—e.g. eating special foods or avoiding others—which will protect the individual against getting epilepsy. The dream of epilepsy appeared to be the archetypal nightmare of the Wapagora. In 81 of the 110 cases epilepsy was known in sisters, brothers, cousins, uncles and aunts. This finding suggests the possibility that, in order to find a marriage partner, the epileptic has to marry another epileptic.

A question of fundamental interest in the study of epilepsy is the extent to which these primitive attitudes to epilepsy survive in Western cultures, and to what extent individuals can be free from prejudice about epilepsy.

It is possible to give some answer to these questions from the serial testing of public opinion about epilepsy in America. Caveness *et al.* (1965) report a national random sample of attitudes to epilepsy in America, compared with the answers to similar questions asked of a sample in 1949. In 1964 95 per cent of respondents knew what epilepsy was, compared with 92 per cent in 1949. Of these, 77 per cent in 1964 and 57 per cent in 1949 would not object to their child playing with an epileptic child. In 1964 79 per cent thought that epilepsy was *not* a form of insanity, compared with 59 per cent in 1954. In 1964 82 per cent said that epileptics should be employed in the general labour market, compared with 45 per cent in 1949. In both surveys, the most favourable responses came from the better-educated, younger, urban-dwelling, higher economic status respondents, living in the northern rather than the southern half of America.

These surveys indicate that favourable change in attitudes to epilepsy can take place, probably as an accompaniment to increasing education of the population. But still in 1964 2 parents in every 10 would not allow their child to play with an epileptic, and 2 respondents in 10 thought that epileptics should not be employed in the labour market.

If there is prejudice against the epileptic in America, there is an even higher amount of prejudice in West Germany. Hauck (1968) carried out a representative survey of attitudes in the German population in 1967, asking similar questions to those used in a 1967 American survey: 27 per cent of Germans and 4 per cent of Americans surveyed thought that epilepsy was a form of insanity; and 37 per cent of Germans and 13 per cent of Americans would object to their child associating with an epileptic child.[1] Schutte (1968) examined the effect that prejudice against epilepsy in West Germany had on the patients themselves: he found that epileptics tended to deny both the fact and the significance of epilepsy, a dreadful diagnosis which had to be resisted at all costs. The effect of this on the patient getting adequate treatment, both in hospital and school, is obvious. Moya and Julian-Ramo (1968) sent postal questionnaires about epilepsy to a random sample of 5,000 in the general population of Spain. Only 461 questionnaires were returned. The authors conclude that there is widespread apathy and ignorance about epilepsy; public opinion, so far as it can be ascertained, associates epilepsy with insanity, unemployability, and exclusion from normal schooling.

The social climate of attitudes to epilepsy can also be judged from attitudes of the popular media. It is obvious from Livingston's handbook for parents of epileptics that the American newspaper and magazine Press will publish sensational articles about anti-social acts said to have been committed by epileptics. In England a novel was published by Heinemann in 1966 entitled *The World of Luke Simpson*. Its theme is the life of a temporal lobe epileptic who makes sexual assaults on small girls. There is a danger, of course, that the general public will associate these two conditions together in an uncritical way. A film shown in London in 1966, from Italy, called *Fists in the Pocket*, depicted the familial association of epilepsy, incest and murder. It is difficult to see how this kind of film could improve the public conception of epilepsy.

The Minister of Health (Robinson, 1966) in an address to the British Epilepsy Association, admitted the existence of irrational attitudes about epilepsy, and said: 'Our job is to replace these unbalanced and ignorant views associated with the term "epilepsy" by attitudes based on fact and clear thinking.'

[1] The latest American figures (W. Caveness *et al.*, *A Survey of Public Attitudes toward Epilepsy in 1969*, Public Health Service, Washington, 1969) indicate that only 9 per cent of a representative national sample would now object to their child playing with a child who had fits.

Work problems

Pinanski (1947) studied the work records of 1,015 epileptics, and found an increase in the percentage of epileptics successfully employed during the war. He found that over-protective and guilty parents often handicapped the ability of the epileptic child to adjust to his first job, so that a social casework intervention might be necessary at this time to assist both parents and children in working out the psychological problems associated with preparing an epileptic for employment.

Lord Cohen (1956) suggested that many epileptics, particularly those with frequent major fits, could be more often employed. The problem of gaining employment for epileptics was principally one of improving the attitudes of the public toward epilepsy:

> The most pressing task of those who seek to ameliorate the lot of the epileptic is *educational*. The public have long cherished the belief that epilepsy is synonymous with mental deficiency and uncontrollable criminal impulses (a view fostered by some of our colleagues in criminal trials) and the epileptic is thus treated as a pariah.

Gordon and Russell (1958) studied the employment problems of 400 randomly selected patients attending the National Hospital, Queen Square. In a time of very low unemployment, approximately 10 per cent of the epileptics were unemployed. This population of epileptics did not include those in permanent institutional care, who are likely to contain those with most frequent fits, low intelligence, and difficulty in social adaption. Only 60 per cent of the epileptics had informed their employers about their illness. The correlates of unemployment were lower intelligence, age 46 or over, *grand mal* fits of temporal lobe origin, frequent fits, and, to a lesser degree, personality disorder. The authors reported that anticonvulsant drugs did not impair the capacity of the patients to work.

Wilson *et al.* (1960), in a study of 42 epileptics, reported a correlation between low intelligence and personality disorder, with poor work adjustment and unemployment. They found that epileptics without personality disorder were liked and accepted in their jobs, leading the authors to suggest that the factor of prejudice does not play a large part in the adjustment of epileptics to work.

Pond and Bidwell (1960), in a study of epileptics in a general practice sample in southern England, reported that 57 per cent of the 157 adult epileptics thus located had serious difficulties with employment because of epilepsy at some time in their career. The employment problems occurred with more frequency in the younger patients, and in the unskilled. An examination by the authors of the

Disabled Persons Register indicated that less than a tenth of adult epileptics were on this register. (By law, firms employing more than twenty persons are required to reserve a percentage of occupations for the registered disabled,[1] so that epileptics thus registered would theoretically find it easier to gain employment.)

Jones (1965) studied the employment problems of epileptics in a steel works in South Wales. He reported that two thirds of epileptics had difficulties in job-finding, twice the number in the population at large. In the steel works he found that many epileptics had to accept jobs below their capacities. The author suggests that a national study relating the intelligence, capabilities and special skills of epileptics to the jobs they actually do, and the difficulties they have in obtaining employment, is called for.

Dennerill *et al.* (1966) compared 43 employed epileptics with 49 who were unemployed. The unemployed had lower intelligence, significantly earlier onset of seizures, poorer response to medication (i.e. more seizures), more organic changes and neurological abnormalities, and significantly more social isolation. This finding suggests the possibility that early brain damage may underly these abnormalities seen in the unemployed epileptics.

In the general practice survey of Pond and Bidwell, a lower social class incidence for the epileptics[2] than the normal population was found, suggesting that the epileptic may drift downward in the social scale because of his inability to find work. Jones's study supports this view. Juul-Jensen (1964), in a Danish study of 956 epileptics, came to a similar conclusion. However, Juul-Jensen reported that unemployment rates for epileptics were the same as those for the general population in Denmark.

The genetic environment of epilepsy

The term 'genetic environment' is used to indicate the existence of disturbed behaviour—mental illness, criminality, alcoholism and psychopathy—in the family members of the epileptic with whom he is likely to come in contact. There appears to be some firm evidence that the genetic environment of the epileptic child, and especially the child in whom epilepsy appears to have a genetic basis, is more adverse than that of the population at large.

Thom and Walker (1922) studied the incidence of mental disorder in the families of 117 epileptics. Twenty-two of the epileptics had

[1] Disabled Persons Employment Act, 1964.

[2] A similar finding has been reported by Michael in a mental health survey of mid-town Manhattan, U.S.A. (1961). Wade (1969), in a survey of epilepsy in England and Wales, also found an overall excess of epileptics in the lowest occupational class.

children with epilepsy. The author noted that in many cases there was a marked incidence of alcoholism, 'insanity', and 'immorality' in the families of the epileptics. However, no controls were used in this study.

Brain (1926) could not find that the incidence of mental disorder in the families of 200 epileptics was any greater than that in the population at large. Dawson and Conn (1929), studying intelligence in 150 epileptic children, could not find any excess over normal population of mental deficiency in the families of these children.

Despite these (and other) negative findings, the familial association of epilepsy and mental disorder does occur in many other studies. Schulz (1928) studied familial mental illness in 515 probands with chorea minor (an illness associated with lesions of the CNS). In the relatives (parents and siblings) an incidence of epilepsy of 0·9 per cent, compared with an expected incidence of 0·3 per cent, was found; the incidence of schizophrenia was 3·8 per cent, compared with the expected 0·85 per cent. The incidence of epilepsy, chorea, alcoholism, personality disorder, and psychosis in the relatives was much higher than that expected in the general population. The association, in particular, of degenerative illnesses of the central nervous system, such as multiple sclerosis and chorea, with schizophrenia, and sometimes with epilepsy, has led a number of authors to suggest that a common hereditary degenerative illness of the CNS underlies all these conditions (Herz, 1928; Tatarenno, 1930; Oppler, 1933; Persch, 1938; Brikmayer and Lenz, 1938; Hochapfel, 1938; Amyot, 1957).

Stein (1933) compared the incidence of mental disorder in 6,752 near relatives of 1,000 institutionalized epileptics with 4,684 near relatives of hospital staff. The author gives the following table:

	Epileptics, %	*Controls, %*	*Ratio of epileptics: controls*
Seizures	3·7	1·3	2·8:1
Feeble-minded	1·9	0·1	19·0:1
Alcoholism	4·2	1·5	2·8:1
Psychosis	0·8	0·4	2·0:1
All neuropsychiatric conditions	16·7	6·0	2·8:1

One caveat must be stressed. These findings apply to institutionalized epileptics, who are specially selected from the population of epileptics as a whole on account of low intelligence, psychosis, difficulties in social adaption, etc. On the other hand, the hospital staff are presumably representative of the general population. Because of this bias in selection, a higher than average incidence of abnormal mental conditions might be expected to occur in the relatives of epileptics; but whether this accounts fully for the findings above is impossible to say.

Conrad (1937) studied the children of 519 epileptic parents, excluding cases in which epilepsy and schizophrenia were coincident. The cases of epilepsy were divided into those with a known organic cause, and those without (idiopathic cases). Two thousand children of the epileptic parents were studied. Epilepsy was found in 7 per cent of the children of the idiopathic group, and in 1 per cent of the symptomatic group. Psychoses occurred in 3·7 per cent of the children of the idiopathic group, but in none of the children of the symptomatic group. Children of the idiopathic epileptics were more abnormal physically and psychologically than other children in every respect; 42 per cent of these children had some kind of mental or physical abnormality.

These findings are important, since the epileptic probands, although hospitalized at the time of the study, were fairly representative of epileptics as a whole, in that they had maintained sufficient social competence to marry and create some kind of family organization. There is a clear implication in Conrad's findings that when epilepsy has a genetic, rather than an acquired, brain-injury basis, it tends to be associated with a high incidence of mental and physical disorder.

Franke (1937) was unable to repeat Conrad's finding, although he was working with much smaller numbers. As Franke says, his failure to validate Conrad's findings does not *contradict* them.

Lennox (1942) studied the incidence of mental disorder in 10,902 relatives of 1,845 non-institutionalized epileptics, thus escaping the bias of Stein's earlier study. The probands were divided into essential (idiopathic) and symptomatic. Lennox showed that the incidence of psychosis and of other neuropsychiatric conditions was much higher in the essential than in the symptomatic group. Mental deficiency in the family of the epileptic was also associated with a familial incidence of epilepsy. The author suggests that low intelligence in epileptics may have a genetic basis. This finding is in contrast to many other studies which have suggested that low intelligence in epileptics is due to early brain damage.

Rey *et al.* (1949), in a study of 59 temporal lobe epileptics, reported that in 32 of them there was a family history of neurosis, psychopathy, psychosis and alcoholism.

Alström (1950) could not show that in the near relatives of the 897 epileptics he studied that the incidence of psychosis was greater than that in the general population.

Pond (1952), in a study of 150 epileptic children, reported that in the brain-injured group, who often showed a focus in the temporal lobe, there was often a bad family history of psychopathy, which was associated with a socially unsatisfactory background.

Ingram (1956), in a study of 25 brain-damaged hyperactive children, 13 of whom were epileptic, reported that a poor family history, with epilepsy, psychopathy, mental deficiency, paranoia, neurosis and behaviour disorder was common. Grunberg and Pond (1957), who found that a poor family history differentiated epileptics with and without behaviour disorder, suggested that mental illness, psychopathy, and alcoholism in close relatives of the child acted as an environmental hazard for the child.

The WHO study group on epilepsy (1957), commenting on recent findings on the family background to children with temporal lobe epilepsy, commented:

> So striking are the associations between severe temporal lobe behaviour disorders and disturbed family background that one is tempted to postulate a genetic or familial factor to account for it. Such an idea is, of course, but a revival of the 'epileptic constitution' but in a new form that may be heuristically more useful.

Why the findings of a poor family background should apply in particular to temporal lobe epilepsy (which, by definition, involves an injury to the temporal lobe) rather than to all epileptics is not discussed.

The WHO report noted that its theory was a revival of the idea of the epileptic constitution. Bleuler (1960), in his *Textbook of Psychiatry*, specifically retains this idea: 'In general, epileptics are found in families which socially can establish themselves only with difficulty. The tendency to vagabondage, begging, personal neglect, prostitution and criminality occurs in patients and in their relatives with more than average frequency.'

Bleuler suggests that the hereditary background of epilepsy means that the epileptic himself is likely to show the abnormal traits of behaviour, on a genetic basis, as well as his family. Given the previous findings of a distinction between symptomatic and idiopathic or essential epilepsy, if this is true then there should be a tendency towards an *inverse* relation of brain damage and disturbed behaviour. This finding emerged clearly in the study of Bridge (1949). However, other studies (reviewed above) have indicated that the brain-damaged is *more* at risk as a behaviour disorder. Gudmundsson (1966), in a study of 987 epileptics, for example, found that psychosis was associated with early brain damage. However, he concluded:

> The conclusions of this investigation suggest that it is not possible to attribute the mental changes to any one cause, but that they are a result of various factors. An important factor is brain damage, though certain inherited defects are also involved, besides socio-psychological influences.

The finding that an abnormal family history is associated with temporal lobe epilepsy (a brain damage type) can be explained from the study of Ounsted *et al.* (1966), which argued that a genetic history of epilepsy often seen in these cases led to fits or states early in life which *in turn* caused temporal lobe damage.

How can the finding—assuming it to be valid—of an abnormal family history in cases where epilepsy has a genetic background be accounted for? A theory will be briefly presented in the present section, and set forth in greater detail later in this study on p. 245 (when the hypothesis of abnormal family history in association with a history of epilepsy, in comparison with brain damage cases, will be tested on a fresh series of epileptic children). The theory makes the following assumptions, which are supported by previous work on epilepsy:

1 There is strong social prejudice against epileptics.
2 Epileptics have difficulty in finding normal marriage partners.
3 Perforce, they often take as marriage partners those in the community with mental and physical abnormality, whom no one else will marry.
4 In this way a number of conditions become linked in the families of these cases.
5 This would explain why an abnormal family history is less often found in cases in which brain damage appears to be the sole or principal aetiological factor in epilepsy.

It is interesting to note that in Sweden, where Alström's study was carried out, epileptics had been forbidden by law to marry for 160 years. This may possibly account for the fact that Alström failed to validate previous findings on the incidence of psychosis in the relatives of epileptics.

Conclusions

The conclusions from the review of literature in this section are:

1 Both in primitive and modern society, the epileptic seems to be the subject of prejudice and rejection.
2 Epileptics have difficulty in finding and keeping work which exceeds the difficulty encountered by the normal population. There is also evidence that those with lower intelligence and frequent seizures have more difficulty in finding and keeping work than other epileptics.

3 Although the finding has not been consistently validated, there is evidence from many studies that, where epilepsy has a genetic basis, a family history of mental illness, alcoholism, criminality and psychopathy is often found, in contrast with the normal population, and with epileptics in whom brain damage seems to be the principal aetiological factor. Some writers have suggested that a common underlying genetic defect of the central nervous system might underlie several of these conditions. An alternative, historical-genetical theory is advanced, which will be discussed in detail later.

14 The problem of prejudice against the epileptic

The literature on epilepsy reviewed above has indicated that prejudice has existed against epilepsy in historical times, in simple societies, and in modern industrial society. Why is it, for example, that 'School teachers commonly show a surprising eagerness to eliminate the affected child from school, and even people with a medical training may show disproportionate emotion when trying to persuade a mother to send her epileptic child to a colony or home' (*Lancet*, 1953)?

If prejudice is defined as a strongly held negative belief or attitude, in the absence of positive grounds for this belief, or in the face of evidence to the contrary, then physicians themselves have been guilty of prejudice against epilepsy. Many authors of papers have attributed negative and anti-social traits to the epileptic when the canons of scientific logic ought to have restrained them from doing so. Time and again, in the literature reviewed above, traits have been attributed to the epileptic on the basis of unspecified methods with unspecified epileptic populations, without accounts of incidence, definitions of terminology, or the use of control groups where this would be appropriate. The number of such studies has decreased in the period after 1947, but they continue to appear. The vogue in the past twenty years among some physicians has been to categorize disturbed behaviour in patients with and without epilepsy as 'epileptic equivalents'. We have argued that the grounds for such an inference are extremely weak. In addition, much pathological behaviour has been attributed to individuals with temporal lobe epilepsy. While some carefully conducted studies have shown that certain psychiatric syndromes are apparently more common in this type of epilepsy, there seems to have been a 'band-wagon' effect, with a rash of studies attributing particular kinds of pathological behaviour to temporal lobe epilepsy on the basis of studies using only a small number of patients or without control subjects. Many studies have assumed a causal connection between epilepsy and disturbed behaviour without considering the range of possible intervening variables.

Some physicians apparently write in the tradition of clinical reporting, in which individual or a small number of cases are presented; in some instances the obvious rarity of such cases (e.g. Gilles de la Tourette syndrome) makes the use of significance testing or control groups inappropriate. Some physicians seem to have made the mistake of assuming that two clinical conditions *in combination* provide a previously unreported or rarely reported syndrome. The papers reporting the combination of temporal lobe epilepsy and the choice of unusual sexual objects are an example of this. What these writers have not discounted is the possibility that these two conditions have coincided *by chance*. The paper by Slater *et al.* (1963) on epilepsy and psychosis is an excellent example of the careful and sophisticated procedures that must be undertaken before any judgment about an integral association can be made. What is necessary, as the paper by Slater and his colleagues shows, is a large number of combination cases for study, and accurate estimates of the incidence of each condition separately in the population at risk. If the chance association has been discounted, an investigation must then be undertaken of possible intervening variables (e.g. genetics and the effect of drugs in the study of Slater *et al.*).

Comfort (1967) has argued, in a historical review of the moral positions taken by physicians, that they have taken a spurious authority from the fact that doctors have undergone a long, technical training for a profession whose practice is a mystery to the layman. Doctors have thus made unwarranted moral pronouncements on social and individual problems which have had an apparent connection with physical conditions.

The attitude of physicians to masturbation is a case in point. In Victorian times surgical measures against masturbation in children was practised: 'By 1880, the individual who wished to tie, chain, or mutilate sexually active children or lunatics, to adorn them with grotesque appliances, and even to castrate them, could find respectable medical authority for so doing.' Other strongly moral and irrational positions have been taken in regard to contraception and venereal disease. The advice of Lord Russell's family-physician (Russell, 1967) that epilepsy would result from the use of contraception is a reflection of the prejudiced attitudes which physicians might express.

There is evidence, then, that in other areas besides epilepsy physicians have been capable of irrationality and prejudice. The writer has gained the strong impression, in reviewing the literature on the connections between organic brain injury and psychosis

(Davison and Bagley, 1970), that studies in this field, including those carried out in the early part of the century, have been carried out with much greater scientific rigour and sophistication than those in the field of epilepsy in the same period. It seems that physicians are most likely to adopt irrational attitudes (like other members of the community) in areas which arouse the passions deeply, such as the problems of sexual conduct and behaviour. Epilepsy appears to be one of these areas.

Szasz (1966), reviewing the progress of psychiatry in the present century, has written:

> In the initial decades of this century much was learned about epilepsy. As a result, physicians gained better control of the epileptic process (which sometimes results in seizures). The desire to control the disease, however, seems to go hand-in-hand with the desire to control the diseased person. Thus, epileptics were both helped and harmed: they were benefited in so far as their illness was more accurately diagnosed and better treated; they were injured in so far as they, as persons, were stigmatized and socially segregated.
>
> Was the placement of epileptics in 'colonies' in their best interests? Or their exclusion from jobs, from driving automobiles, and from entering the United States as immigrants? It has taken decades of work, much of it still unfinished, to undo some of the oppressive social effects of 'medical progress' in epilepsy, and to restore the epileptic to the social status he enjoyed before his disease became so well understood.

In the light of Szasz's criticism of the U.S. immigration policy on epilepsy, it is interesting to note that in 1965 a working party of the British Medical Association recommended that epileptics should not be allowed to immigrate to this country, 'for social and economic reasons'.[1] Lennox and Lennox (1960) have pointed to the irrationality of eugenic and immigration laws which discriminate against epilepsy on the grounds that it is a hereditary illness, when in fact the genetic basis of epilepsy is much weaker than that of many other diseases. The Swedish law against the marriage of epileptics, dating from 1760, was abandoned in the 1920s (Alström, 1950) when it was realized that it was impossible to tell with any certainty whether epilepsy in an individual was caused by an acquired brain injury or by a genetic history for the disease, or both acting in combination. A law forbidding epileptics to marry was effected in Germany in the late 1930s.

[1] Cf. a spokesman of the South African High Commission to *The Times* (28 February 1968), when asked whether his country would admit Asians with British passports: '. . . if British passport holders were hoboes, drug addicts or epileptics we wouldn't let them in . . . .' The spokesman said Asians would be similarly excluded.

The writings of some forensic psychiatrists and criminologists writing about epilepsy display a marked hostility to the epileptic which seems out of proportion to the information available to them. 'Many terrible crimes are committed by epileptics', wrote Bennett in 1965 in a highly regarded medical journal, *Diseases of the Nervous System*. He went on to list these crimes. But the account of any rigorous procedures for establishing the incidence of these crimes in epilepsy, and their connection with epilepsy itself, is lacking. Sethna (1956) wrote with approval of the work of Lombroso, the Italian criminologist who placed strong emphasis on the stigmatization of the criminal from birth and the integral connection of epilepsy in crime. Banay (1961) wrote in a similar vein.

Why do some physicians or scholars still give professional accord to the extraordinary views of Lombroso? Barbara Wootton (1966) reviewed Radzinowicz's *Ideology and Crime* and asked a similar question:

> . . . Equally ludicrous also was the pessimism of those who based their determinist philosophy on what they regarded as the inescapable physical and mental limitations of every individual's personality. Although as Professor Radzinowicz himself admits that Lombroso has become a myth, he apparently feels it necessary to keep this myth alive. So once again we are taken back to the 'gloomy day in December when Cesare Lombroso found in the skull of a brigand a very long series of atavistic abnormalities . . . and realized that the problem of the nature and generation of criminals was resolved for me'. Resolved that is, for Lombroso, yes; but not for Professor Radzinowicz or for the law students of Columbia whom he was addressing. Is it, one can hardly refrain from asking, really necessary to perpetuate this rubbish?

This is a pertinent question. Why has the theory of Lombroso survived, not merely in modern accounts of the development of criminological theory, but in modern theories themselves? Why has the theory of the atavistic connection of crime and the integral connection of epilepsy with that behaviour survived so well, so that it is still presented by some writers in one form or another—for example, as a theory of epileptic equivalents? Lombroso might be said to be the father of the theory of the epileptic equivalent, although the theory was developed in a more clinical form by Maudsley (op. cit.), writing at about the same time.

I would like to suggest that theories with a Lombrosian character have survived because they are emotively satisfying to the individuals who express them: that they are the function of a deep lying prejudice, which is pervasive (or archetypal) in character. This theory must remain extremely tentative, and proof for it is remarkably difficult to obtain. It is possible, as Stevens (1957) has pointed out, writing about the psychophysical law in psychology, that 'a bold and plausible theory that fills a scientific need is seldom broken by the impact of contrary facts and arguments. Only with an alternative theory can we hope to displace a defective one.' The theory of the integral relationship of epilepsy and disturbed, anti-social behaviour is of this kind. It survives criticism and facts to the contrary because it fills a need—in this case a need which is strengthened by emotional as well as epistemological factors.

What is the nature of this hypothetical, innate prejudice against epilepsy? There is evidence of its pervasiveness in different kinds of cultures, and among otherwise rational individuals, such as physicians. The basis of this prejudice is hypothetically that of *fear*—fear of the sudden loss of physical and emotional control. It seems plausible that the prejudices against homosexuality, leading to laws out of all proportion to the possible harmful effects of homosexual behaviour, are due to the fact that every man is afraid of homosexual behaviour because he might easily indulge in it himself: because the desire to engage in homosexual behaviour is deep-rooted, but unconscious. The rigid control of homosexuality is a result of this fear. Freud made a similar case for the rigour with which transgressions of the incest taboo are punished, arguing that the desire for incest is deep-rooted, if unconscious, in every man (cf. Bagley (1969) on the multidimensional nature of the incest taboo).

Hill (1965) writing about the prejudice against coloured people suggests:

> In addition to this social element, there is a strong psychological element underlying this prejudice. It stems partly from a fear of the black man as someone primitive and savage, a man whose reactions to any given situation are unpredictable, a man whose instinctive brutality may at any moment cause him to go berserk and act with irrational savage strength. . . .

There may be some analogies for the epileptic here. He is feared because, without warning and in any situation, he may unpredictably lose control of his movements. It is feared that, like the coloured man, 'instinctive brutality may at any moment cause him to go berserk and act with irrational savage strength'. The epileptic is feared and hated because he does what we are afraid we will do ourselves. He loses control—basic control of his motor movements. He reverts to the 'primitive', so that the punishment of him (by social rejection and ostracism) appears to be justified.[1]

[1] Cf. The Wapagora tribe (Aall-Jilek, *op. cit.*), in which the most feared dream was that of having an epileptic attack.

This theory, as was stressed earlier, is highly tentative, and satisfactory methods for proving it are difficult to obtain. But if the theory is rejected on the grounds of implausibility, and it is still accepted that prejudice against the epileptic is widespread, some other theory must be offered. General theories, such as basic irrationality in human beings or of prejudice in situations difficult to understand, still have to explain why *epilepsy* itself, and not some other condition (e.g. multiple sclerosis or cerebral palsy), is the subject of prejudice. In the case of cerebral palsy, the loss of motor control by the child is mild, constant and predictable because of this constancy. It lacks the sudden nature of the epileptic attack. The prejudiced observer of epilepsy may ask himself the implicit question: 'If he can maintain control of himself for days, weeks, or months, why can't he control himself now?' The victim of cerebral palsy cannot be blamed in this way, for he has never *gained* control of himself, so he cannot lose it. He is not 'morally' responsible. It is interesting to note in this connection that among some early writers a category of 'hysterical epilepsy' was delineated, in which the patient was said to simulate the attack.[1]

Conclusions

1 Prejudice against epilepsy—a strongly held, negative belief, in the absence of supporting evidence or in the face of contrary evidence—seems to be widespread. Among the prejudiced are some physicians and criminologists, particularly those writing in the earlier years of the century.

2 A tentative theory of prejudice against the epileptic is proposed: it is hypothesized that there is a common, but unconscious, fear of a sudden loss of control of the movements of the body, so that individuals who are liable to sudden loss of this control are the subjects of rejection and hostility.

[1] The writer was informed, during a lecture on 'problem children' in a Certificate of Education course, that there were three kinds of epileptic: those with major fits, those with minor fits, and those who simulated fits in order to gain attention. The behaviour of the large majority of epileptic children was said to be truculent and explosive. The writer has subsequently learned the inaccuracy of these statements. Presumably the 300 or more students who gain this Certificate each year at this particular College have not, and may therefore maintain these beliefs as practising teachers.

15 The study of interaction

There appear to be three uses of the term 'interaction' in social and clinical science: (*a*) the study of how relatively uncorrelated variables act together to produce a final outcome;[1] (*b*) the study of how correlated variables act together to produce a final outcome; (*c*) the study of the social relationships of two or more people, and of the influence of these relationships on their behaviour and attitudes. This last approach is exemplified by Rose's monograph (1962), *Human Behaviour and Social Process—an Interactionist Approach.*

The present section is concerned only with the literature on (*a*)—the interaction of relatively uncorrelated variables. This process of interaction may be understood by the example from natural science given by Yates (1958) in a monograph on the techniques of measuring interaction effects. In the experiment described by Yates, a number of fields with homogeneous basic soil were sown with a similar kind and quality of seed potato. After sowing, the following treatments were given to the soil: none; potash; dung; nitrogen; and the various possible combinations of these last three fertilizers, giving a total of eight possible treatments. The potato yield per acre was then measured, and the result analysed by a factorial design. The object of the experiment was to show whether adding one type of fertilizer to another increased the yield of potatoes per acre.

In a later section this method will be applied to a series of epileptic children, in order to see whether hypothetical constraints on behaviour (parental behaviour, environmental hazards, brain damage, etc.) act together to produce differential behaviour 'yields', analagously to the action of the fertilizers on the potato crop.

The difficulties of this exercise will at once be obvious: the measurement involved cannot be undertaken with the accuracy that

[1] This use of the term 'interaction' is similar to that used in analysis of variance terminology (Moroney, 1956, pp.389ff).

the natural sciences can measure such variables as the amount of fertilizer applied per acre; the intervening variables are much more difficult to control—the homogeneity of the potatoes can be assured, but the premorbid personality of the children cannot; and the degree of intercorrelation is not obviously known (as dung and potash may be independent) and a prior analysis of the relative independence of the hypothetically influential variables cannot be undertaken.

Studies or conceptualization of interaction in producing particular outcomes of attitude or behaviour in both epileptics and non-epileptics are reviewed below.

The interaction of constraints on the behaviour of the brain-damaged child

The largest literature on interaction seems to be in this field. Denhoff and Holden (1954), who studied 33 children with cerebral palsy, found that adjustment in school was related not so much to the neurological disorder (as measured by impairment of intelligence and the degree of motor disability) as to the acceptance by the family, teachers and peers of the child's disability. Hersov (1963), who reviewed the literature on psychiatric disturbances in cerebral palsied children, concluded that unrealistic parental expectations, as well as the severity of the disorder, played a part in the emergence of the psychiatric disturbance. Oswin (1967) reached a similar conclusion after an observational study of cerebral palsied children in a special school. Three of Oswin's cases were also epileptics.

The leading exponents of interaction theory suggesting that the interaction of the behavioural individuality of the child at birth with parental behaviour, environment, and acquired brain damage (where this exists) is the major determination of personality are Birch, Thomas and Chess, and their colleagues in New York. The complexity of the factors—social, psychological and organic—which interact to produce behaviour disorder in brain-damaged children have been stressed by Birch and others in a collection of papers reviewing this problem (1964).

Birch, Thomas and Chess (1964) described the behavioural development in three brain-damaged children who were studied in detail from birth. These children were part of a much larger longitudinal study of 128 children without brain damage. The authors were able to show how, over time, the interaction of the original personality, the effect of the brain damage, and the attitudes of parents produce unique behavioural outcomes in each of these three children.

The longitudinal study of the larger number of normal children has been described by Thomas *et al.* (1964). These children were selected for the homogeneity in social characteristics of their parents. A detailed study was made of the child's behaviour through the questioning of parents. The reliability and validity of these methods were established. Detailed questioning over a wide range of areas produced nine temperamental traits on which there was sufficient variation to distinguish the children from one another, and which all children displayed in some form. These traits were:

1 Child's activity level.
2 Rhythmicity.
3 Adaptability.
4 Tendencies to approach or withdraw from environmental stimuli.
5 Thresholds of responsiveness.
6 Intensity of reactions.
7 Quality of mood.
8 Characteristics of distractability or non-distractability.
9 The degree of persistence exhibited by the child in the course of his everyday behaviour.

These traits were found to be persistent during the first two years of life, so that a high score at, say, age 3 months was predictive of a high score at, say, age 2. The problem of the 'halo' effect was avoided by using different interviewers, unaware of previous scores, at the different stages during the two years. The authors give detailed case histories illustrating the scoring of the nine traits, so that the study should be capable of detailed replication by future workers.

A study by Rutter, Korn and Birch (1963) of twins suggested that there was a genetic basis to these traits.

Rutter, Birch, Thomas and Chess (1964) reported that of the 128 children followed from infancy up to their seventh year, 21 had been referred by parents for help with psychiatric problems. A detailed psychiatric study of these 21 children, and a similar study of 71 other children in the series showed significant differences between the two groups. The clinical cases differed significantly from the other children, in that they were more irregular, non-adaptable, intense, and exhibited more negative mood. These temperamental difficulties were present before the onset of the overt symptoms and did not themselves constitute the first signs of behavioural disturbance. There is evidence in this study of an interaction between the child's behavioural individuality and the way in which the parent treats him, so that the best treatment of the child by the parent has to be *specific* to this individuality. This is illustrated in the study of Thomas *et al.* (1965), in which a case is indicated in which the parents applied the same kinds of rearing techniques (e.g. schedule feeding, etc.) to children with *different* basic temperamental patterns, so that one child emerged as a behaviour problem, while the other did not.

Thomas (1965) made an interim report of the history of the 128 children as they approach adolescence. The continued study of these children had confirmed the early pictures of interaction in producing personality.

Wortis *et al.* (1964) concluded, after a review of the literature on brain-injured children, 'There is no clear identification of the behavioural characteristics which are associated with neurological impairment, while the role of social environment in relation to the behaviour of the brain-injured child is still a matter of conjecture'. Wortis and his colleagues set out to test the hypothesis that what in fact happened was that the effect of the brain damage interacted with environmental factors. They studied 250 premature Negro children in New York who, by virtue of the prematurity, were considered to be particularly likely to be brain-injured. An investigation of the behaviour of the child and his mother (by questioning of the mother) was made, as well as an investigation of the extent of 'family disorganization (desertion of father, unemployment, marital or family conflict, alcoholism, mental illness or delinquent behaviour in family members)'. A neurologist investigated the degree of neurological abnormality in the children.

A collation of these measurements was made when the children were aged 2½. The degree of the mother's emotional disturbance in relation to her child was partly correlated with the amount of family disorganization. A high score for deviant behaviour in the children was found to have three significant associations: neurological abnormality; degree of emotional disturbance in the mother; and a high score for family disorganization. These results lead the authors to suggest that these three factors *interact* together to produce the disturbed behaviour in the children; in good surroundings, and with an undisturbed mother, the behavioural adaption of the neurologically-impaired child would be expected to be normal.

The interaction of constraints affecting behaviour in the brain-damaged child has been demonstrated by Patterson *et al.* (1965) in the treatment of two brain-injured hyperactive children. In this experiment the child was rewarded with candy and pennies for successful ten-minute periods of behaviour in which potentially distracting stimuli were ignored. The authors found that as the child became less distractable, the children in his class gave him social approval, thus reinforcing the non-distracted behaviour. This in turn apparently made it easier for the child to ignore distracting stimuli. The interaction of these constraints was successful in reducing the distractable behaviour in the children. This study provides an experimental demonstration of what is apparently the reverse, or 'downward-spiral' in the interaction process, of the interaction of constraints in *producing* behaviour disorder.

Doubros and Daniels (1966) also report the success of operant conditioning techniques in a study of six overactive children.

Wahler *et al.* (1965) describes an experiment with non-brain-damaged children with behaviour disorders, in which the therapist indicated to the mother in the playroom what kind of reaction to initiate to aggression and temper tantrums in the child. In the three cases described, this technique through the control of mother-child interaction was successful in reducing the disturbed behaviour in the children.

Kissel (1967), in a study which makes no reference to the behaviourist literature on the subject, suggests that there is a 'positive spiral in parent-child relationships', so that the treatment of the parents of the child as well as of the child himself means that each individual in the family situation will reinforce the good behaviour of the other in an interactive situation.

A comprehensive theoretical model for children in the educational process has been presented by Hemming (1966). Hemming describes a complex interaction process, in which the individual potentiality of the child interacts with the stimuli presented by him by his home, his school, his peer group, and the more diffuse set of responses offered by the outside social world. As Hemming implies, we can know with some deductive certainty what the inputs of this model must be: yet operationalizing it, to show what the most rational policy for providing optimum situations for the development of learning and mental health in the child are, is an extremely difficult task.

With regard to the epileptic child, it is reasonable to conclude that, as the interaction of constraints in producing behaviour in children with and without brain damage has been demonstrated, these findings may apply to the epileptic child who is a *child* and is also in many cases *brain-damaged.*

Further studies of interaction

There is a vast literature attempting to attribute deviant and pathological behaviour to single causes, or single kinds of causes, so that for some conditions (e.g. crime, mental illness, personality) genetics, or acquired organic injury, or environment have been proposed as being the *only* kind of factor responsible for the condition under study. As Thomas *et al.* (1965) point out, child psychiatry is still dominated by the view that social factors and, in particular, the way a mother treats her child are the sole causes of disturbed behaviour in the child.

A similar situation exists in the study of schizophrenia, so that proponents of the genetic-organic school are in direct epistemological conflict with the environmental school of schizophrenia. But why should these factors be *sole* causes? May not each of these schools have *part* of the truth? This view has been put forward by Bellak (1958):

> Schizophrenia is . . . a syndrome characterized by a final common path of a disturbance of the ego, with a primary aetiology of chemogenic, histogenic, genogenic, or psychogenic nature and a combination thereof, different in each individual case, but probably identifiable as clusters in subgroups.

Thoday (1965) and Ecland (1967) have pointed out that in fields such as intellectual attainment, genetics and environment may be said to interact together. These are recent views, and there is a weighty literature from psychologists and geneticists on the one hand, and sociologists on the other, each ignoring or denigrating the work of the other disciplines.

Thoday suggests that many of these studies have been misconceived in trying to find a *single* cause for the phenomenon in question: his conclusion is similar to that of Bellak:

> Unique genotype and unique environment are interacting in the development in unique ways; and though we must classify individuals into groups for scientific, administrative or educational purposes, we ignore this uniqueness to our great loss and at our peril. . . . Geneticism and envii onmentalism must both die a rapid death. Let us begin to realise that the question, 'is this character inherited or is it acquired?' can never have an answer other than 'No', because the question has no meaning. Let us take into account, in social and educational theory, policy and polemic, the biological fact of the uniqueness of the individual, implying as it does that the needs of each individual are unique and that it is *just* to treat different people differently so long as each is treated as well as possible. All men are different from conception.

If we substitute the term 'appropriate' for the word 'just', it is also clear that Thoday's views are similar to those of Thomas and his colleagues on child-rearing: since children are endowed with a behavioural uniqueness, the behaviour of parents towards them ought to be appropriate to that behaviour.

Interaction with the emergence of personality in epileptic children

A number of writers have stressed that the emergence of disturbed behaviour in epileptics may be due to a process of interaction of diverse factors which affect personality. Bridge (1934 and 1949) presents case histories to show the appearance of fits in a child elicits prejudiced behaviour on the part of the environment, which provokes aggressive behaviour in the child, thus confirming the stereotype of the epileptic child. Further rejection because of this merely makes the behaviour worse, and may increase the frequency of fits as well. When fits are controlled, the child is no longer rejected and his disturbed behaviour disappears.

Diethelm (1948) studied in detail the behaviour of epileptic children, and suggested that the wide variety of behavioural pictures seen might be due to the interaction of the child's previous personality with the factors associated with the onset of epilepsy. Guinena (1953) has illustrated how this interaction can take place by means of case histories of young epileptics.

Pond (1957), after reviewing studies of the connection between epilepsy, or an epileptic EEG, and psychopathic behaviour, arrived at the conclusion that 'Order is brought into this difficult field of behaviour disorders only by taking particular cases and trying to see how much of his or her behaviour may be explicable by the physiological mechanisms known to occur in proven epileptics'.

Pond (1961) further suggested that the study of the psychiatry of the epileptic and the brain-damaged child involved the study of the physiological effects of epilepsy and brain damage with other modifying factors, including the before-injury personality of the child and the after-injury treatment and environment.

Ounsted *et al.* (1966), in a study of children with temporal lobe epilepsy, found a number of diverse factors which correlated with behaviour disorder, and concluded: 'There is no single, causal relationship of disordered behaviour and any other factor'.

Gudmundsson (1966), in a study of all the locatable epileptics in Iceland, made a similar conclusion:

> The conclusions of this investigation suggest that it is not possible to attribute the mental changes to any one cause, but that they are the result of various factors. An important factor is brain damage, though certain inherited defects are also involved, besides socio-psychological influences.

Further studies indicating that behaviour disorder in epilepsy may be due to the interaction of a number of factors are reviewed above in the the section on 'Psychiatric Aspects on Epilepsy since 1947 (pp. 26–50).

The methodology of interaction studies

The studies reviewed above have all relied on a hypothetico-deductive method, inferring that interaction takes place, (*a*) from the study of individual cases and (*b*) from the finding that a number of factors are associated with the disturbed behaviour, but are not associated with one another. Thus, Wortis and his colleagues base their views of interaction on inference from a correlation matrix, in which disturbed behaviour was correlated with neurological abnormality, family disorganization, and the mother's emotional disturbance. Neurological abnormality showed no correlations with the latter two variables; between the last two variables there was a partial correlation.

The methodology of interaction studies in the sociological field is not very far advanced. Coleman (1964), in a textbook of methods of mathematical sociology, points out that there is no general model available for the study of interaction effects:

> . . . An example will make this clear. In a study of male juvenile delinquency in Nashville, Tennessee, it was found that there was a general relation between social class and delinquency, and between race and delinquency. But this relation was not constant; the lower-class Negro boys were more delinquent than the additive model would predict. There was an apparent interaction between social class and race to produce this deviation (p. 239).

It might be possible to solve this problem by measuring the *combined* statuses of class and race, and measuring their relationship with delinquency. The writer (Bagley, 1965) was faced with a similar problem in a study of juvenile delinquency in twenty-two geographically similar, isolated English towns. In this study a significant correlation (—0·6) was found between an index of social class and delinquency rates, so that towns with high social class had low delinquency rates. An additional correlation of —0·58 was found between expenditure on youth services and juvenile delinquency, so that towns which had a high expenditure on youth services had a low delinquency rate. Expenditure on youth services had no correlation with social class in a town.

An attempt was made to show that when social class was combined with youth expenditure the juvenile delinquency rate could be more accurately predicted. Two methods were used. The percentage which each town contributed to the total (*a*) of the social class index for the twenty-two towns and (*b*) of the youth expenditure for the twenty-two towns was added for each town. The resulting indices (which then totalled 200) were correlated with the delinquency rates. A second method used was to add the ranks of each of the twenty-two towns for youth expenditure and social class; the correlation of this index with the delinquency rates was then calculated. Both of these methods gave the same result: the combined index of social class and youth expenditure showed a correlation with the delinquency rates of

—0·75. The line of best fit between the delinquency rates and the combined index was a straight one, suggesting that there were no effects of extra sensitivity, which Coleman indicated might be present in the Tennessee delinquency study. However, the above method might show up this sensitivity: if Negroes belonging to the lowest social class are more likely to commit delinquency in (say) a logarithmic proportion to Negroes of higher social class, this relationship should emerge in the form of *curve* as the line of best fit. An alternative method is the interaction table (described below), which should show whether the combination of race and low social class had a particular relationship to delinquency.

The second method for studying interaction is the 2^n table, a method used for experimental design in the chemical sciences (Bennett and Franklin, 1954).[1] At the time of writing the above study of delinquency, the writer was unaware of this method of studying interaction, which has the merit of simplicity and clarity. The method involves the dichotomization of a final outcome, and then analysing the dichotomization of a number of other variables in terms of the outcome studied.

Applied to the twenty-two towns, the delinquency rates have been ranked, and the first 11 ranks assigned to a 'high delinquency' category and the last 11 ranks to a 'low delinquency' category. The same dichotomization procedure has been used for the social class index and the youth expenditure. The procedure is indicated in the following table:

Table 4 The interaction of social class and youth expenditure in a delinquency study

Social class	−11		+11	
Youth expenditure	−6	+5	−5	+6
Proportion with high delinquency rate	5/6	3/5	3/5	0/6

Minus sign indicates a score in the low category; plus sign in the high category. Two social class ranks tied at the eleventh position, and have been randomly assigned to the high/low categories.

It will be seen that where social class and youth expenditure are both low five out of the six towns with these attributes have a high delinquency rate; where social class and youth expenditure are both high, none of the six towns has a high delinquency rate. Towns

[1] Cf. Coleman (1964), who stresses the similarity between some of the statistical techniques used in chemistry, and in sociology (pp. 112ff.).

where only one of youth expenditure, or social class, occupy an intermediate position.

A number of methods are available for testing and analysing these results, including complex factorial designs (Yates, 1958; Maxwell, 1961), in which the mathematics, even by conventional statistical standards, become extremely difficult. The simplest and most direct method is to see if any combination of constraints has added to the risk of a particular outcome by comparing one cell with another by the x-squared method.

One of the difficulties of this method will be apparent from this analysis: the more complex the dichotomization, the smaller the number in the final cell, so that significance testing becomes difficult. A fairly large sample is needed before the complex range of associations can be demonstrated to any significant degree.

As an experimental design, the above studies relied on *ex post facto* methods, so that the only manipulation of variables available was a statistical one. In a study of biases in voting behaviour (Bagley, 1966) an analysis of election results suggested that there were two factors which biased electors' choice when presented with a conventional ballot paper: names high in the alphabet were chosen more often than names low in the alphabet; and central positions were chosen more often than top or bottom positions. These two effects were posited as independent variables. An experimental design was set up, with three kinds of simulated ballot papers: effect *A* most likely (clearly differentiated alphabetical names); effect *A* technically impossible, but effect *B* possible (all names similar); and both effects *A* and *B* possible (putting the names high in the alphabet in the middle positions). It was hypothesized that when both the bias effects coincided, as in the third design, the resulting positional bias on the simulated ballot papers would be greater than in the first two situations. The results (when the simulated ballot papers were given to three groups of subjects) supported this hypothesis.

A programme for the detection of interaction effects, for use with social survey data, has been written for the I.B.M. 7090 by Sanquist and Morgan (1964). This programme establishes relationship among up to thirty-seven variables. Regarding one of the variables as a dependent variable, the analysis employs a non-symmetrical branching process, based on variance analysis technique, to subdivide the sample into a series of sub-groups which maximize the ability to predict the values of the dependent variables. Assumptions of linearity and additivity are not made. This programme may be extremely useful for studying interactions in the field of human behaviour, but no empirical examples of its use are yet to hand.

A combination of the factorial and experimental method has been used by Whimbey and Denenberg (1966) in an experiment which the authors title, 'Programming Life Histories'. In this experiment a homogeneous group of infant rats was exposed to sixteen different patterns of experience. These patterns were made up of the various combinations of four possible treatments which related to (*a*) type of mother; (*b*) presence or absence of handling in infancy; (*c*) type of rearing environment in the pre-weaning stage; (*d*) type of post-weaning environment. Twenty-three conventional tests of behaviour for rats were administered to the sixteen groups. The scores were factor-analysed, and six factors extracted. Three of these factors could be clearly labelled as 'emotional reactivity', 'consumption-elimination', and 'field exploration'. This study showed, conclude the authors, that stable and relatively permanent individual differences can be produced by the combination, or interaction, of factors in the environment.

The importance of the interaction studies for the study of epilepsy

The theory of interaction suggests that outcomes in the field of biology (including human behaviour) rarely have a single cause. More often, the final outcome is the result of the interaction of a number of variables. If any problem in the behavioural sciences is to be solved, the investigator must take into account the full range of hypothetical variables, and the influence of each upon the final outcome, as well as on one another.

Considered thus, interaction theory seems little more than common sense. Yet it is remarkable how often in the past both theories and empirical descriptions of particular events have been framed in terms of a single variable or kind of variable. The different approaches to the cause of suicide (sociological, psychological, biological), each ignoring the findings of the other workers, is a case in point (Bagley, 1968). Stott (1964), writing about delinquency research, has suggested, '. . . our present disagreements about delinquency constitute an epistemologically intolerable situation'. The same may be said of theories about the cause of behaviour disorder in epilepsy which stress organic, psychological, or social factors as being the principal or only causal ones, to the exclusion of other factors. But other kinds of factors can not be excluded unless they have been adequately conceptualized, measured, and their relationship with the disturbed behaviour examined, and shown to be negligible.

It may be that many studies which have found that organic factors play a part in influencing behaviour disorder in epileptic children may be correct; and it may be that studies emphasizing social and psychological variables are correct also. But if the behaviour disorders have a *multiple* causation, it is also possible that some factors which influence the behaviour disorder may not clearly emerge, since the behaviour disorder can only be understood by considering the operation of a number of different factors together. If this is so, the lack of agreement between many studies of epilepsy which have studied only isolated factors may be more easy to understand.

Conclusions

1 Recent work on the development of behaviour in both brain-damaged and non-brain-damaged children supports the view that personality is the result of the complex interaction of social, psychological and biological variables.

2 These findings should logically apply to epileptic children. A number of authors have made the hypothesis of interaction for epileptic children after the study of case histories, and on the basis of the fact that in larger numbers of cases there are variables which correlate with behavioural outcome, but not with one another. However, no specific test of interaction has been made in a series of epileptic children.

3 The possibility that interaction theory applies to many fields of behaviour is considered.

4 The methodology of interaction studies has been considered. The methods so far developed have been: (*a*) generalizations from studies of individual cases; (*b*) generalizations from correlation studies; (*c*) the use of interaction tables; (*d*) experimental studies, which may use a variety of methods for demonstrating interaction, of which the interaction table is probably the best.

5 The theory of interaction may be of great importance in studying behaviour disorders in epileptic children, in which organic, psychological and social factors may possibly interact together to produce a final behavioural outcome. The neglect of organic, or psychological, or social factors by previous writers on behaviour disorder in epileptics may account for the lack of agreement between their findings, although other factors—differences in method and different patient populations—may also have contributed to this.

Part three
Results and hypotheses

16 The categorization of behaviour

The literature on the categorization of behaviour in children who do not have epilepsy will be considered first, and compared later in the chapter with the literature on the categorization of behaviour in epileptic children.

Behaviour in children without epilepsy

A frequently quoted study, and probably the earliest systematic attempt to categorize disturbed behaviour in a large number of children, is that of Hewitt and Jenkins (1946). These two authors recorded the characteristics (behaviour, as well as social background, and parental behaviour) of 500 Michigan children seen at a child guidance clinic, on cards. Three pictures emerged from the machine analysis of these cards: (*a*) 'Unsocialized aggressive behaviour'; (*b*) 'Socialized delinquency'; (*c*) 'Over-inhibited behaviour'.

In a further description of these 500 children, Jenkins and Glickman (1946) pointed out that these three categories were 'ideal types', so that only a minority of the children were 'perfect' fits in the behavioural categories. The authors present a further analysis of 5,000 children in which the three ideal types again emerged, as well as three others—the brain-injured child; the paretic child; and the schizoid child. The characteristics of the brain-injured children were described by the following intercorrelated traits: In boys: a change of personality or behaviour after brain injury; a diagnosis of encephalitis; irritability; changeable moods; 'queerness'; emotional instability; contrariness; nervousness; irregular sleep habits or insomnia. For girls the traits were: restlessness; a diagnosis of encephalitis; distractability; nervousness; violence; change of personality from a specific time or episode; temper tantrums; restlessness in sleep; disturbing influence in school; changeable moods.

Field (1967) has repeated the original Hewitt and Jenkins study, following as closely as possible the methods used in the original study. The subjects in Field's study were a quota sample of 274 13-year-old boys in approved schools in England and Wales. Using Hewitt and Jenkins' original criteria and method of classification, 4·7 per cent fell into the category of unsocialized aggression, 23·4 per cent into the category of socialized delinquency, and 14·6 per cent into the over-inhibited category. The proportions in the Hewitt and Jenkins study were 10·4, 14·0, and 14·6 per cent respectively. The remainder of the cases in both studies fell into a mixed category, being the largest single group in both studies. The lack of agreement about the proportions falling into the three categories is not particularly optimistic for the potential usefulness of this kind of categorization. In addition, Field could not validate the association of environmental and parental traits posited by Hewitt and Jenkins.

Jenkins (1966) has undertaken a further analysis, by computer, of a sample of 500 child guidance clinic cases.[1] In this study, five behavioural groups emerged:

1 A Shy-Seclusive group, being shy, timid, having no close friends, apathetic, under-active, depressed, and sensitive; typical age 9 to 14; $n=61$.

2 An Overanxious-Neurotic group, having sleep disturbances, fears, crying easily, over-imaginative, marked inferiority feelings, and nervousness; typical age, 9 to 12; contains a high proportion of girls; $n=43$.

3 A Hyperactive-Distractable group, with hyperactivity, lack of concentration, mischievousness, inability to get on with other children, over-dependent, bashful; typical age 9 to 11; $n=76$.

4 An Undomesticated group, showing negativism, defiance of authority, vengefulness, sullenness, malicious mischief, and temper outbursts; typical age 11 to 14; $n=58$.

5 A Socialized Delinquent group, with stealing, running away from home, truancy, and association with undesirable companions; typical age 12 to 15; a low proportion of girls; $n=53$.

The first two groups are called 'inhibited' and the last two 'aggressive'. Individuals were classified by the existence of three or more traits belonging to one particular group. The classification accounted for 291 of the 500 children, the remainder having a mixture of traits.

The two poles of aggression and inhibition or anxiety, have emerged in a number of other studies of child behaviour and maladjustment.

Burt and Howard (1952) factor-analysed data relating to 394

[1] It seems possible, from the text of this study, that this is a re-analysis of the original 500 cases in the 1946 study.

English children attending child guidance clinics. A behavioural factor emerged, which was represented at one pole by 'general emotional instability and excessive extraversion', and at the other pole by 'excessive introversion, often accompanied by anxiety states, conflicts, or feelings of inferiority'.

Lewis (1954) applied Hewitt and Jenkins' classification procedures to 500 British children taken into care. This author found 52 children who were unsocialized aggressives, 57 were 'socialized delinquents' and 80 were 'over-inhibited'. This left a large number of children falling into a mixed category.

The Underwood Committee (1955) on Maladjusted Children in England and Wales reported that 'the lines of classification in use in child guidance clinics in this country' divided maladjustment into three major categories:

1 Nervous disorder (fears, withdrawal, depression, excitability and over-activity, apathy, obsessions, hysterical fits, loss of memory).
2 Habit disorders (speech difficulties, sleep-terrors and difficulty, tics and nail-biting, feeding difficulties, incontinence, nervous pains and paralysis, physical symptoms).
3 Behaviour disorders (defiance, disobedience, school-refusal, temper, aggressiveness, jealousy, demands for attention, stealing, lying, truancy, sexual difficulties).

Three further categories were listed: organic disorders (including epilepsy); psychotic disorders; and educational and vocational difficulties.

This categorization is based on *a priori* conceptualization rather than on any empirical study (e.g. by factor analysis) of behavioural traits. The division of nervous and habit disorders is difficult to understand. Why, for example, should fears during sleep be in a different category to fears during the day? Why should a 'nervous pain' be a habit disorder and not a nervous disorder? Why is 'excitability and over-activity' included in the same category as 'withdrawal and depression'? It seems unlikely, considering the matter *a priori*, that the excitable and over-active child will at the same time be withdrawn and depressed. What is the justification for classifying epilepsy as an organic disorder not, apparently, connected with the behavioural categories shown by non-epileptic children?

Bennett (1960), in a study of an English child guidance clinic population, asked the psychiatrists dealing with the cases to define those who, in their opinion, were clearly 'delinquent' or clearly 'neurotic'. Fifty age and sex matched children from each group were compared, and the behavioural characteristics of each group described.

The delinquent children were found to show the following traits which clearly differentiated them from the neurotic children: stealing;

lying; truanting; wandering from home; aggressive and destructive behaviour; quarrelsomeness; disobedience and defiance; unmanageableness; open hostility to parents and teachers; open cruelty to animals or younger children; not responding to ordinary punishment; membership of a tough or aggressive gang; verbal aggression, or using bad language.

The neurotic children showed a significant excess of the following traits: fears and phobias; anxiety and worry; over-sensitiveness; tearful and easily upset; nightmares and bad dreams; babyish and dependent; not joining in other children's play; passive, no initiative or ambition; timid; hesitant; awkward, ill-at-ease; feels inferior, depressed; obsessional symptoms; hysterical symptoms.

The category of delinquent children appears to include both the 'unsocialized aggressive' and 'socialized delinquents' defined by Hewitt and Jenkins. The neurotic group appears to be similar to Hewitt and Jenkins' 'over-inhibited' group.

Eysenck (1960) reports the results of a factor analysis of a child guidance population. Two clusters of traits appeared, having positive or negative relationship with a factor termed 'introversion-extraversion'. The first cluster, termed 'personality problems', had the following traits in descending order of their positive association with the 'introverted' pole of the factor: psychoneurotic; sensitive; absent-minded; day-dreams; seclusive; depressed; inefficient; inferiority feelings; 'queerness'; changeable; nervous; mental conflict; intelligent; emotionally unstable; irritable; spoiled; masturbation; irresponsible.

The following traits were termed 'conduct problems', and are listed in descending order of their association with the extraverted pole of the factor: stealing; truanting; lying; destructive; swearing; disobedient; disturbing influence; fighting; violent; rude; egocentric; temper tantrums; unpopular; bossy; lacks interest; sexual delinquency.

Eysenck and Rachman (1965) suggest that the origin of these two kinds of symptoms is based on the type of response which an organism gives to a stimulus. The organism is categorized by two polar personality types, extraversion and introversion. In the face of a stimulus (e.g. stress) the organism acts in a characteristic way by 'externalizing' symptoms (aggression) of 'internalizing' them (neuroticism, anxiety). If this suggestion is correct, it may explain why writers (e.g. Field, and Hewitt and Jenkins) have failed to find any consistent relationship between *types* of stress and the kind of disturbed behaviour seen in the child. This point will be taken up later in the discussion of the relationship of parental attitudes to children's behaviour.

Mulligan (1964) studied the incidence and types of maladjustment in a national sample of 5,302 children in England and Wales born in the first week of March 1946, excluding illegitimate children and twins. Checks were made of the children at ages 6, 11 and 15 to find those children attending a child guidance clinic. In this way, 105 boys and 95 girls were obtained, and these children were compared with carefully matched controls.

A questionnaire was given to the teachers of the children. This questionnaire elicited information about nervous and aggressive traits, and showed that children with high scores for symptoms of the nervous type tended to be low on the aggressive items, and vice versa.

The application of the questionnaire to all the children in the national sample showed an incidence of 'serious' maladjustment of 8·1 per cent, which agreed closely with previous estimates of the total incidence of maladjustment in children.

A further study of delinquents in this national study showed that three times as many delinquents as non-delinquents had been classified as very aggressive. There was also a relationship between marked aggression and recidivism.

Rutter (1965) reviewed the attempts at classification in child psychiatry, and suggested that the following groups might be indicated, on the grounds of their long-term prognosis, response to treatment, and the clustering of the symptoms making up the classificatory group observed in some statistical studies. Epidemiological, aetiological, and age and sex factors were also taken into account in proposing eleven types of psychiatric disorder in children: (1) Neurotic disorder. (2) Anti-social or conduct disorders. (3) A mixed group, in which neither neurotic nor anti-social symptoms predominate. (4) Developmental disorders—such as enuresis and speech abnormalities. (5) The hyperkinetic syndrome—distinguished by its response to treatment and its association with neurological abnormality. (6) Child psychosis occurring before puberty. (7) Psychosis occurring at or after puberty, similar to adult schizophrenia. (8) Mental subnormality. (9) Educational retardation as a primary problem. (10) Depression. (11) Adult-type neurotic illness.

As Rutter points out, 'this outline of a classification is purely phenomenological . . . '; distinguishing syndromes by aetiology and prognosis obviously separates hyperkinesis and mental subnormality from conditions of behaviour whose genesis and treatment are different. From the point of view of the phenomenology of behaviour, however, there is no *a priori* reason why hyperkinetic children of low intelligence should not display behaviour defined by the first two major clusters of behaviour—neurotic or conduct disorders.

Stone and Rawley (1965) report the results of a factor analysis of a group of American children with behaviour disorders. Two groups emerged from this exercise: a personality-problem factor (implying an excessive inhibition of impulses); and the other a conduct-problem factor (implying an excessive expression of impulses).

Achenbach (1966) carried out a factor analysis of the symptoms of 600 American children referred for psychiatric investigation. Two major factors emerged, similar to those reported by Stone and Rawley—an internalizing versus an externalizing factor, the latter being associated with anti-social behaviour. Factoı analysis, as the author points out, classifies symptoms, not individuals, and the problem of deciding to which category any individual should be assigned remains. Achenbach suggests that a procedure similar to that of Hewitt and Jenkins may be used, and a child should be placed in a particular category if 60 per cent or more of his symptoms are made up of items from that category. The author suggests that the internalized disorders are the result of over-learning signals for the inhibition of behaviour, and externalization due either to the lack of signals, or the under-learning of them. This conceptualization is in accord with Eysenck's description of the learning capacities of extravert and introvert personality types.

Conners and Greenfield (1966) suggest that hyperkinetic impulsive disorders were a category of behaviour disorder in children, and were distinct from the anxious, over-inhibited disorders. A factor analysis of the symptom scale of a sample of 316 American child guidance clinic patients, compared with 367 normal children, supported this hypothesis. Separate factors of anxiety and restlessness, hyperactive and aggressive symptoms emerged. In addition, 15 hyperkinetic children were selected, and compared with 14 neurotics, for involuntary left-hand startle. The hyperkinetic group showed poorer voluntary control over the magnitude of this startle.

This is an interesting study, since it poses the question of the relationship of other kinds of behaviour to hyperactive or hyperkinetic behaviour. As the authors point out, 'these children are likely suspects for underlying central nervous system defects or maturational deficits in central inhibitory mechanisms'. The Underwood Committee suggested that over-activity was a symptom of nervousness, correlating with symptoms such as fears and depression. The factor analysis of Conners and Greenfield clearly does not confirm this view. As these authors point out, hyperactivity is associated with the aggressive pole of behaviour, which in their own and in previous factor analyses had shown an inverse relationship to the traits of anxious and over-inhibiting behaviour.

Hutt and Hutt (1964), in an experimental study of hyperactive children (some of whom were also epileptic), suggested that the test performance of these children categorized them as 'extreme extraverts'. In the light of the suggestions made by previous authors on the responses of the extraverted child, it is easy to understand why the hyperactive child emerges in the aggressive cluster of behavioural symptoms.

Kaufman (1962) had made the interesting suggestion that very high levels of anxiety may precipitate acts of extreme aggression, such as murder or arson. When the very anxious child becomes aggressive, he suggests, he may be entering a state of psychic disintegration, or psychosis. Ten case histories are given in support of this view.

The practical implication of this suggestion is that children with a mixed disorder containing elements of both anxiety and aggression are likely to be the most disturbed of all, perhaps being borderline or actual psychotic cases. It is interesting to note that in Mulligan's national study the mixed group emerged as a special category in relation to the depression of intellectual test scores, which was directly related to the degree of maladjustment—thus implying that the children with mixed disorders were the most disturbed of all.

Oswin (1967) has categorized the behaviour problems of cerebral palsied children on the basis of an *a priori* conceptualization into 'outward' and 'inward' behaviour problems. The basis of this division seems to be the manifestation of the behaviour. 'Outward behaviour problems' were suggested as: destructiveness; distractability; castastrophic reactions; spitting; crying; hyperactivity (chattering and noisiness); excitability; spitefulness; swearing; unco-operativeness; giggling; disinhibition. 'Inward behaviour problems' were: emotional instability; perseveration; unco-operativeness; withdrawingness; laziness; fluctuating learning performances; social immaturity; extreme goodness; fear, depression; learning disorders; distractability.

These divisions seem to be eccentric. Unco-operativeness is listed in both categories. If 'outward' means detectable in the external behaviour of the child, then traits such as learning disorder, perseveration and social immaturity, which all entail behaviour external to the child, might logically have been included in the first category. The definition of hyperactivity as 'chattering and noisiness' is unusual, since, although hyperactivity may contain this behaviour, there are many kinds of behaviour entailed by hyperactivity other than this. Since distractibility has been linked in the literature with hyperactivity, the placing of these two traits in opposite categories is difficult to understand.

The conclusions from this review of the literature are:

1 The categorization of disturbed behaviour in children has not been an easy task. This task has been made more difficult by workers who have included environmental factors in the analysis of behaviour, under the assumption that specific kinds of behaviour are related to specific kinds of environment. This kind of exercise has met with little success. A possible reason for the variability of findings may be

that children react in characteristic ways to different kinds of stress in the same environment so that two children will react differently to the same kind of stress.[1]

2 Despite this difficulty, two distinct kinds of behavioural clusters have emerged in several studies. These have been behaviour of an aggressive or externalized type as opposed to behaviour of an anxious or internalized type.

3 Despite the evidence from factor analyses, some workers still, apparently, rely on an idiosyncratic classification of traits of abnormal behaviour.

4 There is a suggestion that children with mixed disorders may be the most disturbed of all. This hypothesis requires further investigation.

The categorization of behaviour disorder in epileptic children

Turner (1927) divided the behaviour of epileptic children into three kinds: normal; neurotic (nervous, anxious-minded and easily worried apprehensive, fearsome); and anti-social (being egotistical, self-opinionated, lazy, asocial, and pugnacious). This last group weie those traditionally said to be showing the 'epileptic personality'.

The ways in which later writers about childhood epilepsy have categorized the behaviour of these children have been presented in tabular form in ch. 5, 'Psychiatric Aspects of Epilepsy since 1947' (pp. 26–50). It will be seen that a number of authors have categorized the children into aggressive and neurotic gıoups. Two other groups are occasionally put forward—a specific organic syndrome, such as hyperactivity, and mental defect.

These last two categories create a number of problems. Is hyperactivity a separate behavioural category in epilepsy or should it be contained within the aggressive category? The work of Ounsted and his colleagues, for instance, has shown that the hyperactive child may display catastrophically aggressive behaviour. Conners and Greenfield (op. cit., above, p. 134) have shown that hyperactive children fell into an aggressive group in a factor analysis of non-epileptic children. It seems reasonable to suppose that hyperactive, epileptic children will do likewise. The work of Hutt and Hutt (1964) on the extraverted nature of hyperactive children lends support to this view.

In the case of mental defect, this category is not one of behaviour, but of performance on standardized tests of intellect. It is difficult to see why the aggressive-anxious categorization of behaviour should not be applied to children whose intelligence is high enough for them to remain in the community.

[1] Cf. the study of Thomas *et al.* (1964) cited in the section on 'interaction', pp. 114-25

There do not appear to be any studies of careful statistical detail which have investigated the actual kinds and categories of behaviour in epileptic children. The studies which have attempted a categorization of behaviour seem to have relied on observational methods. Where a classification of behaviour is used for further analysis, the methods are not usually described. Nuffield's study (1961) was more systematic than most. He assigned a score on a 3-point scale to traits which previous work had characterized as aggressive or neurotic. However, whether the final categorization of children by this method had any relation to *reality*, the study did not show. The classification of cases in this way must be checked by a more careful numerical technique, such as a factor analysis, before reliable generalizations of the categories of behaviour that epileptic children display can be made. Such an exercise has not been reported in the literature.

The problems to be solved in a study of the behaviour of epileptic children seem to be:

1 Can a detailed numerical study of behaviour in epileptic children show that the aggressive-anxious typology of behaviour seen in non-epileptic children applies to epileptic children?

2 How does hyperactivity relate to the other behavioural traits in epileptic children?

3 Is there any special reaction of epileptic children with low intelligence? It should be mentioned in this context that a study by Rutter (1964) of maladjusted children, including some epileptics, could find no relationship between type of disorder and intellectual level. There have, however, been a number of studies of epileptic children (reviewed above, pp. 45–52) which have suggested a link between low intelligence and aggression, or other disturbed behaviour.

The measurement of behaviour in the 118 epileptic children

There are a number of ways in which the extent of disturbed behaviour in children can be investigated: by questioning the parents about the child's behaviour, which Thomas *et al.* (1967) suggest as the most reliable method; a direct interview with the child, or the use of a projection test with him; questionnaires completed by teachers (e.g. Mulligan, 1964); and the observation of the behaviour of the child in a controlled situation, such as a playroom or hospital ward.

The method used in the present study has been the interview with parents. This was carried out by a psychiatrist, who completed a standard item sheet in common use in child psychiatric practice in England. A separate interview with the parents was carried out by a psychiatric social worker. This was a lengthy, discursive interview which made a systematic inquiry into a wide range of aspects of the child's life, including his behaviour. In addition, the psychiatrist also interviewed the child himself.

When all 118 children had been investigated in this way, a list of thirty-nine items of possible disturbed behaviour was drawn up, so that each item could be evaluated on a four-point scale according to the categories: 0, never; 1, some sign; 2, definite sign; 3, marked.

The judgment about what constitutes a trait, and the degree to which it is manifested, is an evaluative one. This is true of all the methods that have been used to study behaviour in children. An attempt to control the possible error inherent in this procedure was made through the 'socialization' of two workers (the writer and a psychiatric social worker) in the norms of judgment of a larger group of workers (two psychiatrists, a further psychiatric social worker, a clinical psychologist, and the two workers already mentioned). Specimen case histories were selected at random, and each worker separately scored the thirty-nine items of behaviour according to his interpretation of the information in the case history and item sheet. The scores of each worker were compared, and reasons for disagreement discussed. This procedure was continued until an inter-rata reliability of +0·07 between the six workers was obtained.

The first two workers mentioned above then scored the behaviour of each of the 118 cases, using the two sources, the interview by the psychiatrist, and the discursive history taken by the social worker. The two workers independently made a judgment of the score on each behavioural item. In cases of conflict, the information was re-examined until agreement was reached. Where there were insufficient grounds for a judgment to be made, the code for 'no information' was completed. The completed schedules of behaviour for the 118 cases were punched on seven-hole paper tape. This information was analysed in the manner described below.

The thirty-nine items, in the order in which they were recorded, were: Eating disturbance; abdominal pain, nausea, or vomiting from anxiety; nightmares; night terrors; sleep-walking; restless sleep; nocturnal enuresis (distinct from enuresis occurring during fits); diurnal enuresis; encopresis; nail-biting and -picking; thumb sucking; tics; masturbation; head banging; breath holding; lisping, stammer; hyperactive, impulsive, distractable; temper tantrums; aggressive fantasy and play; aggressive outbursts against others; anxiety symptoms or panic attacks; sibling jealousy; truanting from school; refusal to go to school; lying; stealing; destructiveness and/or cruelty; initiatory fighting; disapproved sexual acts; attention-seeking; disobedience of authority; wandering from home; obsessional symptoms; psychotic symptoms; depression; agitation; paranoid symptoms; increasing memory deterioration; fears. This last item was based on an average score from a judgment about fears of any particular phenomena.

It should be mentioned that at the time the investigation and the scoring of items was undertaken both the writer and his associate, as well as the larger group of professional workers, were unaware of the literature on categorization in child psychiatry which has been reviewed above. This work was undertaken before the appearance of Rutter's influential paper on categorization (1965). In part, this *naïveté* was contrived. The workers were anxious to avoid any sort of halo effect, and to approach the problem as open-mindedly and as empirically as possible. It was for this reason that the behavioural traits were broken down as much as possible, to avoid- overinclusiveness in the judgments made.

This kind of naïve, empirical approach can have its dangers. Some conceptualization of the subject matter is necessary before even the most simple kinds of measurement can be undertaken. The conceptual system that the research team operated under was the view that the field of psychiatric disturbance in epileptic children was overburdened with *a priori* notions and unsupported assumptions about the behaviour of these children, and that a much more empirical approach to the problem was urgently needed.

The analysis of the thirty-nine items of behaviour

A number of factor analyses have been carried out which have apparently shown two major types of maladjustment in children. The fact that similar results have emerged from independent analysis suggests that this finding has definite validity. Yet the validation of this finding seems to be despite, rather than because of, the statistical procedures used.

First of all, the relationships between symptoms in previous studies all appear to have been calculated by product moment correlations and factors extracted from the resulting matrix. Maxwell's criticism of this method as applied to data which have an evaluative basis, and are often based on the measurement of a dichotomy (e.g. present/not present—0/1) is relevant:

> . . . in a correlation model of this kind the assumption is implicitly made that the variables involved are distributed in a multivariate normal distribution. However, such an assumption is rarely true where dichotomous variables are concerned, and tetrachoric correlations at all times are very unreliable (Maxwell, 1961, p. 87).

A similar criticism is made by Gower (1966):

> Recently there has been widespread interest in the possibility of

> using numerical methods as an aid to classification. Sokal and Sneath (1963, p. 178) give references to investigations using a variety of different numerical methods; these methods all begin with a multivariate sample, but so far as is known each individual may come from a different biological population or all individuals may come from the same population. An additional complication is that many or all of the variates may be qualitative, so that product moment correlations between variates may be inappropriate (p. 325).

Gower reviews some of the multivariate techniques of classification and continues:

> One of the by-products of most standard multivariate statistical techniques is a representation of the multivariate sample in a small number of dimensions. There is a growing tendency to use these techniques formally on association matrices to derive multi-dimensional representations of the sample, although the standard underlying assumptions are not even approximately satisfied. In particular the association matrix is a n $\times$ n matrix formed from the comparison of all pairs of individuals, i.e. a so-called Q matrix, while standard techniques postulate a v $\times$ v dispersion or correlation matrix, i.e. a so-called R matrix, formed from comparison between the variates. Despite this the techniques have been used successfully, in the sense that the expected relative magnitudes of inter-individual distances have been recovered (p. 326).

Gower sets out the criteria for a method of principal components analysis, which is based on the analysis of a Q matrix, rather than of the *R* matrix, on which Thurstone's original technique of factor analysis (1947) is used.

Coleman (1964), discussing the usefulness of multivariate techniques in sociology, comments:

> A modification of factor analysis, the *Q* techniques, appears to be quite a useful tool in inferring individual attributes. This is an inversion of the usual factor analysis, in which correlations between pairs of individuals over a number of tests replace the usual correlations between pairs of tests over a number of individuals. Because the investigator has control over the nature of the tests, though not over the nature of the individuals, he he can vary the tests so that statistical independence and meaningful independence do reasonably well coincide.

Gower's important paper (1966) clarifies the use of the Q matrix in classification work. His method of principal components analysis:

> grew from a dissatisfaction with the many reported applications of factoı analysis and principal component analysis of *Q* matrices found in classification work, particularly in the biological literature. The interpretation of such methods can be better understood by examining the distances, suitably defined, between the individuals, and we have given a method for finding co-ordinates for each individual referred to principal axes which preserve these distances. To distinguish the method from classical principal components analysis it might be more useful to refer to a principal co-ordinates analysis.

The reader is referred to Gower's two papers (1966) and (1967) for the mathematical explanation and proof of the techniques.

In terms of our present data, this technique will consider the scores of each of the 118 children on each of the thirty-nine tests. An average similarity for each test with each other test is obtained, and represented as a *Q* matrix. From this matrix, latent vectors are extracted which account for the maximum amount of variance in the data. The technique is essentially one of data reduction.

A programme for the type of analysis described by Gower has been written for the Orion Computer at the Rothamsted Experimental Station, to which the data on the children's behaviour has been submitted. The *Q* matrix was calculated in the programme by the procedure of calculating the percentage similarity of each test with every other test for each child. The possible scores on each test are 0, 1, 2 or 3, so the possible associations are 0, 0·33, 0·66 or 1. When this had been done, the average similarity of each test with every other test was calculated, and latent vectors extracted from the resulting matrix.

The results of this procedure showed that two latent vectors accounted for a little under half the variance of the data. The distribution of the items of behaviour in relation to these two vectors has been plotted in Diagram A.

The first vector relates to the amount of information available for the item, so that the more information available for an item, the further to the right along the horizontal axis it will be. The second vector relates to an aggression-anxiety dichotomy. Items positively associated with this vector appear to be of an aggressive nature (initiatory fighting; destructive; aggressive fantasy; hyperactive, impulsive, distractable; aggressive outbursts; disobedience; temper tantrums, etc.), while items negatively associated with this vector are of an anxious nature (anxiety symptoms; fears, abdominal pain, nausea, and vomiting from anxiety; restless sleep; eating disturbance; nail-biting and -picking; depression; nightmares, etc.).

The closer the symptoms are to the horizontal axis, the less clearly

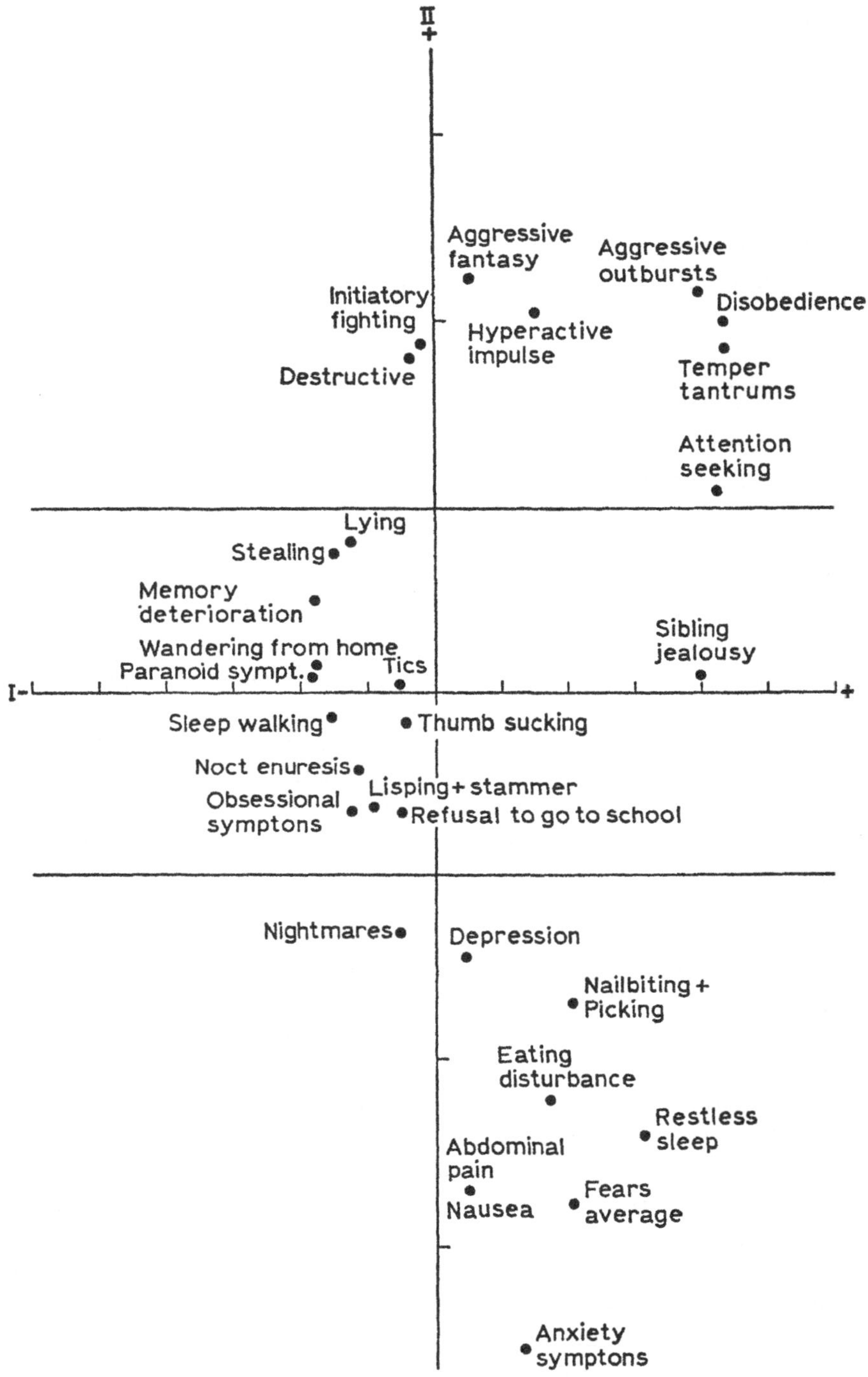

The two components of behaviour disorder in epileptic children

they characterize the extreme poles of the aggressive-anxious vector. The fact that these items are also those on which relatively little positive information is available (i.e. in a fairly high proportion of cases these items are scored 'never' or 'no information') is convenient. Because of this, items to the left of the diagram can be said to be of less significance than those to the right. Since the 'polar' symptoms of the aggressive-anxious dimension are predominantly on the positive side of the 'information' dimension, this fact lends added weight to the significance of the aggressive-anxious dimension. The only exception is the symptom of sibling jealousy, which is frequently noticed and has a positive association with the aggressive side of the dimension. This positive association, however, is very slight.

Ten of the items of child behaviour occurred with very low frequency, and would be represented on Diagram A far to the negative end of the 'information' dimension. Because of the low frequency of these items, they have not been included in the subsequent diagnostic classification.

The ten items are: head banging; breath holding; truanting from school; masturbation; disapproved sexual acts; psychotic symptoms; encopresis; diurnal enuresis; night terrors; agitation.

The results of this component analysis are important. They show that, using a technique of analysis that is apparently less beset with error than some techniques which have previously analysed this kind of evaluative data, that the behaviour of epileptic children can be divided into two clear categories, aggressive and anxious. These categories are similar to those observed in previous factorial studies of disturbed behaviour in non-epileptic children. Hyperactivity is clearly associated with the aggressive symptoms.

The classification of individuals and of symptoms

It is important to know, for the purposes of further analysis, how individual cases stand in relation to the classification of symptoms. This involves the problem of finding an adequate cut-off point to distinguish the aggressive and the anxious symptoms, in Diagram A, above. Symptoms close to the horizontal axis occur with fairly low frequency, so the significance in relation to the vertical axis (the aggressive-anxious axis) is in question. In fact, these central symptoms are the ones which are the least clinically explicable as either aggressive or anxious symptoms.

An arbitrary cut-off point has been chosen at points on either side of the horizontal axis which excludes items relating to the vertical axis at less than a level of $+0{\cdot}05$, or $-0{\cdot}05$. The aggressive symptoms categorized by this procedure are, in descending order of their relationship to the aggressive-anxious axis: Aggressive fantasy;

aggressive outbursts; hyperactivity; disobedience; initiatory fighting; temper tantrums; destructiveness; attention-seeking; lying; stealing (ten symptoms). The anxious symptoms are: Anxiety symptoms and panic attacks; abdominal pain, nausea, and vomiting from anxiety; fears; restless sleep; eating disturbance; nail-biting and picking; depression; nightmares; refusal to go to school; lisping and stammer; obsessional symptoms (eleven symptoms).

All of these symptoms seem clinically explicable as anxious or aggressive symptoms, in the categories to which they have been assigned. However, two traits which have traditionally been associated with aggressive or conduct disorder—wandering from home and sibling jealousy—have been excluded by this procedure. Since all of the excluded symptoms, with the one exception of sibling jealousy, occur with low frequency, the effect of this exclusion on the final analysis—supposing that the excluded symptoms may have some significance—will be small.

Previous workers have had difficulty in assigning individuals to diagnostic categories (e.g. aggressive or anxious), even though a list of traits making up these categories has been agreed upon. Some workers (e.g. Hewitt and Jenkins) have used the method of assigning an individual to a diagnostic group if 60 per cent or more of his symptoms coincide with those in a particular diagnostic group. This method has left many individuals in unclassified or 'mixed' categories.

A further problem, from the point of view of the present series, is the fact that a proportion of the cases will show no psychiatric disturbance at all, since the cases were referred on neurological rather than psychiatric grounds. It thus has to be decided which cases are normal, as well as to which category the disturbed cases belong.

A possible solution to this problem for the present population is to divide the data into four cells, according to the occurrence of cases above or below the median aggressive score and above or below the median anxious score. This would give four categories: below the median for both aggression and anxiety (normal); above the median for anxiety, but not for aggression (anxious); above the median for aggression, but not for anxiety (aggressive); and above the median for both aggression and anxiety (mixed).

The results of this compartmentalization or categorization are given in Table 5. Cases which have anxiety scores equal to or below the median score of 5 and aggression scores equal to or below the median score of 6 have been placed in the top left-hand cell and classified normal. Cases which are high on the aggression score have been classified aggressive in the top right-hand cell; high on the anxiety score, in the bottom left-hand cell, as anxious; and cases high on both the aggression and anxiety scores as mixed, in the bottom right-hand cell.

The average scores on the anxiety and aggression scales for the four behavioural groups are given in Table 6, and the distribution of total behaviour disorder scores (anxiety plus aggression scores) are given in Table 7. It will be seen that of the three 'disturbed' groups, the anxious children have the lowest total behaviour disorder scores and the mixed children the highest.

Previous estimates of the incidence of psychiatric disturbance in children in the general population have suggested a figure of between 5 and 10 per cent (Mulligan, 1964). However, the incidence of psychiatric disturbance in the present series of epileptic children seems to be much higher than this, although no direct comparison with a normal control population is available.[1] Consider what a score of, say, 15 on the behaviour disorder scale means. In order to have a score of 15, the child must have a 'marked' manifestation of 5 of the 21 traits of abnormal behaviour which make up this classification, or

Table 5 The classification of behaviour disorder in 118 epileptic children

	Equal to or below median aggression score	*Above median aggression score*	
Equal to or below median anxiety score	Normal 35	Aggressive 30	65
Higher than median anxiety score	Anxious 28	Mixed 25	53
	63	55	118

Table 6 average scores of four diagnostic groups for anxiety and aggression in 118 epileptic children

Group	*Anxious symptoms, mean score*	*Aggressive symptoms, mean score*	*N*
Normal	2·73	2·85	35
Anxious	10·35	2·89	28
Aggressive	3·5	14·16	30
Mixed	11·7	9·84	25
Total	—	—	118

[1] But see the addendum to this chapter on p. 147.

Table 7 Total behaviour disorder scores in four categories of epileptic children

Total behaviour disorder score	*Diagnostic group*			
	Normal	*Anxious*	*Aggressive*	*Mixed*
0– 4	29	0	0	0
5– 9	5	3	1	0
10–14	1	16	9	1
15–19	0	6	8	8
20–4	0	2	7	10
25–9	0	1	4	1
30–4	0	0	0	4
35–9	0	0	1	0
40–4	0	0	0	1
Totals	35	28	30	25

Note: Total behaviour disorder score arrived at by adding the anxious and aggressive scores.

a combination of 'marked' (scored 3), 'definite sign' (scored 2) and 'some sign' (scored 1) in combination in more than 5 traits. In clinical terms this would almost inevitably be considered to represent a serious psychiatric disorder in the child. For example, a child with a score of 15 might have marked manifestation of temper tantrums, aggressive outbursts against others, stealing, initiatory fighting, and attention-seeking; or a marked manifestation of anxiety symptoms, depression, fears, obsessional behaviour, and nightmares; or a marked display of attention-seeking, aggressive fantasy and play, and a definite sign of hyperactivity, together with a definite sign of abdominal pain, nightmares, and depression, and some sign of nail-biting and picking.

Nearly half the children in the present study have a score as large as or greater than 15. Just over a quarter have scores which are higher than 20, and 6 children have scores higher than 30. This indicates a very high degree of disturbance indeed. In the control group study, reported later in this study, behaviour controls were obtained for the epileptic children categorized as aggressive, anxious and mixed from the non-epileptic population at a child guidance clinic. It was found very difficult to find children in this child guidance population who were as disturbed as the most disturbed 10 children in the epileptic series.

In the chapters that follow, four kinds of analysis of the variation of other variables in terms of psychiatric disorder will be made: a comparison of the four behavioural groups in the epileptic children; a comparison of the low anxiety scores versus the high anxiety scores; a comparison of the low aggressive scores versus the high aggressive scores; and a comparison of the low total scores versus the high total scores.

Conclusions

The conclusions of this chapter are:

1 The literature on classification of disturbed behaviour in children suggests that two major syndromes exist, those of anxiety and aggression.
2 Some writers have suggested that these two syndromes of behaviour are present in epileptic children, although this has not been systematically investigated.
3 Behaviour in the 118 epileptic children in the present study has been investigated by two workers making independent ratings of thirty-nine items of disturbed behaviour, evaluated on a 4-point scale.
4 The resulting scores have been submitted to a component analysis, specifically designed for classifying evaluative data. This analysis confirms that the disturbed behaviour of the epileptic children falls into two major categories, anxious and aggressive.
5 The extent of behaviour disorder in 109 of the 118 epileptic children has been assessed by scoring a brief questionnaire of items of behaviour which has been tested on general population and clinic children. This procedure suggests that about 43 per cent of the children have a psychiatric disturbance as great as that which would be seen in a child guidance clinic. This estimate agrees with that seen by writers studying special populations of epileptic children.
6 There are grounds for supposing that the epileptic children contain some cases who are much more disturbed than non-epileptic children seen at a child guidance clinic.

A comparison of the epileptic children with the behavioural norms of a non-epileptic population

After the preceding chapter on the categorization of behaviour had been completed, and much of the subsequent analysis in the following chapters undertaken, a paper appeared (Rutter, 1967) which gave a short questionnaire relating to children's behaviour for which population norms were known, and which had been validated by examining the extent to which answers to various questions about behaviour (on a schedule completed by teachers) predicted the diagnostic groups to which the children had been assigned after a standard psychiatric interview.

The instrument was developed by Rutter in an epidemiological study of child psychiatric disorder in the Isle of Wight and in Aberdeen. Teachers were asked to complete twenty-six questions according to the responses 'doesn't apply' (0), 'applies somewhat' (1), and 'certainly applies' (2). The psychiatric examination of children having high scores on these items indicated that children with a score of nine or more differentiated children attending a psychiatric clinic from those in the normal population.

The twenty-six items on which the teachers were asked to rate the child were:

1 Very restless. Often running about or jumping up and down. Hardly ever still.
2 Truants from school.
3 Squirmy, fidgety child.
4 Often destroys own or others' belongings.
5 Frequently fights with other children.
6 Not much liked by other children.
7 Often worried; worries about many things.
8 Tends to do things on his own; rather solitary.
9 Irritable. Is quick to 'fly off the handle'.
10 Often appears miserable, unhappy, tearful, or distressed.
11 Has twitches, mannerisms, or tics on the face or body.
12 Frequently sucks thumb or finger.
13 Frequently bites nails or fingers.
14 Tends to be absent from school for trivial reasons.
15 Is often disobedient.
16 Has poor concentration or short attention-span.
17 Tends to be fearful or afraid of new things or new situations.
18 Fussy or over-particular child.
19 Often tells lies.
20 Has stolen things on one or more occasions.
21 Has wet or soiled himself at school this year.
22 Often complains of pains or aches.
23 Has had tears on arrival at school *or* has refused to come into the building this year.
24 Has a stutter or stammer.
25 Has other speech difficulty.
26 Bullies other children.

This schedule has been completed for 109 of the epileptic children, for whom reports from teachers were available, in the following way. At the time the children were first investigated a questionnaire was sent to the child's teacher, asking for information in a number of areas, including behaviour of the child. The question was open-ended, the teacher being asked to describe in detail any disturbed behaviour in the child. These data were coded by a clinical psychologist who had no knowledge of the ratings of behaviour made by the writer and his associate. An additional source of information used in completing Rutter's schedule was the information about the child's behaviour in school from the psychiatrist's item sheet.

On Rutter's scale, a score of 9 or more discriminated a child who had a psychiatric disorder as great as that of a child attending a child guidance clinic. In the total population of 10- and 11-year-old children resident in the Isle of Wight, there were 7·2 per cent (157) children with scores of 9 or more on Rutter's schedule.[1] In the present series, 43·2 per cent of children have a score of 9 or more. This result suggests that the epileptic children in the present series have an incidence of psychiatric disorder which is considerably higher than that found in the population at large. This conclusion is qualified by the fact that the present series contains children who were slightly older than those on whom the general population norms were arrived at, and the schedule was not filled in directly by teachers.

This estimate of the incidence of psychiatric disorder (43·2 per cent) agrees fairly well with that made by a number of writers. Bridge (1949) gave an estimate of 46 per cent as the incidence of psychiatric disorder in epileptic children attending a pediatric hospital; Halstead (1957) gave an estimate of 51 per cent for epileptic children in normal and special schools; Lennox and Lennox (1960) gave an estimate of 50 per cent in an all-age sample; Gudmundsson's and others' unselected samples of epileptic children in the general population have suggested a lower incidence (Henderson (1953) 12 per cent; Pond *et al.* (1960), 25 per cent). The recent study by Rutter *et al.* (1966) of children in the Isle of Wight does suggest, however, that the incidence of psychiatric disorder in epileptic children is considerably in excess of the 7 per cent incidence in non-epileptic children.[1]

It should be noted that the children in the present study were neurological rather than psychiatric referrals, so that the high incidence of psychiatric disorder would not immediately be expected. It may be that parents whose children are psychiatrically disturbed over-stress the physical (neurological) factors to the referring authorities. It is also possible that neurological factors (e.g. brain damage, type of fit, etc.) underlie psychiatric disorders, accounting for the incidence of this kind of disorder in a neurological

[1] Rutter (personal communication, 1966) suggests that nearly 40 per cent of the epileptic children in the Isle of Wight survey had a psychiatric disorder as great as that in the 7 per cent of children attending child guidance clinics. Cf. Graham and Rutter (1968): the incidence of psychiatric disorder in children with 'neuroleptic conditions' (i.e. including cerebral palsy, etc.) in the Isle of Wight survey is 34 per cent.

population. The connection of these factors with psychiatric disorder will be investigated later in this study.

Conclusion

A behaviour schedule for which general population norms are known has been applied to 109 of the 118 epileptic children. In the general population 7 per cent of children have a score of 9 or more, and have a degree of psychiatric disturbance as great as that in children attending child guidance clinics. In the present series of epileptic children, 43·2 per cent have a behaviour disorder at this level, suggesting that the incidence of behaviour disorder in these epileptic children is much greater than in the population at large.

17 A controlled study

How do environmental, familial, and developmental factors distinguish epileptic children from similar children (i.e. matched controls) without epilepsy? How do these factors distinguish between epileptic children who are disturbed and those who do not show behavioural disturbance?

A partial answer to these questions was provided by Grunberg and Pond (1957), who compared 53 epileptic children with conduct disorders with 53 epileptic children who were behaviourally normal. Thirty-five of the disturbed epileptic children were compared with 35 non-epileptic children with a similar kind of (conduct) behaviour disorder. The term 'conduct disorder' included the traits of severe and frequent temper tantrums, destructiveness, fighting, truanting and wandering, lying and stealing. The two groups of 53 epileptic children were not matched, except that children with I.Q. below 65 were not included. The two groups of 35 children (epileptic and non-epileptic) were matched for age, sex and intelligence, but not for social class.

The two sets of groups were compared for twelve organic, genetic and environmental items. The total incidence of the items in the groups (rather than the incidence in matched pairs) was compared. The two disturbed groups (epileptic and non-epileptic) were found to have a similar incidence of disturbed maternal attitudes towards the child, and of breaks and changes in the child's environment, as well as a similar incidence of parental disharmony, paternal attitude disturbed, and restriction at home. A similar incidence of adverse conditions (psychosis, neurosis, psychopathy) in family members was found in the two disturbed groups. However, disturbed and non-disturbed epileptics showed significant differences on all the environmental factors, and a lower incidence of psychopathy in family members. These results led the authors to conclude that social factors played an important part in conduct disorder in epileptic children.

This study seems to have influenced clinicians in the field of child psychiatry. Rutter (1966) for example, considered an unspecified number of epileptic children in his study of the effect of parental illness on child behaviour, on the grounds that social factors were of major importance in behaviour disorder in epileptic as well as non-epileptic children. Implicit in this assumption is the view that organic factors (e.g. type of epilepsy) play only a minor role in the outcome of the disturbed behaviour. However, in the light of some of the previous literature (e.g. Nuffield, 1961), this view does not seem to be entirely justified.

The present study has been undertaken in an attempt to replicate the Grunberg-Pond study, but with some extensions: including anxious and mixed disorder children, as well as ones with an aggressive (conduct) behaviour disorder, using a more exact control procedure and comparing a wider range of items, the measurement of which was undertaken by a small group of clinicians in a homogeneous setting.

Controls, matched for the kind of behaviour presented and without epilepsy, were obtained for the eighty-three disturbed epileptic children in the present series from a child guidance clinic serving a catchment area in north-west London, within the hospital catchment area. A child psychiatrist working at this clinic also saw the epileptic children, and item sheets were completed for both kinds of children.

The characteristics of the child guidance population, numbering nearly 400, had been recorded on punched cards, and these were utilized in the matching procedure. At first an attempt was made to find exact matches for all psychiatric symptoms as well as for demographic factors. However, it proved impossible to match the epileptic children with non-epileptics symptom for symptom. Instead, the child guidance population was divided into three groups—aggressive, anxious, or mixed—according to the occurrence of symptoms on the punched cards.[1] From these three groups, an epileptic child was matched with a diagnostically similar child; however, the *exact* extent and nature of all the symptoms were not matched. Particular difficulty was encountered, in the initial comparison, of finding non-epileptic children who were as disturbed, in extent and range of symptoms, as the most disturbed (about 30) epileptic children.

The epileptic and non-epileptic children were exactly matched for sex; social class was matched by using three groups: Registrar General's Classes I and II; Class III; and Classes IV and V. This corresponds to a classification of professional and managerial;

[1] The traits considered were those which emerged in the cluster analysis reported in the previous chapter.

skilled working-class and clerical; and semi-skilled and unskilled. It was not possible to match age exactly, because the epileptic children had a modal grouping in the 12 to 14 age group, while the child guidance clinic children's ages were more evenly spread. However, children attending the three types of school, infant (4–6), junior (7–10), and secondary (11–16), were matched. Any child in his first year at a new school was matched with a similar child. Only children were exactly matched with only children. Rutter (1964) indicated that intellectual level was not a significant factor in childhood psychiatric disorder, and this variable was in consequence not controlled. It is to some extent accounted for, however, by the variable of social class.

Controls for the 35 normal epileptic children in the series were obtained from the 83 disturbed epileptics, using the methods described above. The similarity of age groupings in the diagnostic groups assisted this matching procedure; social class, too, does not differentiate the diagnostic groups. In addition, the two groups of epileptics (normal and disturbed) were matched for the number of years since the onset of epilepsy. Children with an interval of 0, 1, 2, 3 or 4 years since the onset of epilepsy were exactly matched; where the interval was greater than this, a difference of 1 year was accepted for matching—for example, an interval of 7 years could be matched with one of 6, 7 or 8 years. Brief reports of data on the control group have appeared elswhere (Bagley, 1970; Bagley and Evan-Wong, 1970).

A comparison of the incidence of 34 developmental, environment and familial factors in the matched pairs is given in the table on pp. 155–8. The first figures give the total incidence of the item, and the figures in parentheses the number of cases in which the item occurred in the subject and *not* in his control. Significance testing has been applied to the comparison of those cases in which the item occurred in a case, but not in its control. The value of χ^2 has been calculated by the method given by McNemar (1955), with corrections for continuity. As Maxwell (1961) points out, this procedure is more accurate than that of testing the total incidence of items in the diagnostic group and its control group as a whole (the method employed by Grunberg and Pond). The method of comparing total incidence rather than that in matched pairs slightly over-emphasizes the real difference between the matched groups.

The items in the table on pp. 155–8 were taken from the item sheets completed by a single psychiatrist (in the case of the epileptic children), and by this psychiatrist and his consultant colleagues and registrars working for them in the case of the clinic children. A relative homogeneity of methods may be assumed.

Discussion

Before an item can be considered of aetiological importance it must distinguish between the disturbed epileptics and the epileptics without behaviour disturbance. If the item does not distinguish between epileptic children and behaviourally similar disturbed, non-epileptic children, the item may be considered to be of a type which may be involved in the aetiology of behaviour disorder as such, perhaps independently of the fact of epilepsy. Such a differentiation does not, of course, guarantee causality.

The following items have a significantly higher incidence in the disturbed than in the normal epileptics, but a similar incidence in the disturbed groups, epileptic and non-epileptic: the accumulated index of environmental hazards (items (14)–(20)): gross marital disharmony; the accumulated index of family pathology (items (26)–(28)); and the existence of neurosis in family members.

The following items distinguish both the disturbed and the normal epileptics, and the epileptic and non-epileptic disturbed children to some degree, and may be considered as being specific to the epileptic behaviour disorder: early feeding difficulty; and the accumulated index of disturbed behaviour in relatives (psychosis, or neurosis, or behaviour disorder, or psychopathy). A further three items: persistent hyperactivity from an early age; separation from the father before age six; and disturbing relatives in the house; may be added to this list, since these items distinguished disturbed epileptic children from non-disturbed epileptic children at a significant level, and show a trend towards doing so in the comparison between the disturbed and the normal epileptics.

The following items distinguished the epileptics from their non-epileptic controls, but not the two matched epileptic groups, and must therefore be consideıed as endemic to epilepsy, but not to behaviour disorder: severe maternal illness during pregnancy; prolonged or difficult labour; the accumulated index of pregnancy and birth difficulties; serious physical illness up to the age of six; epilepsy in family members. All of these items are of probable aetiological significance for the epilepsy.

It is interesting to note the fact that abnormal behaviour in family members differentiates the disturbed epileptics from the disturbed non-epileptic children. In the Grunberg and Pond study these factors did not distinguish the two disturbed groups, although they did distinguish the disturbed and the normal epileptics. Apart from this fact, however, the results of this study confirm the findings of Grunberg and Pond. The finding that social and environmental factors are an important factor in the background of aggressive or conduct behaviour disorder in epileptic children also holds for

Table 8 Developmental, parental, environmental and familial factors in epileptic children and controls

Column headings:

a	Anxious epileptics	$n=28$
b	Anxious controls	$n=28$
c	Aggressive epileptics	$n=30$
d	Aggressive controls	$n=30$
e	Mixed epileptics	$n=25$
f	Mixed controls	$n=25$
g	All disturbed epileptics	$n=83$
h	All disturbed controls	$n=83$
i	Normal epileptics	$n=35$
j	Disturbed epileptic controls	$n=35$

First figures indicate total incidence of item in each group. Figures in parentheses (on which significance testing has been carried out) indicate that number of cases in which the item occurred in the case, but not in the matched control.

*=significant at the 5 per cent level.
†=significant at the 1 per cent level.
‡=significant at the 0·1 per cent level.

Item	*(a)*	*(b)*	*(c)*	*(d)*	*(e)*	*(f)*	*(g)*	*(h)*	*(i)*	*(j)*
1 Threatened miscarriage of child	4 (3)	2 (1)	2 (2)	1 (1)	0 (0)	0 (0)	3 (2)	0 (0)	0 (0)	2 (2)
2 Severe maternal illness during pregnancy	8 (8)	0 (0)*	7 (7)	1 (1)	6 (6)	1 (1)	21 (21)	2 (2)‡	3 (3)	5 (5)
3 Prolonged or difficult labour	9 (8)	4 (3)	11 (9)	6 (4)	8 (8)	4 (4)	28 (25)	14 (11)†	14 (6)	12 (4)

Table 8 (*cont.*)

Item	(*a*)	(*b*)	(*c*)	(*d*)	(*e*)	(*f*)	(*g*)	(*h*)	(*i*)	(*j*)
4 Prematurity (birth weight less than 5½ lbs)	5 (4)	3 (2)	3 (3)	2 (2)	3 (3)	2 (2)	11 (10)	7 (6)	3 (3)	5 (5)
Number having (1) *or* (2) *or* (3) *or* (4)	16 (12)	7 (3)*	16 (10)	10 (4)	14 (12)	5 (3)*	46 (34)	22 (10)‡	17 (7)	19 (9)
5 Feeding difficulty	6 (6)	0 (0)*	10 (9)	1 (0)†	4 (4)	0 (0)	20 (19)	1 (0)‡	3 (1)	11 (9)
6 Toilet training difficulty	6 (6)	3 (3)	4 (4)	3 (3)	4 (2)	4 (2)	14 (12)	10 (8)	6 (6)	4 (4)
No. having (5) *or* (6)	10 (7)	3 (0)*	11 (8)	4 (1)*	5 (2)	4 (1)	26 (17)	11 (2)†	9 (7)	12 (10)
7 Precocious motor and/or speech development	2 (1)	5 (4)	3 (3)	1 (1)	5 (4)	2 (1)	10 (8)	8 (6)	1 (0)	6 (5)
8 Undue slowness in speaking, standing or walking	3 (3)	3 (3)	6 (6)	2 (2)	2 (2)	1 (1)	11 (11)	6 (6)	6 (6)	4 (4)
9 Persistent hyperactivity from an early age	0 (0)	0 (0)	7 (7)	0 (0)*	4 (4)	0 (0)	11 (11)	0 (0)†	9 (0)	3 (3)
10 Serious physical illness before age 2	7 (6)	2 (1)	7 (7)	5 (5)	6 (6)	3 (3)	20 (19)	10 (9)*	9 (7)	11 (9)
11 Serious physical illness, 2–6	8 (7)	3 (2)	12 (12)	2 (2)*	8 (6)	5 (3)	28 (25)	10 (7)†	9 (8)	8 (7)
No. with (10) *or* (11)	13 (11)	5 (3)*	17 (14)	6 (3)*	10 (7)	7 (4)	40 (32)	18 (10)‡	13 (10)	16 (13)
12 Separation from mother before age 4 (2 weeks or more)	17 (8)	16 (7)	19 (7)	20 (8)	18 (7)	16 (5)	54 (22)	52 (20)	22 (9)	22 (9)
13 Separation from father before age 6	15 (7)	14 (6)	20 (15)	15 (10)	20 (15)	8 (3)†	55 (37)	37 (19)*	20 (7)	25 (12)

Table 8 (*cont.*)

Item	*(a)*	*(b)*	*(c)*	*(d)*	*(e)*	*(f)*	*(g)*	*(h)*	*(i)*	*(j)*
14 Disturbing relatives in house	5 (5)	1 (1)	8 (8)	0 (0)*	7 (7)	1 (1)	10 (10)	2 (2)‡	6 (5)	9 (8)
15 Grandparent(s) living in home	7 (6)	5 (4)	3 (3)	1 (1)	6 (4)	5 (3)	16 (13)	11 (8)	1 (1)	6 (6)
16 Care of child mainly or partly delegated	3 (3)	5 (5)	3 (2)	5 (4)	3 (3)	2 (2)	9 (8)	12 (11)	3 (3)	5 (5)
17 Overcrowding (3 or more per room)	4 (3)	5 (4)	4 (4)	2 (2)	5 (5)	2 (2)	13 (12)	9 (8)	3 (3)	7 (7)
18 Lack of play space	2 (2)	4 (4)	3 (3)	0 (0)	5 (5)	1 (1)	10 (10)	5 (5)	1 (1)	4 (4)
19 Relative poverty	5 (5)	2 (2)	2 (2)	1 (1)	4 (4)	0 (0)	11 (11)	3 (3)	3 (3)	3 (3)
20 Frequent changes of home environment	1 (1)	2 (2)	4 (4)	3 (3)	4 (4)	0 (0)	9 (9)	5 (5)	2 (2)	4 (4)
No. having 2 or more (14)–(20)	9 (7)	7 (5)	9 (9)	5 (5)	13 (11)	5 (3)	31 (27)	17 (13)*	4 (4)	16 (15)*
21 Illegitimate child	2 (2)	2 (2)	2 (2)	6 (6)	0 (0)	3 (3)	4 (4)	11 (11)	1 (1)	2 (2)
22 Adopted child	1 (1)	0 (0)	4 (3)	3 (2)	0 (0)	2 (2)	5 (4)	5 (4)	1 (1)	1 (1)
23 Stepfather or stepmother	0 (0)	1 (1)	1 (1)	3 (3)	1 (1)	3 (3)	2 (2)	7 (7)	0 (0)	0 (0)
24 Foster-parents	2 (2)	1 (1)	3 (3)	0 (0)	0 (0)	1 (1)	5 (5)	2 (2)	0 (0)	1 (1)
25 Institutional upbringing in first 4 years of life	1 (1)	0 (0)	0 (0)	3 (3)	0 (0)	1 (1)	1 (1)	4 (4)	0 (0)	0 (0)
No. having 1 or more (21)–(25)	7 (7)	2 (2)	5 (4)	10 (9)	3 (3)	5 (5)	15 (14)	17 (16)	1 (1)	3 (3)

Table 8 (*cont.*)

Item	(*a*)	(*b*)	(*c*)	(*d*)	(*e*)	(*f*)	(*g*)	(*h*)	(*i*)	(*j*)
26 Gross marital disharmony	4 (2)	7 (5)	8 (6)	5 (3)	5 (4)	6 (5)	17 (12)	18 (13)	0 (0)	7 (7)*
27 Broken home	2 (2)	3 (3)	8 (6)	7 (5)	6 (4)	6 (4)	16 (12)	16 (12)	4 (4)	6 (6)
28 Father's main interest outside home	0 (0)	5 (5)	4 (3)	5 (4)	4 (4)	0 (0)	8 (7)	10 (9)	9 (0)	4 (4)
No. with 1 or more (26)–(28)	6 (2)	12 (8)	13 (6)	14 (8)	9 (5)	10 (6)	28 (13)	36 (21)*	4 (2)	14 (12)*
29 Psychosis in siblings, parents, grandparents or parental siblings	5 (4)	2 (1)	1 (1)	0 (0)	2 (2)	0 (0)	8 (7)	2 (1)	4 (4)	2 (2)
30 Neurosis in above relatives	8 (5)	9 (6)	9 (9)	3 (3)	7 (6)	8 (7)	24 (20)	20 (16)	3 (2)	14 (13)†
31 Epilepsy in above relatives	11 (11)	2 (2)*	13 (13)	3 (3)	7 (7)	1 (1)	31 (31)	6 (6)‡	13 (11)	11 (9)
32 Behaviour disorder in above relatives	3 (3)	2 (2)	3 (3)	0 (0)	5 (5)	2 (2)	11 (11)	4 (4)	2 (2)	3 (3)
33 Mental defect in above relatives	1 (1)	0 (0)	4 (4)	2 (2)	1 (1)	0 (0)	6 (6)	2 (2)	0 (0)	1 (1)
34 Psychopathy, criminality, or alcoholism in above relatives	5 (4)	4 (3)	3 (3)	4 (4)	5 (5)	1 (1)	13 (12)	9 (8)	3 (3)	3 (3)
No. having relatives with psychosis *or* neurosis *or* behaviour disorder *or* psychopathy, etc.	15 (8)	12 (5)	15 (9)	7 (1)*	15 (10)	8 (3)	45 (27)	27 (9)†	8 (5)	18 (13)*

anxious, or neurotic epileptic children, who were not considered in Grunberg and Pond's study.

Conclusion

The comparison of 83 disturbed epileptics with matched controls with behaviour disturbance, but without epilepsy, and 35 epileptics without behaviour disorder with matched controls with epilepsy and disturbed behaviour suggests that social factors (disturbed environment, family pathology, and neurosis in family members) may be of aetiological significance for behaviour disorder in epileptic children, since these factors distinguish normal epileptics from epileptics with behaviour disorder, but do not distinguish the disturbed epileptics from their disturbed, non-epileptic controls.

18 Epileptic fits and behaviour disorder

The literature on the relationship of epileptic fits and disturbed behaviour in adults and children (reviewed above, pp. 26–50) has not produced consistent findings. Some studies have found a relationship between the years since the onset of fits and the occurrence of behaviour disorder; but an inverse relationship between the duration of epilepsy, and the occurrence of psychiatric disorder has also been found. Other studies have found no relationship between duration of epilepsy and disturbed behaviour.

The problem is not a simple one, but has three facets: the *number of years* since the first appearance of fits; the *kind of fits* displayed; and the *frequency* with which they occur.

These three aspects of epileptic fits have been examined in the 118 epileptic children in the present series, and the relationship with the four diagnostic groups tested.

Three hypotheses are tested:

(*a*) There will be a positive relationship between the time that has elapsed since the onset of the first fit and the existence of disturbed behaviour in the epileptic child.

(*b*) There will be a positive relationship between the amount of disturbance of motor behaviour and consciousness caused by an epileptic fit and the disturbance of behaviour in the child, so that fits with the most outwardly manifested signs (falling to the ground, convulsions of arms and legs, biting of tongue, incontinence, prolonged unconsciousness) will be more alarming to the child's parents and peers and will thus be accompanied by more disturbance in the child than minor fits (with brief loss of consciousness without the patient falling, and with none or only minor motor disturbance), which are less alarming to the child and to his parents, teachers and peers.

(*c*) There will be a positive relationship between the number of

Table 9 Time since first fit and psychiatric diagnosis in 118 epileptic children

Years since first fit	*Normal*		*Anxious*		*Aggressive*		*Mixed*		*Low total scorers*		*High total scorers*	
	n	*cum. p.*	*n*	*cum. p.*	*n*	*cum. p.*	*n*	*cum. p.*	*n*	*cum. p.*	*n*	*cum. p.*
0–1	11	0·31	10	0·36	5	0·17	5	0·2	18	0·28	13	0·24
2–3	4	0·43	9	0·68	6	0·37	7	0·48	15	0·52	11	0·44
4–8	10	0·71	5	0·86	13	0·8	7	0·76	16	0·78	19	0·78
9–14	10	1·0	4	1·0	6	1·0	6	1·0	14	1·0	12	1·0
Totals	35		28		30		25		63		55	

Note: Time data divided as nearly as possible at median and quartiles.
Significance: Kolmogorov-Smirnov one-tailed test:

Comparison	χ^2 (2 d.f.)	*Significance*
Normal-anxious	3·86	Less than 0·25, greater than 0·1
Normal-aggressive	1·27	Greater than 0·5
Normal-mixed	0·71	Greater than 0·5
Low scorers-high scorers	0·65	Greater than 0·5

Note: *cum. p.* In this and subsequent tables refers to cumulative proportion

fits in recent months and the disturbance of behaviour in the child.

The comparison of the time that had elapsed since the appearance of the first fit and the diagnostic group of the child is set out in Table 9.

There is a complete lack of association between the time since the first fit and the type and extent of behaviour disorder. There is a slight but non-significant trend for the fits to have been manifest for a *shorter* time in the anxious than in the normal group. It must be concluded that the evidence does not bear out the first hypothesis, there being no observable relationship between behaviour disorder and the time that has elapsed since the onset of epilepsy.

In order to test the second hypothesis, about the relationship between the outwardly alarming manifestations of the fit and the existence of psychiatric disturbance, the manifestations of the fit displayed by each child were ranked in four categories, according to the degree of external manifestation of the fit. Where the child at times displayed different kinds of fit, the type of fit ranked as containing the most marked external manifestations was used in the following analysis.

A detailed description of the fit was made for the purpose of this research by a neuropsychiatrist using all the medical information available about the child, except the data from the electroencephalograph. These data have been analysed separately, and will be discussed in a later chapter.

The types of fit were ranked in the following way:

1 *Petit mal* fits, involving a brief loss of consciousness, but without any loss of motor control, and very often unnoticeable in, for instance, the classroom.

2 Minor fits with some motor involvement, psychomotor fits, Jacksonian focal attacks, and atypical minor forms involving a brief loss of consciousness and some motor involvement.

3 Minor major attacks, involving unconsciousness for a short time and falling to the ground, but without any of the characteristics of the *grand mal* fit. Such cases are differentiated from the classic *grand mal* fits by the absence of convulsions, the absence of movement of the arms and legs, and the absence of incontinence. The patient loses consciousness and falls to the floor, but the attack rarely lasts more than a minute.

4 Major attacks with the usual accompaniment of this type of fit—convulsions of hands and legs, clenching of teeth, perhaps incontinence, and prolonged unconsciousness.

The results of comparing the degree of external manifestations of the fit with the diagnostic category to which the child belongs are given in Table 10.

It will be seen that the distribution of the fit rankings are signifi-

Table 10 Manifestation of fit and psychiatric diagnosis in 118 epileptic children

	Normal		*Anxious*		*Aggressive*		*Mixed*		*Low total scorers*		*High total scorers*	
Rank of outward manifestations of fit	*n*	%	*n*	%	*n*	%	*n*	%	*n*	%	*n*	%
1 (*petit mal*)	6	17·1	1	3·6	0	—	1	4·0	6	9·5	2	3·6
2 (minor forms)	4	11·4	6	21·4	8	26·6	11	44·0	10	15·9	19	34·5
3 (minor major)	11	31·4	3	10·7	5	16·7	4	16·0	14	22·2	9	16·4
4 (major forms)	14	40·0	18	64·3	17	56·6	9	36·0	33	52·4	25	45·4
Totals	35		28		30		25		63		55	

Note: Arrangement of data treated as nominal rather than ordinal (Siegel, 1956, pp. 21–33), and tested by the χ^2 method· Cochran's Rule is used for small numbers (Siegel, 1956, p. 46).

Significance:

Comparison	χ^2 (3 d.f.)	*Probability level*
Normal-anxious	7·81	Equal to 0·05
Normal-aggressive	8·71	Less than 0·05, greater than 0·02
Normal-mixed	9·94	Less than 0·05, greater than 0·02
Low scorers-High scorers	6·14	Less than 0·1, greater than 0·05

cantly different when the normal and disturbed groups are compared.

These results, although having some significance, are not immediately explicable in terms of the hypothesis tested, since the greatest difference is provided by the comparative dearth of minor forms of epilepsy (ranked 2) in the normals, and an excess of *petit mal* (ranked 1) and of minor major forms (ranked 3), with only a small under-representation of major forms (ranked 4) in the normals.

The data were re-examined to see if the differences between the diagnostic groups could be fully explained by the existence of minor forms of epilepsy (ranked 2) accompanying major forms (ranked 4) rather than minor major (ranked 3). The fit manifestations were reclassified, using the existence or absence of minor fits (other than *petit mal*) as the crucial point of distinction rather than the degree of outward manifestations of the fit. This reclassification showed that it was relatively rare for children with minor major epilepsy to also have minor fits on occasions, but that children who had major fits quite often had minor fits as well. The results of comparing the new classification by diagnostic groups is given in Table 11.

The rearrangement of the fit manifestation data using the existence or absence of minor fits as a crucial point of classification generally increases the significance of the difference between the diagnostic groups. The existence of major fits now only contributes to the difference between the normal and the anxious groups. The existence of the minor forms (minor motor fits) of epilepsy clearly contributes to the difference between the normal and the aggressive and the mixed groups. The anxious children have an incidence of minor motor fits which is in fact fairly similar to that in the normal children. The failure of the fit manifestations to clearly differentiate between the low and high total scorers can be accounted for by the fact that the majority of the anxious children with major fits have total scores below the median of the combined behaviour disorder scores, and the fact that the anxious children with high total scores, unlike the aggressive and mixed children, do not in the main display minor motor forms.

The difference in fit manifestation pattern between the anxious children, and the aggressive and mixed groups combined has been tested. The data (which is taken from Table 11) give a value of χ^2 (3 d.f.) of 9·96, which is significant at the 2 per cent level. In Table 9 there was a slight trend for the anxious children to have a more recent onset of fits than the other groups. The data from Table 9 and Table 11 suggest the hypothesis that *anxiety* in epileptic children may be related to major fits of recent onset. However, the evidence in the present series for this proposition is at a fairly low level of

Table 11 The incidence of minor forms of epilepsy by diagnostic groups in 118 epileptic children

Type of fits	*Normal*		*Anxious*		*Aggressive*		*Mixed*		*Low total scorers*		*High total scorers*	
	n	%	*n*	%	*n*	%	*n*	%	*n*	%	*n*	%
(*a*) *Petit mal* only	6	17·1	1	3·6	0	—	1	4·0	6	9·5	2	3·6
(*b*) Minor major (with or without (*a*))	11	31·4	3	10·7	4	13·3	3	12·0	14	22·2	7	12·7
(*c*) Major (with or without (*a*) and/or (*b*)	7	20·0	12	42·8	3	10·0	4	16·0	17	26·9	9	16·4
(*d*) Minor forms (with or without any of (*a*), (*b*), or (*c*))	11	31·4	12	42·8	23	76·7	17	68·0	26	41·2	37	67·2
Totals	35		28		30		25		63		55	

Note: Data treated as nominal; Cochran's Rule for χ^2 used.

Significance:

Comparison	χ^2 (3 d.f.)	*Probability level*
Normal-anxious	8·25	Less than 0·05, greater than 0·02
Normal-aggressive	13·52	Less than 0·005, greater than 0·001
Normal-mixed	7·98	Less than 0·05, greater than 0·02
High scorers-low scorers	7·67	Less than 0·1, greater than 0·05

Table 12 Frequency of fits and psychiatric disturbance in 118 epileptic children

Highest frequency	*Normal*		*Anxious*		*Aggressive*		*Mixed*		*Low total scorers*		*High total scorers*	
	n	*cum. p.*	*n*	*cum. p.*	*n*	*cum. p.*	*n*	*cum. p.*	*n*	*cum. p.*	*n*	*cum. p.*
1 a day or more	4	0·11	2	0·07	9	0·3	4	0·16	7	0·11	12	0·22
1 a week or more	8	0·34	6	0·28	4	0·44	7	0·44	15	0·35	10	0·44
1 a month or more	10	0·63	6	0·50	7	0·68	5	0·64	16	0·6	12	0·62
1 or more in 3 months	4	0·74	5	0·68	7	0·91	2	0·72	10	0·76	8	0·76
1 or more in 6 months	3	0·83	3	0·78	0	0·91	4	0·88	4	0·86	6	0·87
Less than 1 in 6 months	6	1·0	6	1·0	3	1·0	3	1·0	11	1·0	7	1·0
Totals	35		28		30		25		63		55	

Note: Inclusion in a category indicates a higher frequency than in the category below and a lower frequency than in the category above.

Significance: Kolmogorov-Smirnov one-tailed test:

Comparison	χ^2 (2 d.f.)	*Probability level*
Normal-anxious	1·05	Greater than 0·5
Normal-aggressive	2·59	Less than 0·3, greater than 0·2
Normal-mixed	0·6	Greater than 0·5
Low scorers-high scorers	1·42	Less than 0·5, greater than 0·3

significance, and it must be tested on a larger group of anxious epileptic children and appropriate controls.

The relationship of minor motor fits to behaviour disorder (especially of an aggressive or mixed kind) is more difficult to explain in 'external' terms, and it may be that neurological factors underlie this type of behaviour. This hypothesis will be explored further in later chapters.

Is there a connection between the *frequency* of fits and behaviour disorder? A count has been made of the frequency of all types of fits occurring during the six months prior to the examination of the child by the psychiatrist. The results are given in Table 12.

It will be seen that there is no relationship between fit frequency and psychiatric disorder in these epileptic children. Although the aggressive group has a frequency of fits occurring once a day or more, which is somewhat higher than that of any other group, the normal group has a higher frequency than the aggressive group of fits occurring once a week or more (but not as often as once a day). In the aggressive group, the three highest frequency categories occupy 67·6 per cent of the total; in the normal group the three highest frequency categories occupy 62·8 per cent of the total: these differences are too slight to be significant.

It is concluded that the third hypothesis—that the more frequent the fits the more likely an epileptic child will be disturbed—is not sustained.

Conclusions

1 The hypothesis that behaviour disorder is connected with the time since the onset of fits has been tested with the 118 epileptic children. This hypothesis cannot be sustained.

2 The hypothesis that behaviour disorder is associated with the degree of outward manifestation of a fit has been tested with the epileptic children by ranking the fits observed into four categories according to the degree of outward manifestation of the fit (*petit mal* ranked 1, *grand mal* ranked 4). Significant variations are observed, with some excess of *grand mal* fits in the anxious children, but a predominance of minor motor fits (ranked 2) in the disturbed cases, in comparison with the normal children. The data has been recategorized, making the existence or absence of minor fits (ranked 2) a crucial point of classification. Aggressive and mixed children are seen to have an excess of minor fits, and a relative dearth of all other foıms, in comparison with normal children. It is concluded that there is a significant association between the existence of minor fits and behaviour disorder in the child of an aggressive or mixed mind.

3 The significance difference between anxious and normal children

according to fit manifestations (using minor motor forms as a crucial point of classification) is based to a large extent on an excess of *grand mal* (major) epilepsy in the anxious cases. There is also a significant excess of this kind of fit in the anxious cases when they are compared with the aggressive and mixed cases. It might be possible to explain the anxiety—in part, at least—as a reaction of fits which individuals in the child's environment view with alarm. There is also a slight suggestion in the data that the anxious children have fits of more recent onset than children in other behavioural categories. The hypotheses implied by these data require fuller investigation with a larger group of anxious, epileptic children.

The association of minor motor fits with behaviour of the aggressive or mixed type is more difficult to explain in environmental terms, and it may be that neurological factors underlie—in part, at least—this type of behaviour. This hypothesis will be explored more fully in later chapters.

4 The hypothesis that behaviour disorder is associated with the frequency of the fits (in the six-month period before the child was seen at the hospital for intensive psychiatric examination) has been tested. No relationship can be found between the two factors, and the hypothesis is thus not proven with these data.

19 Environmental hazards and behaviour disorder

Although some writers on epilepsy in childhood have argued that factors in the environment are important for the emergence of behaviour disorder in epileptic children, other writers have failed to show that there is a connection between these factors and the behaviour disorder. Other writers have ignored the factor of environment, and have argued that the behaviour disorders are caused by brain damage or neurological or constitutional factors.

In the present study, the number of hazards in the environment of each child has been assessed by establishing the existence or absence of the following factors: items (14) to (20) in the control group study (overcrowding, poverty, disturbing relatives, etc.), except that additional sources of information (the social worker's report) were used to supplement this information. In addition, the item 'frequent changes of home environment' was broken up into separate items, so that each substantial change in home or family environment was considered as an item. Included under this heading were migration from one country to another; death or desertion of a parent; placement in a new family setting, such as the taking of the child into care because of the eviction of the family or the illness of the mother.

Environmental factors were conceptualized as factors involving possible *indirect* stress for the child, so that direct interaction between the child and his parents was not considered as an environmental factor. The parental attitudes and behaviour are considered in another section. Discord between the parents was included as an environmental hazard, but discord between the parents about child management was specifically excluded. The evidence for the existence of discord between parents was taken from the psychiatrist's item sheet.

The results of the comparison of the number of environmental hazards according to diagnostic group are given in Table 13. The

Table 13 Environmental hazards and behaviour disorder in 118 epileptic children

No. of environmental hazards	*Normal*		*Anxious*		*Aggressive*		*Mixed*		*Low total scorers*		*High total scorers*	
	n	*cum. p.*	*n*	*cum. p.*	*n*	*cum. p.*	*n*	*cum. p.*	*n*	*cum. p.*	*n*	*cum. p.*
0	15	0·43	7	0·25	6	0·2	3	0·12	24	0·38	7	0·13
1–2	12	0·77	5	0·43	6	0·4	7	0·4	16	0·63	14	0·38
3–5	4	0·88	10	0·79	12	0·8	8	0·72	15	0·87	19	0·73
6 or more	4	1·0	6	1·0	6	1·0	7	1·0	8	1·0	15	1·0
Totals	35		28		30		25		63		55	

Notes: Data for environmental hazards divided as near to the median and quartiles as possible.

Significance: Kolmogorov-Smirnov one-tailed test:

Comparison	χ^2 (2 d.f.)	*Probability level*
Normal-anxious	7·26	Less than 0·02, greater than 0·01
Normal-aggressive	8·88	Less than 0.01, greater than 0.005
Normal-mixed	8·02	Less than 0·02, greater than 0·01
Low scorers-high scorers	7·57	Less than 0·02, greater than 0·01

number of environmental hazards clearly differentiates the 35 normal cases from the three groups of disturbed epileptics. These environmental hazards may well be of aetiological significance in the behaviour disorder.

An analysis of the associations of the number of environmental hazards has shown that a heredity of epilepsy in near relatives (siblings, parents, grandparents, parental siblings) is related to a high number of environmental hazards (Table 14).

Table 14 Environmental hazards and heredity for epilepsy

No. of environmental hazards	*No heredity of epilepsy*		*Heredity of epilepsy*		*Total*
	N	%	*N*	%	
0–2	45	60·8	15	38·4	60
3 or more	29	39·2	24	61·6	53
Totals	74		39		113

Information not available for heredity in five cases.

Significance: χ^2 (1 d.f.) = 5·06
P less than 0·05, greater than 0·02.

There is a significant relationship between heredity for epilepsy and a high number of environmental hazards (which in turn is associated with behaviour disorder in the child). Why should this be so? Some previous studies (reviewed earlier) have suggested that there is a relationship between a heredity for epilepsy and a history of mental illness and abnormal behaviour in family members, conditions which themselves may have a genetic basis. Grunberg and Pond (1957) suggested that this disturbed behaviour in other family members acted in itself as an environmental hazard.

If these relationships hold good for the present data, there should be a relationship between a history of epilepsy in close relatives and the multiple existence of the conditions of neurosis, psychosis, behaviour disorder, and psychopathy, criminality or alcoholism in near relatives (parents, siblings, grandparents, parental siblings). In the 113 children in the present series, for which information about a heredity for epilepsy is available, 19 had 2 or more near relatives displaying one of the disturbances of behaviour listed above. Fourteen of the children (73·3 per cent) also had a relative with epilepsy. Ninety-four children did not display this 'multiple heredity' for disturbed behaviour, and 34 (36·2 per cent) of these children had a relative with epilepsy. These differences are significant at the 1 per cent level (χ^2 (1 d.f.)=9·1).

It is of interest that the opposite kind of relationship with the number of environmental hazards has been found in those cases in which there is the possibility of early brain injury (because of threatened miscarriage, severe maternal illness during pregnancy, prolonged or difficult labour, prematurity, meningitis, encephalitis, or post-natal head injury); in these cases there is a *negative* relationship between a history of events likely to have caused brain injury and the number of environmental hazards. This relationship is explicable if one considers that brain injury and a heredity for epilepsy are usually considered to be separate or alternative factors in the aetiology of epilepsy. The data are set out in Table 15.

Some hypotheses about the nature of association of poor environment and the existence of abnormal behavioural conditions in family members of the epileptic will be advanced in Chapter 25.

The relationship between the number of environmental hazards and the distribution by social class has been tested to see if the environment of those cases whose parents occupy the Registrar General's Categories IV and V (semi-skilled and unskilled) have a higher number of environmental hazards than those children with parents in the business and professional classes (Registrar General's Categories I and II). The results are set out in Table 16. The results support the hypothesis of a relationship between low social class and a high number of environmental hazards.

Table 15 Environmental hazards and a history of possible brain damage in 118 epileptic children

No. of environmental hazards	*No history of possible brain damage*		*History of possible brain damage*		*Total*
	N	%	*N*	%	
0–2	19	37·2	42	62·7	61
3 or more	32	62·7	25	37·3	57
Totals	51		67		118

Significant differences:

Median test—χ^2 (1 d.f.) = 7·5
P less than 0·01, greater than 0·005.

Table 16 Social class and environmental hazards in 118 epileptic children

No. of environmental hazards	*Social class*					
	I and II		*III*		*IV and V*	
	n	%	*n*	%	*n*	%
0–2	23	74·2	32	47·1	6	31·6
3 or more	8	25·8	36	52·9	13	58·4
Totals	31	—	68	—	19	—

Significant differences: Overall distribution of table, χ^2 (2 d.f.) = 10·26
P less than 0·005, greater than 0·001.

Conclusions

1 Adverse factors in the environment clearly distinguish between epileptic children with and without behaviour disorder of all kinds, anxious, aggressive and mixed. It may be that these adverse factors play a part in causing this behaviour disorder.
2 There are significantly more adverse factors in the environment of those cases in which a near relative has epilepsy. Epilepsy in near relatives is associated with the multiple occurrence of adverse behavioural conditions in those relations. This adverse behaviour itself may well be connected with the creation of an adverse environment for the epileptic child.
3 There are significantly fewer adverse factors in the environment of those cases in which there is a history of events which may be associated with brain injury in the child.
4 There is a positive, significant association between the number of environmental hazards and low social class in the parents of the epileptic child.

20 Brain injury, the evidence from the EEG and behaviour disorder in epileptic children

The relationship of brain injury and behaviour disorder in epileptic children has been a subject for controversy in earlier studies. Brain injury has been found to have a positive relationship with disturbed behaviour, a negative relationship, or no relationship at all.

The present inquiry has measured brain injury in two ways. An index of possible brain injury has been taken to be a history of an event (threatened miscarriage during pregnancy; maternal illness during pregnancy; bleeding during pregnancy; toxaemia of pregnancy or hypertension; prolonged or difficult labour; prematurity—birth weight less than 5½ lb.; rhesus incompatibility; neo-natal anoxaemia; neo-natal fits, twitching, or pallor; encephalitis; cerebral vascular accident; head injury) which previous studies have shown to have an association with injury of the central nervous system. This index was referred to above in the section on environment (pp. 109–73), when it was shown to have a significantly negative relationship with the number of environmental hazards (which had a significantly *positive* relationship with a history of epilepsy in family members).

A second index of brain damage has been taken from the EEG. The original EEG records of 90 of the children were available, and were interpreted 'blindly' by a physician experienced in this field.[1] The blind reading consisted of an interpretation of the record with no other information available except the age of the child.

The two indices of possible brain injury are compared in Table 1. Although these two indices were made by independent workers using independent sources of information, there is a highly significant, positive agreement between them. The most disagreement occurs in

[1] This exercise was undertaken at a late stage in the research, and it was found that a number of the earlier records had been routinely discarded by the electroencephalographic department.

the third cell, in which the historical data indicate a possible brain injury and the EEG data do not. The EEG data in fact provide a more conservative index of possible brain injury.

In a further 26 cases the judgment about possible brain injury was taken from the report of the electroencephalographer, who had access to some of the clinical information relating to the child. In a further two cases, the existence of an EEG record having been performed at any hospital could not be traced.

Table 17 A comparison of historical and EEG data indicating brain injury in 90 epileptic children

	EEG data		
Historical data	*Brain injury unlikely*	*Brain injury likely*	*Totals*
Brain injury unlikely	28	6	34
Brain injury likely	24	32	56
Totals	52	38	90

Significance: χ^2 (1 d.f.) = 11·85
P less than 0·001.

The conservatism of the EEG record for indicating the possibility of brain injury is illustrated by the following case: at the age of three months the child had encephalitis. Minor fits had their onset shortly after the child's recovery. A subsequent neurological examination suggested that the boy was brain-damaged, a diagnosis confirmed by A.E.G. The EEG record, however, showed no neurological abnormality.

The final index of the existence of possible brain injury has been taken from two sources: the existence of a history of an event (as defined above) likely to be associated with brain injury; and the indication of brain injury from the EEG record.[1] As was seen in Table 17, there is a good agreement between these two indicators of brain damage, so that in the large majority of cases where the historical data are positive the EEG data will be positive also.

The verbal-performance discrepancy (and other I.Q. test data) was not considered in making the judgments about the existence of brain injury. However, a number of writers (e.g. Halton, 1966) have stressed that a large difference between verbal and performance I.Q.

[1] Cf. the use by Pond (1965) of multiple indicators of brain damage (historical data; physical signs; A.E.G.; E.E.G.) in a study of psychiatric disorder in brain-damaged children: '. . . the commonest causes of brain damage in the child psychiatric population are the events around the time of birth, whether by anoxia or by physical damage with forceps, etc.'

Table 18 Verbal-performance discrepancy on the W.I.S.C. and brain injury in 109 epileptic children

Verbal-performance discrepancy	*Brain injury unlikely*		*Brain injury likely*	
	n	*cum. p.*	*n*	*cum. p.*
0–4	21	0·4	9	0·6
5–9	15	0·7	6	0·26
10–14	11	0·92	13	0·48
15–19	3	0·96	12	0·69
20–4	1	1·0	11	0·88
25–9	0	1·0	4	0·95
30+	0	1·0	3	1·0
Totals	51		58	

Test details not available in nine cases.

Significance: Kolmogorov-Smirnov one-tailed test.
χ^2 (2 d.f.) = 19·9
P less than 0·001

is a possible indicator of brain damage. Table 18 shows that this is true for the present series.

In the section on fits (above, pp. 160–8) it was found that the existence of minor fits with motor involvement was a good predictor of behaviour disorder of an aggressive or mixed kind. It is clinically feasible that brain damage underlies this type of fit; a test of this hypothesis (Table 19) shows that there is in fact a significant association between brain damage and minor motor fits.

Since minor fits were associated with disturbed behaviour, we would expect brain damage to show this relationship as well. The hypothesis is tested in Table 20. It will be seen that, although the existence of brain damage differentiates normal and aggressive cases at a high level of significance, no other comparison is significant, and the possible existence of brain damage differentiates the low and high total scorers at only the one in ten level of probability of chance occurrence.

Two possibilities seem likely: that the index of brain damage has only a limited validity for predicting organic cerebral damage; or else only that kind of brain damage which leads to the occurrence of minor motor fits is likely to be associated with behaviour disorder. If the latter is the case, whether the brain damage or the fits themselves are causally involved in the behaviour disorder, or some other, unknown factor linked with these variables, is difficult to tell from the evidence available.

Table 19 Brain damage and minor fits with motor involvement in 118 epileptic children

Type of fit	*Brain injury unlikely*	*Brain injury likely*	*Totals*
Petit mal, minor/ major, or major	36 (64·3%)	19 (30·6%)	55
Minor, with motor involment	20 (35·7%)	43 (69·3%)	63
Totals	56	62	118

Significance: χ^2 (1 d.f.) = 15·77
P less than 0·001

It should be noted that the anxious cases differ significantly from the aggressive cases in the incidence of brain damage at the 1 per cent level (x^2=6·92, 1 d.f.). The mixed cases occupy an intermediate position, the incidence of brain damage showing no significant variation from that in any other group. The rank order of the data in this, as in many other comparisons of data in this study is: (1) aggressive; (2) mixed; (3) anxious; (4) normal.

Behaviour disorder and EEG categories

In the 116 cases in which EEG results are available (a 'blind' reading of the original EEG record in 90 cases, and the electroencephalographer's typed report in a further 26 cases) the results have been assigned to six categories. In the 90 'blind' readings this categorization was done by the physician without recourse to any other information. It is possible that in the remaining 26 cases the report was made in the light of other clinical information about the child (e.g. fit pattern). However, since the EEG was carried out as part of a neurological rather than a psychiatric investigation, it is unlikely that the electroencephalographer would have any information about the child's behaviour.

The six EEG categories are as follows:

Normal. Perhaps some abnormalities, but within normal limits for the child's age. *N*=31.

Epileptic. A definitely abnormal record, specific for epilepsy rather than brain damage (other than 3 per second spike-and-wave). *N*=12.

Petit mal. Bilateral, symmetrical 3 per second spike-and-wave patterns. *N*=11.

Immature. A normal record, but typical of a child three or more years younger. *N*=6.

Table 20 Brain injury and behaviour disorder in 118 epileptic children

Brain injury	*Normal*		*Anxious*		*Aggressive*		*Mixed*		*Low total scorers*		*High total scorers*	
	n	%	*n*	%	*n*	%	*n*	%	*n*	%	*n*	%
Brain injury unlikely	21	60·0	16	57·0	7	23·3	11	44·0	34	54·0	21	38·2
Brain injury likely	14	40·0	12	43·0	23	76·7	14	56·0	29	46·0	34	61·8
Totals	35		28		30		25		63		55	

Significance: χ^2 test:

Comparison	χ^2 *(1 d.f.)*	*Probability level*
Normal-anxious	0·52	Less than 0·5
Normal-aggressive	8·86	Less than 0·005, greater than 0·001
Normal-mixed	1·5	Less than 0·25, greater than 0·1
Low scorers-high scorers	2·94	Less than 0·1, greater than 0·05

Table 21 Disturbed behaviour and EEG categories in 116 epileptic children

Behavioural category	*EEG Category*					
	Normal	*Epileptic*	*Petit mal*	*Immature*	*Generalized brain damage*	*Temporal lobe focus*
Normal	6	6	7	2	8	6
Anxious	11	3	1	1	7	5
Aggressive	7	1	2	1	9	9
Mixed	7	2	1	2	7	5
Totals	31	12	11	6	31	25

Note: EEG results not available in two cases.

Significance: Because of the many cells in which the incidence was less than five, a comparison of the distribution of all EEG categories between normal-anxious, normal-aggressive, and normal-mixed cases could not directly be made. Instead, these comparisons were made for each *pair* of EEG catagories. Only one result emerged at beyond the 5 per cent level of significance—the comparison of normal and anxious cases for the incidence of the Normal EEG category ($\chi^2=3{\cdot}87$; P less than 0·05, greater than 0·02). However, since partitioning the data in this way may increase the risk of a significant result occurring by chance, this result must be treated with caution.

The comparison of low scorers and high scorers is treated in a continuation of the present table:

Behavioural category	*EEG Category*						
	Normal	*Epileptic*	*Petit mal*	*Immature*	*Generalized brain damage*	*Temporal lobe focus*	*Totals*
Low total scorers	17	8	8	3	16	11	63
High total scorers	14	4	3	3	15	14	53
Totals	31	12	11	6	31	25	116

Significance: χ^2 (5 d.f.) 1·39, greater than 0·5

Generalized Brain Damage. An abnormal record with either generalized abnormalities indicative of brain damage, or the location of these abnormalities in one hemisphere. Four cases in which there appears to be a location of these abnormalities in frontal lobe have been included in this category. $N=31$.

Temporal Lobe Focus. A brain-damaged group, with an abnormal EEG focal in a temporal lobe. $N=25$.

The distribution of these six EEG categories, according the classification of behaviour into 'normal', 'anxious', 'aggressive', and 'mixed' cases, is given in Table 5.

Only one comparison (a higher incidence of the 'normal' type of EEG in the anxious compared with the normal cases) gives a result which can be accepted even at a moderate level of confidence. The association of disturbed behaviour with a temporal lobe focus does not appear in these data—by the present method of analysis, at least.

Discussion

The association of temporal lobe focus and disturbed behaviour has occurred in some studies (e.g. Nuffield, 1961), but has remained elusive in other, equally well conducted studies (e.g. Small *et al.*, 1962 and 1966; Stevens, 1966; Wilson and Harris, 1966). Rodin *et al.* (1964), who studied epileptic patients by a factor analytic method, found an association between psychiatric disorder in ninety patients, and temporal lobe seizures. This correlation, although significant, was of a low order, leading the authors to comment on the controversial studies in this field. They suggest that there might be a definite association between *some kinds of* temporal lobe disorder and psychiatric disturbance, occurring in only a minority of cases.[1] This low but significant association, they suggested, might account for the fact that separate studies had at times validated, and at others had failed to validate this association.

One possible association of temporal lobe damage (Ounsted, 1955, Ingram, 1956; Ounsted *et al.*, 1966) is hyperkinesis, a syndrome which recent studies have shown to be associated with aggressive behaviour. Ounsted showed that hyperkinesis occurs in about 10 per cent of epileptic children. Hyperkinesis in the present series will be discussed in the following chapter.

Brain damage, not merely of the temporal lobes, has been implicated in previous studies as a factor in hyperkinesis, so that it might be expected that brain damage which includes temporal lobe damage, but also some other types of damage to the brain, might be associated

[1] Cf. the factor analysis reported in Ch. 28 of the present study, which suggests that a special sub-syndrome of temporal lobe psychiatric disorder may exist.

with aggressive behaviour. This relationship occurs in the present study at the 1 per cent level of significance (*vide supra*, p. 178).

Conclusions

1 Brain damage in the present series has been measured in two ways: according to a positive history of events likely to be associated with brain injury (birth injury, encephalitis, head injury, etc.), and the evidence from the EEG (which were read 'blind' by an independent electroencephalographer in 90 cases). These two separate indices have positive and highly significant association with one another, although the EEG index is more conservative, there being some cases in which other evidence (AEG, neurological examination, etc.) clearly indicated the existence of brain damage, when the EEG did not. Accordingly, brain damage has been assumed to be likely when *either* the historical index *or* the EEG index is positive. This combined index has a highly significant, positive association with a third factor—verbal-performance discrepancy on the WISC—which previous writers have suggested is an indicator of brain damage.

2 The final index of brain damage has a highly significant, positive association with a history of minor fits with motor involvement. This latter variable was previously seen to have a strong association with behaviour disorder of the mixed and aggressive kinds.

3 The likelihood of brain damage discriminates the normal from the aggressive children at a highly significant level, but it does not discriminate normal from anxious cases, which have a similar incidence of the likelihood of brain damage. The mixed cases are in an intermediate position.

4 Six EEG categories have been derived from the data available for 116 cases. In 90 of the cases this categorization was made from a 'blind' reading of the EEG record. No clear differences emerge when the EEG categories are compared with the behavioural categories, although there is some suggestion that a normal EEG is associated with anxiety when compared with behaviourally normal epileptics.

5 The data indicate that brain damage, rather than temporal lobe damage in particular, is associated with aggressive behaviour.

21 The hyperactive group

Hyperactivity in epileptic children has been described by a number of writers studying different patient populations (*vide supra*, pp. 86–92). What is the incidence of hyperactivity in the present neurological series of epileptic children?

Eleven children obtain a maximum score of 3 ('marked'), on the behavioural ratings for 'hyperactive, impulsive, distractable'. Fourteen children scored 2 on this trait ('definite sign') and nineteen scored 1 ('some sign'). These data suggest that hyperactive behaviour in these epileptic children can be represented as a descending continuum, with a small minority of the total in the series (9·4 per cent) displaying hyperactivity to a marked degree. This incidence of serious hyperactivity is very similar to that given by Ounsted (1955) for serious hyperactive behaviour in epileptic children.

What are the characteristics of these children? Since the children scoring 3 on this trait are similar in all respects to those scoring 2, they have been combined for the purpose of analysis. Twenty of these 25 cases are thought to be brain-injured (according to the historical and the EEG data), compared with 43 of the remaining cases in the series. This suggests an association between hyperactivity and brain damage at the 0·05 per cent level ($\chi^2=9{\cdot}02$, 1 d.f.).

No single EEG group can be implicated as being associated with hyperactivity, and of the two categories which have been taken to imply brain damage (generalized damage and temporal lobe focus), each is as likely as the other to be associated with hyperactivity. These findings agree with those of Ingram (1956).

Nineteen of the 25 hyperactive children have an IQ equal to or below the median for the whole series, compared with 40 of the remaining 91 cases (IQ being unknown in two cases). This difference is significant at the 0·05 per cent level ($\chi^2=8{\cdot}06$, 1 d.f.). This finding agrees with that of Ounsted *et al.* (1966).

Nineteen of the 25 hyperactive cases are male, compared with 54 of the 93 remaining cases in the series. This difference, while in the direction predicted by earlier studies (for hyperactivity to be associated with male sex) is not significant.

All but one of the 25 hyperactive children have a score on the aggressive symptoms that is above the median aggression score for the whole series. This is to be expected, since the cluster analysis reported above showed that hyperactivity was strongly correlated with a number of aggressive traits. The eleven children who have a maximum score on the item measuring hyperactivity in all but two cases have total behaviour disorder scores of over 20 (i.e. above the third quartile for the series) and comprise some of the most seriously disturbed children in the study.

Conclusions

Hyperactivity in the present series is apparent to at least some degree in 44 of the 118 children. However, in only 11 children is the trait 'marked' according to the ratings used. This gives an incidence of serious hyperactivity of 9·4 per cent similar to that observed by Ounsted (1955) in epileptic children. There is a highly significant, positive association between brain damage and hyperactivity. No particular location of brain damage (e.g. in the temporal lobe) can be associated with hyperactivity. There is a significant relationship between lower intelligence and hyperactivity. There is a slight trend towards an association between male sex and hyperactivity.

22 Parental attitudes and behaviour

The quantitative appraisal of the quality of family interactions is one of the most difficult areas of measurement in social science. This difficulty is illustrated by studies of epilepsy which have sought to show the existence of disturbed parental attitudes as an aetiological factor in behaviour disorder. A judgment about parental behaviour and attitudes inevitably involves value presumptions, and no study of the parents of epileptic children has attempted to place the making of these judgments on a systematic basis. Studies usually make an overall judgment, such as 'parental attitude disturbed', without specifying clearly what this means or how this judgment was arrived at. The studies which have reported the influence of parental attitudes on behaviour in epileptic children have been reviewed above. The conclusion from this review was that, notwithstanding the difficulty of measuring parental attitudes, some studies have apparently shown an association between disturbed behaviour in the parents and behaviour disorder in the child. Both 'rejection' and 'over-protection' on the part of parents have been implicated.

The measurement of attitudes and behaviour in the parents of 118 epileptic children

The available methods for studying how parents behave towards their children seem to be: (*a*) By a questionnaire given to the parent. This usually consists of items describing parental behaviour or feeling, which the respondent checks according to the degree of his agreement or disagreement with the statement. For example, in the Schaefer Parental Attitude Inventory (Schaefer *et al.*, 1959) the parent is asked to agree, strongly or mildly, or disagree, strongly or mildly, to statements such as, 'A child will be grateful later on for strict training'.[1] (*b*) A direct observation of parent-child interaction.

[1] Cf. also the questionnaire used in an English context by Gibson (1968).

This method is beset with the difficulty of the effect of the observer on the behaviour of the parent. (*c*) A questionnaire to the child about how his parents treat him (Siegelman, 1965). This method is ingenious, but involves the difficulty that the child's disturbance itself may affect the way he reports his relationship with his parents. (*d*) The behaviour and attitudes of the parent towards his child may be elicited by detailed questioning of the parent by a worker using a systematic schedule, a method whose reliability and validity with the parents of very young children has been shown by Thomas *et al.* (1964).

An initial approach to the problem of measuring the attitudes and behaviour of the parents of the 118 epileptic children was made by giving the mothers of the children a copy of Schaefer's Parental Attitude Research Instrument to complete. A number of limitations in this approach emerged. Firstly, despite repeated requests, over a third of the mothers did not fill in the questionnaire (a bulky document requiring responses to 115 statements about parental behaviour and attitudes). Analysis of the non-responders showed them to be of two types—parents of the most disturbed children and parents from the lower social classes. Secondly, it became manifest from an analysis of the responses that mothers were putting up 'formalized' responses, which weıe at variance with information gathered about their behaviour and attitudes from other sources.

These conclusions were very similar to those drawn by Becker and Krug (1965), who reviewed published and unpublished reports of the use of Schaefer's P.A.R.I. These authors observed that '... The parents might respond in terms of cultural norms, professional opinion, empirical facts, or beliefs about what is best for others, none of which have anything to do with what the parent actually does with his own child'.

An alternative method of assessing parental attitudes and behaviour had been developed in another study by a worker from the psychiatric department of the hospital (Ryle and Hamilton, 1962), and it was decided to use a development of the method used by these authors. This method is that of the extended interview with the parent (a version of (*d*), above) and has been used in various settings (e.g. Zweig, 1965; Heimler, 1967). The method of the extensive, depth interview has also been developed by Brown and Rutter (1966) for the measurement of family activities and relationships. The judgment of different, trained and experienced workers about the extent of such items as 'Disagreement over the care of the child' and 'behaviour prohibited to the child' in Brown and Rutter's study of thirty families had correlations in excess of $+0{\cdot}6$.

The interviews with the parents of the epileptic children were carried out by three psychiatric social workers. Two of these workers between them carried out over 90 per cent of the interviews. Information on a wide range of data was obtained by means of a lengthy face-to-face interview, systematically covering standard areas of behaviour. The data thus obtained were recorded without any attempt at interpretation at this stage. It is reasonable to suppose that the workers were successful in by-passing the formal defence that the mothers might have erected.

The problem of extracting information from these interviews according to a formal scale remained. The items and scales to be used and the meanings to be attached to the questions asked were decided by a group of professional workers in this field—two psychiatrists, a clinical psychologist, two psychiatric social workers, and the writer. This was the same group which at an earlier stage in the research had agreed on the norms of judgment of child behaviour. The two areas of the work—judgment about child disturbance and judgment about parental behaviour and attitudes—were kept strictly separate. However, in some cases the information used for assessing child behaviour also gave some indication of the quality of the parental attitudes, and vice versa, so that the possibility of 'contaminated' judgment cannot be entirely ruled out. All that can be said about this kind of bias is that the workers involved were aware of the dangers of making circular judgments, and the utmost rigour was used to try to avoid contâminated judgments.

The following list of 18 items of parental attitude and behaviour was drawn up, the items being selected because the group considered that the semantic label of the behaviour in question had common meaning to the group of workers involved, and which it was considered possible to make a judgment upon, in the light of the information available. The 18 items are:

1 Degree to which mother manifests anxiety, regardless of cause.

2 Degree to which mother is unable to cope with her problems.

3 Degree to which mother has a 'psychiatric' depression.

4 Degree to which mother expresses criticism of child (in interview).

5 Degree to which mother is over-ambitious for child (in full context of his abilities).

6 Degree to which mother shows preference for child's siblings.

7 Degree to which mother nags child and overtly expresses irritation.

8 Degree to which mother and father are conflicting authorities on child management.

9 Degree to which father punishes child.

10 Degree to which the father is controlling and rigid.

11 Degree to which father is critical of child.

12 Degree to which mother shows guilt about her handling of the child's illness.

13 Degree to which mother is over-protective of child in relation to his epilepsy.
14 Degree to which mother is non-supporting, or cannot support, the child in the difficulties surrounding his illness.
15 Degree to which mother cannot understand the implications of the child's epilepsy.
16 Degree to which mother overemphasizes the implications of child's epilepsy.
17 Degree to which the father is non-supporting of child in the difficulties surrounding his illness.
18 Degree to which mother shows guilt about the cause of the child's illness.

The items were evaluated on a 5-point scale: 1, not at all; 2, some but apparently little; 3, clearly present, but not obviously marked; 4, marked; 5, very marked.

The group of workers selected a number of case histories at random, and each of the six workers completed a schedule for the first case without knowing the judgments of the other workers. The judgments were compared and the reasons for disagreement discussed. In this way common norms for evaluating the data were arrived at. Further case histories were evaluated by each of the six workers in this way, until the correlation of the judgments of any one worker reached a correlation agreement of +0·7 with those of any other worker.

From the outset there was good agreement between the workers on the meaning of the items involved, and the relevance of particular pieces of information in the case histories, so that the +0·7 level of agreement was reached after the consideration of seven case histories.

When this stage of inter-rater agreement had been arrived at, the writer and his associate (the psychiatric social worker who had completed the majority of the case histories) then undertook the scoring of the parental attitudes and behaviour for all the 118 cases. The two workers made their judgments separately, and where there was a disagreement discussed the interpretation of the evidence until agreement was reached. The commonest kind of disagreement was because the two workers wished to score an item in separate but adjacent categories, e.g. disagreement over whether an item was 'marked' or 'very marked'. Disagreement other than that over adjacent categories was rare.

The data was not interpreted in a psychoanalytical sense, so that an overt action on the part of the mother (e.g. affection) was not interpreted to be something other than affection (e.g. hostility according to some psychoanalytical interpretations of particular situations). In making the judgments, however, the circumstances of the whole case were taken into account. For example, deciding on the 'Degree to which mother manifests anxiety, regardless of cause' involves a consideration of all the factors which might cause her to be anxious.

The completed schedules of parental behaviour and attitudes were then analysed in terms of the four diagnostic groups. An average score on the 18 items was obtained. Cases in which the child had no sibling were not scored in Item 6. Occasionally an item was not completed when it was considered that insufficient information was available for a judgment to be made.

The results of comparing the mean of the average score on the 5-point scale (1 to 5) for 18 items of parental attitudes and behaviour according to diagnostic group are given in Table 22.

It will be seen that the incidence of high adverse scores on the items of parental behaviour and attitudes strongly differentiates the normal and aggressive groups, and the mixed and normal groups to a lesser degree.[1] The anxious children, while having higher adverse parental scores than the normal children, are not so clearly distinguished. In fact, the parental scores of the anxious children more closely resemble those of the normal than of the aggressive groups, the difference between the distribution of the parental attitude scores for the aggressive and anxious groups being significant at the 1 % level. It is interesting that the mixed group, who have the highest total behaviour disorder score, do not have the highest number of disturbed parental attitudes. It is the parents of the aggressive children who display markedly more disturbed attitudes than any other group.

These results can be interpreted in four ways:

1 The significant differences are an artefact of the measurement situation, such as the possibility of contamination discussed above. Again, it must be said that the workers who made the measurements were aware of this problem, and were at pains to avoid making contaminated judgments. The actual patterning of the data does in fact support the view that no contamination took place. If the workers 'unconsciously' attributed high adverse parental attitudes to the parents of the most disturbed children, the most disturbed children (the mixed group) should have the highest incidence of disturbed parental attitudes. This is not the case. In addition, higher scores for the anxious group than those which actually occurred would be expected.

2 Disturbed parental attitudes are a cause of behaviour disorder in epileptic children, and particularly of aggressive behaviour disorder.

[1] Cf. Hauck (1969), who found that 'authoritarianism and autocracy' in parents had an adverse effect on clinical recovery in a series of 160 epileptic children.

Table 22 The incidence of disturbed parental attitudes according to behavioural groups in 118 epileptic children

Parental attitudes	*Normal*		*Anxious*		*Aggressive*		*Mixed*		*Low total scorers*		*High total scorers*	
score	*n*	*cum. p.*	*n*	*cum. p.*	*n*	*cum. p.*	*n*	*cum. p.*	*n*	*cum. p.*	*n*	*cum. p.*
Less than 1st quartile	19	0·54	8	0·29	1	0·03	4	0·16	25	0·4	7	0·13
Less than Median, more than Q1	8	0·77	7	0·54	4	0·17	5	0·36	15	0·63	11	0·33
Less than Q3 more than Median	4	0·89	10	0·89	11	0·5	8	0·68	12	0·82	19	0·67
More than 3rd quartile	4	1·0	3	1·0	14	1·0	8	1·0	11	1·0	18	1·0
Totals	35		28		30		25		63		55	

Note: Q1 of the parental score for the 118 cases (taking the average score on all eighteen items) is 2·059; Median, 2·372; Q3, 2·703.

Significance: Kolmogorov-Smirnov one-tailed test:

Comparison	χ^2 *(2 d.f.)*	*Probability Level*
Normal-anxious	3·86	Less than 0·25, greater than 0·1
Normal-aggressive	23·26	Less than 0·001
Normal-mixed	9·8	Less than 0·01, greater than 0·005
Low scorers-high scorers	10·57	Less than 0·01, greater than 0·005

This view is the one most conventionally held in other areas of child psychiatry, in which much importance is attached to the way in which parents treat children.

3 Parental attitudes and behaviour are disturbed because their children's behaviour is disturbed. The cause of this behaviour disturbance lies in some other factor (e.g. brain damage or other organic factors). On this hypothesis, the *parents* react adversely to their *children's* behaviour.

4 Parental attitudes and behaviour and disturbed behaviour in the child interact in a complex way. In terms of the interaction theory outlined earlier, there is a 'spiral' process: the child is initially disturbed, either because of organic factors or factors in his environment. *Because of this*, the parents react adversely to the child (e.g. rejection or control because of his changed behaviour). The child, in turn, reacts adversely to this behaviour in the parents, thus presenting a more seriously disturbed picture.

Discussion

Two factors besides disturbed parental attitudes have been identified as having a significant association with behaviour disorder in the epileptic children: a high number of environmental hazards; and the existence of minor fit forms, with motor involvement.

To elucidate the possible relationships between these variables, first of all the association of the existence of a high or low parental score and the existence of a high or low number of environmental hazards (dividing the data in each case as nearly as possible at the 50th percentile) has been examined (Table 23).

It will be seen that there is a significant association between the

Table 23 Disturbed parental attitudes and behaviour and environmental hazards in 118 epileptic children.

Parental attitudes	*Environmental hazards*		*Totals*
	Low	*High*	
Low	38	20	58
High	23	37	60
Totals	61	57	118

Median test:

χ^2 (1 d.f.) = 5·43

P less than 0·02, greater than 0·01

two variables.[1] When the number of adverse parental attitudes and behaviour items are high there tends to be a high number of environmental hazards.

Two points must be considered: Firstly, the association with behaviour disorder of disturbed parental attitudes and behaviour is much stronger than the association of environmental hazards. Normal children are distinguished from disturbed epileptic children by environmental hazards at the 2 per cent level; normal and disturbed children are distinguished by parental attitudes and behaviour at the 0·1 per cent level. Secondly, there are 23 cases in which adverse parental behaviour and attitudes are high, but in which the number of environmental hazards is low, so that the existence of environmental hazards is only a *partial* explanation of the existence of high adverse parental scores.

Are adverse parental behaviour and attitudes associated with the existence of minor fits with motor involvement (which we saw earlier to have a significant association with behaviour disorder in the epileptic children)? Are, in fact, the parental attitudes and behaviour *reactions* to behaviour disorder which has a basis in neurological factors?

The association between the existence of minor fits with motor involvement and adverse parental behaviour and attitudes has been tested in Table 24. It will be seen that there is no relationship between the two factors.[2]

This lack of association is important, since it leads to the two following assumptions:

(*a*) If disturbed parental behaviour and attitudes are a reaction to disturbance in the child which has been caused by some other factor, and not primary or causal in itself, then an association should occur between disturbed parental attitudes and behaviour and the existence of minor fits with motor involvement. This is not the case.

(*b*) If the association of disturbed parental attitudes and behaviour and disturbed behaviour in the children is an artefact of the measurement procedure, by which a child displaying behaviour disorder (from whatever cause) tends automatically to have disturbed attitudes and behaviour assigned to his parents, there should be an association of parental attitudes and disturbed behaviour disorder when minor fits are associated with behaviour disorder. This is not the case; there is no association of adverse parental attitudes and the existence of minor fits. This lack of association

[1] Although environmental hazards have a significant, positive association with low social class, the distribution of social class for the parental attitude and behaviour scores, is not significantly different from random.

[2] There is a completely random association between time since first fit and the disturbed parental attitude score.

Table 24 Disturbed parental attitudes and behaviour and fit manifestation in 118 epileptic children

Parental attitude and behaviour score	*Type of fit* (*a*) *Petit mal alone*		(*b*) *Minor major*		(*c*) *Major*		(*d*) *Minor with motor involvement*		*Totals*
	n	%	*n*	%	*n*	%	*n*	%	
Low	6	75·0	10	47·6	13	50·0	29	46·0	58
High	2	25·0	11	52·4	13	50·0	34	54·0	60
Totals	8		21		26		63		118

Note: Parental attitude and behaviour score divided as near to the 50th percentile as possible.
χ^2 (3 d.f.)=1·16
P less than 0·8, greater than 0·7, not significant

suggests that there has been no contamination of the measurement of parental attitudes and behaviour, and child behaviour.

An interaction hypothesis

There is an association between a high number of environmental hazards and a high score on the scale of adverse parental attitudes and behaviour, but the parental score is a better discriminant of behaviour disorder than the environment hazards score.

A hypothetical process involved in the interaction of these two variables may be as follows: each variable by itself can cause behaviour disorder in the epileptic child, and in a number of cases these two constraints do occur independently, and are associated with behaviour disorder. However, when parents have to bear with environmental difficulties (poverty, overcrowding, disturbing relatives, marital difficulties, etc.), they are less likely to react to epilepsy in their child in a rational or undisturbed manner than if they did not have environmental difficulties to cope with as well. If environmental hazards and parental attitudes and behaviour are *relatively* unrelated precipitants of behaviour disorder in epileptic children, when adverse environment and adverse parental attitudes occur *together*, the epileptic child should be more likely to be disturbed than if only one of these constraints on behaviour had existed.

A similar hypothesis can be made for the coincidence of minor fits with motor involvement (which are associated with behaviour disorder in the child independently of poor environment) with adverse parental behaviour and attitudes. If the three constraints on the behaviour of the child are relatively independent, then there should be a higher incidence of behaviour disorder in children who have two constraints upon them rather than one or none, and the highest incidence of behaviour disorder in those children who have all three constraints on their behaviour.

In order to try to provide a test of the interaction hypotheses, the data have been put in a 2^3 interaction table, dividing the data (environmental hazards; parental attitudes and behaviour; fit manifestation; and child behaviour disorder) as nearly as possible at the 50th percentile into 'high' and 'low' categories. The model for the interaction table (which is used for experimental designs in chemistry—Bennett and Franklin, 1954; and in biology—Yates, 1958) has been taken from Maxwell (1961), and the significance of the result tested by χ^2 method.

The following hypotheses are tested:

1 There will be a higher incidence of behaviour disorder when both environment hazards and disturbed parental attitudes and behaviour are high than when environmental hazards alone are high.

Table 25 The interaction of fit manifestation, environment and parental attitudes, and their association with behaviour disorder in 118 epileptic children

Total no. of children	*118*							
Adverse parental attitudes	*Low, 58*				*High (P), 60*			
Adverse environment	*Low, 38*		*High (E), 20*		*Low, 23*		*High (E), 37*	
Fits (Minor + motor involvement/other)	*Other* 21	*Minor (F)* 17	*Other* 8	*Minor (F)* 12	*Other* 11	*Minor (F)* 12	*Other* 15	*Minor (F)* 22
Normal	16	7	3	1	3	1	2	2
Anxious	4	5	4	2	3	0	5	5
Aggressive	0	1	0	4	3	8	4	10
Mixed	1	4	1	5	2	3	4	5
Total behaviour disorder scores:								
Low	17	10	7	6	6	5	6	6
High	4	7	1	6	5	7	9	16
% High	18·1	41·2	12·5	50·0	45·4	58·33	60·0	72·7
Combinations	*O*	*F*	*E*	*EF*	*P*	*PF*	*PE*	*PEF*

2 There will be a higher incidence of behaviour disorder in those cases with two constraints on behaviour (e.g.) fit manifestation and adverse environment) than in those cases in which there is only one constraint (e.g. fit manifestation); the highest incidence of behaviour disorder will be in those cases in which all three constraints on behaviour are present.

The interaction table for the testing of these hypotheses is presented in Table 25.

Hypothesis 1: Does the interaction of adverse parental attitudes and poor environment produce a higher incidence of behaviour disorder than in those cases in which only environmental hazards are high? In making this comparison, the occurrence of fit forms need not be considered, since the occurrence of minor fits with motor involvement shows a random pattern when compared both with high and low environmental hazards and with high and low parental scores.

In 20 cases in which environment alone is high, seven cases have a 'high' behaviour disorder (i.e. total behaviour disorder score, 14 or more). In the 37 cases in which both environmental hazards and parental scores are high, 25 have a 'high' behaviour disorder score.[1] This difference is significant at the 2 per cent level ($\chi^2=5{\cdot}59$, 1 d.f.) It is concluded that the hypothesis is sustained: the interaction of adverse parental attitudes with poor environment does significantly add to the risk of becoming a behaviour disorder.

Hypothesis 2a: Is there a higher incidence of behaviour disorder when there are two constraints on behaviour rather than one, and when there are three constraints on behaviour rather than two?

In every case this prediction is correct. The yield in terms of adverse behaviour is higher in *EF* than in *E* or *F;* higher in *PF* than in *P* or *F;* higher in *PE* than in *P* or *E;* and higher in *PEF* than in *EF*, *PF*, or *PE*. A more precise test of this hypothesis is given in Table 26.

Hypothesis 2b: Does the addition of high environmental hazards, high adverse parental behaviour scores, and minor fits with motor involvement significantly increase the risk of cases showing a high behaviour disorder score?

The influence of parental factors has been examined by comparing the cells in which *P* is not a constraint (*O*, *F*, *E*, *EF*) with those in which it is (*P*, *PF*, *PE*, *PEF*). This comparison of not *P*/*P* gives the incidence of high behaviour disorder of 18/58 (for not *P*) and 37/60 (for *P*). This difference is highly significant, at the 0·001 per cent level ($\chi^2=11{\cdot}12$, 1 d.f.).

The influence of environmental factors has been examined by comparing the cells in which *E* is not a constraint (*O*, *F*, *P*, *PF*) with

[1] These figures are derived from the comparison of *E* + *EF*.
Cf. *PE* + *PEF* in Table 25.

Table 26 Comparison of psychiatric groups according to three constraints on behaviour in 118 epileptic children

Number of constraints	*Normal*		*Anxious*		*Aggressive*		*Mixed*		*Low total scorers*		*High total scorers*	
	n	*cum. p.*	*n*	*cum. p.*	*n*	*cum. p.*	*n*	*cum. p.*	*n*	*cum. p.*	*n*	*cum. p.*
0 (0)	16	0·46	4	0·14	0	—	1	0·04	17	0·27	4	0·07
1 (*F*+*E*+*P*)	13	0·83	12	0·57	4	0·13	7	0·32	23	0·63	13	0·31
2 (*EF*+*PF*+*PE*)	4	0·94	7	0·82	16	0·67	12	0·8	17	0·9	22	0·71
3 (*EPF*)	2	1·0	5	1·0	10	1·0	5	1·0	6	1·0	16	1·0
Totals	35		28		30		25		63		55	

Note: Data derived from the interaction cells in Table 25.

Significance: Kolmogorov-Smirnov one-tailed test:

Comparison	*Chi-squared* (*2 d.f.*)	*Probability Level*
Normal-anxious	6·32	Less than 0·05, greater than 0·02
Normal-aggressive	31·65	Less than 0·001
Normal-mixed	15·16	Less than 0·001
Low scorers-high scorers	12·02	Less than 0·005, greater than 0·001

those in which it is (*E*, *EF*, *PE*, *PEF*). The comparison of not *E*/*E* gives the incidence of high behaviour disorder of 23/61 (for not *E*) and 32/57 (for *E*). This difference is significant at the 5 per cent level ($\chi^2=4{\cdot}02$, 1 d.f.).

The influence of minor fits with motor involvement has been examined by comparing the cells in which F is not a constraint (*O*, *E*, *P*, *PE*) with those in which it is (*F*, *EF*, *PF*, *PEF*). The comparison of not *F*/*F* gives the incidence of high behaviour disorder of 19/55 (for not *F*) and 36/63 (for *F*). This difference is significant at the 2 per cent level ($\chi^2=6{\cdot}02$, 1 d.f.).

It is concluded that hypothesis 2*b* is sustained: when high environmental hazards, or when high parental score, or when the existence of minor fits with motor involvement are added to the existence of the other possible combinations of constraints, the yield in terms of high adverse behaviour scores is significantly increased. The lowest adverse behavioural yield is in those cases in which none of these factors is a constraint; the highest yield is in those cases in which all three factors are present. These data suggest that the higher the number of adverse constraints on behaviour that exist, the more likely the child is to display a behaviour disorder.

The interaction of further variables associated with behaviour disorder will be examined in a subsequent chapter (pp. 254–64).

Addendum: an independent test of the reliability of the parental ratings

Since the above work was carried out, an independent test of the reliability of the judgments of attitudes and behaviour of the parents of the epileptic children has become available. Data from a questionnaire to the child's teacher are available in 81 cases. (In the remaining cases the child had left school, or the school did not complete the questionnaire or the relevant sections of it, or the parents refused permission for the school to be contacted.) One of the questions asked teachers to give a descriptive account of the parents' attitude and behaviour in relation to the school and to the child. These accounts were coded by a clinical psychologist into three categories, 'positive' (code 1), 'neutral' (code 2) and 'negative' (code 3). This psychologist had no knowledge of the ratings made by the writer, of the child's behaviour, and of the behaviour and attitudes of the parent.

The median test has been applied to the two judgments about parental attitudes (Table 27). There is reasonable agreement between the two ratings, significant at the 2 per cent level. This level of agreement is encouraging, considering the fact that the information given by teachers refers to different situations (i.e. events involving the school) and is based on a less detailed and systematic observation than that used in the ratings of parental attitude and behaviour made by the writer.

Table 27 A comparison of two types of measure of parental attitudes

Clinical rating	*Teacher's rating*		*Totals*
	Low	*High*	
Low	27	14	41
High	15	25	40
Totals	42	39	81

Note: 'Low' categories in both ratings indicate a score equal to or below the median score for the rating; in both cases 'high' is in the direction of adverse parental attitudes.
Significance: Median test:
X^2 (1 d.f.) = 6·52
P less than 0·02, greater than 0·01

Conclusions

1 The measurement of parental attitudes and behaviour, and of the quality of family interactions, is one of the most difficult areas of measurement of social science. The history of studies of the influence of the family in behaviour disorder in epileptic children illustrates this problem. However, recent work on the measurement of family activities, relationships and attitudes by the method of detailed and systematic discussive questioning of parents has shown promising results.
2 A method for quantifying the evaluations of parental behaviour and attitudes in epilepsy by a team of clinical workers has been developed. This involves the recording of a detailed and systematic case history by a psychiatric social worker; from this history a schedule of 18 items of disturbed parental behaviour and attitudes towards the epileptic child has been recorded. This procedure has good inter-rater reliability.
3 The total disturbed parental behaviour and attitude scores obtained discriminate strongly between normal and disturbed epileptic children. Disturbed parental attitudes and behaviour are particularly marked for aggressive children. The parents of the anxious children, however, more closely resemble those of the normal children, rather than those of the aggressive children. The parents of

the mixed children are more like those of the aggressive children, than the normal or anxious children.

4 The possibility has been considered that the high scores for disturbed parental attitudes and behaviour which the parents of the disturbed children obtain is an artefact of the measurement situation, in which children with behaviour disorder are automatically assigned a high parental score. The evidence, however, does not support this view, since the patterning of the parental attitudes does not show the consistently high parental score for disturbed children that one would expect if the scores were an artefact of the measurement situation. In addition, a substantial number of children with minor fits with motor involvement are disturbed; but the parental attitude scores in these cases have a distribution which is no different from that in the whole series. The random patterning of parental scores in these cases also suggest that the parental attitudes and behaviour are not themselves caused by disturbed behaviour in the child.

5 There is a significant association between disturbed parental attitudes and behaviour and a high number of environmental hazards. However, in a substantial number of cases environmental hazards are low, and parental attitudes scores are high, so that high environmental hazard scores cannot adequately predict a high parental score. In fact, the association of parental attitudes with disturbed behaviour is much stronger than that of a disturbed environment.

6 The independence of parental attitudes and behaviour, adverse environment, and minor fits with motor involvement as constraints upon the behaviour of the epileptic child has been demonstrated by putting the data in an interaction table. It has been shown that when two constraints are combined, the adverse behavioural yield is higher than in those cases where there is only one constraint. The highest yield of all is in those cases where all three constraints are present.

7 The evidence seems to suggest that adverse parental behaviour and attitudes may *cause* disturbed behaviour in the epileptic child. It seems possible, too, that when there are a high number of hazards in the environment (poverty, overcrowding, marital difficulties, etc.) the parents of the epileptic child are proportionately more likely to display disturbed attitudes and behaviour than if there were no environmental hazards.

23 The epileptic child and the school

The following section reviews the literature on the relationships between intellect and educational retardation and other factors in the life of the epileptic child, including psychiatric disturbance. In the course of this review, some of the literature on the connections of psychiatric disturbance and intelligence and retardation[1] in non-epileptic children will be considered, and the relevance of these studies for epilepsy discussed.

Much has been written about epilepsy by clinicians, for clinicians. There do not appear to be any post-war articles in English *educational* journals about the educational and psychological needs and dispositions of the epileptic child. There do not seem to be any books on the education of the epileptic child. The shelves of the Institute of Education library of the English University[2] contain books about the education of deaf and partially deaf children, blind and partially blind children, children with cerebral palsy, and brain-injured children. Three books have appeared which discuss the education of the brain-injured child—Strauss and Lehtinen (1947), Strauss and Kephart (1955), and Cruickshank (1966). All are American. None of them considers the problems of the epileptic child, and in two of these works the term 'epilepsy' nowhere occurs. This omission is surprising, in view of the fact that epilepsy is an outcome of a not inconsiderable proportion of children with brain injury.[3]

[1] The term 'retardation' is used here to indicate the gap between the child's mental age, as revealed by standardized tests of intelligence, and the child's attainment age, as revealed by standardization tests of attainment in reading, spelling or arithmetic.
[2] This generalization is based on an inspection of the catalogues of the Institutes and Departments of Education of the Universities of London, Exeter and Bristol.
[3] Cf. the small attention paid to the education of epileptic children in the British literature on education and handicap reported by Pritchard (1963).

Intellectual factors and behaviour disorder in epileptic children

A detailed 'Review of the Literature on the Relationship of Epilepsy and Intelligence in School children' has been made by Keating (1960). In view of the comprehensiveness of this review, only studies appearing after the period Keating considered (before 1959), and papers not mentioned by him, or of special theoretical importance, will be discussed here.

The main conclusions from Keating's review were:

1 From such studies as have been made we get a very indefinite picture of the level of intelligence of epileptics and its relation to epilepsy.

2 Whilst there is little evidence to show that epileptics *per se* have a lower degree of intelligence than non-epileptics, certain groups of epileptics—notably institutionalized cases—reveal mental shortcomings and in some cases progressive deterioration ending in extreme dementia. The nature and aetiology of these cases invites research.

3 Largely owing to the extreme seizure-tolerance variation shown by difficult individuals, there is as yet insufficient evidence to show to what extent and in what manner the incidence of epilepsy is responsible for mental deterioration, though it would appear that convulsions, especially if frequent, severe and of long standing do in fact cause actual cell damage in the C.N.S. and in the brain.

4 Although it may be accepted that drowsiness and apathy induced by most anticonvulsant drugs disappears on reduction or withdrawal, it is obvious that intensive temporary effects are produced during the often prolonged periods of medication.

5 There is as yet no recognizable connection between the EEG pattern of the normal or epileptic subject and any measure of mental capacity.

There is a further tendency in the literature (noted in the earlier review of the literature on behaviour disorder in epilepsy) to ascribe lower intelligence to aggressive epileptic children, lower intelligence to temporal lobe cases, and higher intelligence to *petit mal*, and to anxious cases. These findings, however, have not been made with any consistency. The paucity of valid findings in this area was noted by Halstead (1957) in a review of the literature on the 'ability and behaviour of epileptic children'.

General intelligence in epileptics

Vislie and Henriksen (1958), in a study of 142 adolescent and adult epileptics, found a mean I.Q. (Raven's matrices) of 96. There was a non-significant tendency for cases with lower intelligence to have had an onset before the age of nine years, and the cases with higher intelligence to have an onset after this age.

Chaundry and Pond (1961) compared 28 epileptic children who showed intellectual deterioration (more than 20 I.Q. points in three years) with 28 epileptic children with a similar incidence of brain damage, who did not show any such deterioration. No difference was found between the two groups with respect to site and extent of brain damage, age at brain damage, age at onset of epilepsy, amount and duration of anticonvulsants, and associated emotional and behavioural problems. However, significant differences were found between the two groups with respect to the number of seizures, the poorer response to medication, and the more generalized abnormalities, and focal signs, on the EEG. The authors draw attention to cases in which the child's intelligence deteriorates, and then improves, returning more or less to its original level. This latter finding indicates that other factors besides tissue damage (e.g. disturbed EEG) may be responsible for the deterioration.

Keith (1963) found that in a series of 296 epileptic children a greater number were 'retarded' than 'dull-normal' or 'average' on the Stanford-Binet test of intelligence. There was a clear relationship between low intelligence and an early age of onset of epilepsy. In addition, 73 per cent of children in whom epilepsy was symptomatic of organic brain damage showed low intelligence, compared with 22·2 per cent of those in whom the aetiology was idiopathic (i.e. unknown). These findings suggest a link between the three factors of brain damage, early onset of epilepsy and lower intelligence.

Gudmundsson (1966), in a study of 987 epileptics of all ages in the general population of Iceland, found the following incidences of 'normal intelligence':

Category	*% with normal intelligence*
Petit mal	90·0
Grand mal	75·5
Petit mal + grand mal	72·0
Grand mal + focal	50·0
Focal motor + sensory	65·0
Psychomotor	78·0
Aetiology unknown	74·8
Aetiology doubtful (probably organic)	63·4
Aetiology known (organic)	51·5

The cases in which an aetiology of organic brain damage was known had an earlier age of onset of epilepsy and a higher proportion of cases with disturbed behaviour.

Ounsted *et al.* (1966), in a study of 100 children with temporal lobe epilepsy, found that the average I.Q. was only slightly below average. However, there was a relationship between the frequency of temporal lobe attacks and lower intelligence, and there was a significant relationship between 'acute cerebral insult' or *status epilepticus* occurring early in the child's life and lower intelligence. The authors could not show that anticonvulsant drugs had any effect on learning or intellect in the epileptic children.

Studies in particular aspects of cognitive functioning in epilepsy

Bradley (1947) and 1951) reported that epileptic children were liable to display a specific syndrome involving (1) erratic variability in mood or behaviour, (2) hypermotility, (3) irritability, (4) short and vacillating attention span, and (5) a rather selective difficulty in mathematics as a school subject. This last item does not appear to have been studied by any subsequent writers on epilepsy.

Davies-Eysenck (1952) studied 161 children and young adults attending the National Hospital. The average IQ on the progressive matrices test was 94, which was significantly below a normal population score. Compared with controls, the epileptic children took a significantly longer time to complete the matrices test.

Milner (1954) reviewed 111 studies dealing with the intellectual functions of the temporal lobe. He concluded that temporal lobe damage (which might, but by no means always, be accompanied by epilepsy) caused intellectual changes. In the monkey bilateral removal of the temporal lobes severely hampered visual learning and retention; in man, too, temporal damage or lobectomy curbs the understanding of complex pictorial material. There appears to be a 'focus' on the ventral surface of the temporal lobe. If this is damaged, visual defects of the type described above occur. There is some evidence that epileptic fits may affect this visual area.

Parsons and Kemp (1960) studied 46 adult male epileptics, matched for age, duration of epilepsy, and psychological state. Psychomotor epileptics had a higher IQ than epileptics with generalized abnormalities on the EEG the latter having performance scores significantly lower than verbal, a deficit not found with the psychomotor cases.

Matthews and Kløve (1967) compared patients with psychomotor fits with other kinds of epileptics on a battery of tests, the groups being matched for age and previous education and age at brain damage. All groups (major motor and mixed seizure of known and unknown aetiology and psychomotor fits of known origin) *except* the psychomotor cases of unknown origin showed a significant impairment on the tests when compared with matched control subjects without epilepsy. The psychomotor cases of unknown aetiology performed significantly better than the major motor cases of unknown aetiology.

Beck (1959) compared sixty 'convulsive organic' children with seventy-one 'non-convulsive organic' children. The first group showed fewer W.I.S.C. gains on retest and more variability on sub-tests. The second group showed more unrecognizable Bender *Gestalt* figures.

Nuffield (1961) studied the intelligence of 288 cases of epilepsy seen at the Maudsley Hospital. The mean IQ was 89, a figure similar to the mean of 91 in 100 child psychiatric referrals without epilepsy. Nuffield found a *slight* relationship between aggression and lower intelligence. Neurosis and intelligence were not associated. Rutter (1964) studied the intelligence according to psychiatric diagnosis of 306 children seen at the Maudsley Hospital, including an unstated number of epileptic children. No significant variation in intelligence was found when the psychiatric diagnostic groups (neurotic behaviour disorder, neurotic illness, conduct behaviour disorder, and mixed behaviour disorder) were compared by intelligence. The intelligence distribution of the disturbed children was significantly lower than the standard normal distribution; however, this difference was thought to be because of the policy of the referring agencies, rather than a difference connected with the psychiatric disorder itself.

Milstein and Stevens (1961), who studied nine adolescent and adult epileptics, found that a diffuse, synchronous spike-and-wave and slow wave EEG was apparently associated with learning handicap, although the small numbers in this study did not make the relationship entirely clear.

Hutt *et al.* (1963) studied four epileptic children with unexplained learning difficulties. They found that stimulation with a flickering light systematically caused paroxysmal EEG discharges, and that in *two* subjects this stimulation significantly affected the memory for the recall of digits. The author concluded: 'These findings confirm previous observations indicating that short-retrograde amnesia may be observed in association with *petit mal* seizures in children'.

Jus and Jus (1963) also reported that retrograde amnesia was associated with *petit mal* fits.

Tizard and Margerison (1963) studied 3 per second spike-and-wave activity (the *petit mal* EEG pattern) in two epileptic patients. They found that alertness, including response time, increased as the spike and wave activity (not necessarily involving a fit) diminished. During these discharges, both patients were slower and made more mistakes.

Kimura (1964) investigated variations in the time taken to put a disordered series of letters into a required pattern in 89 epileptics with a diagnosis either of centrencephalic (3 per second spike-and-wave epilepsy) or of focal epilepsy. The mean ordering time was significantly longer for the 23 centrencephalic subjects, compared with the subjects with focal epilepsy. Some of the centrencephalic subjects had motor movements secondary to the *petit mal* seizures. The ordering time of these subjects resembled those of the focal group, and was significantly different from the group with *petit mal* seizures alone.

Tucker and Forster (1950) described a case in which *petit mal* occurred in *status* (another attack occurring before recovery from the previous one was complete, proceeding to a series of such attacks). This case was mis-diagnosed as a psychic state, in which the subject's inability to concentrate in school was remarked upon.

Williams (1963) wrote of the epileptic child:

> In his work his efficiency may be lowered, particularly through the occurrence of *petit mal*, and it must be remembered that even two absences may prevent the child from maintaining the the understanding of the theme of a lecturer, as we all know to our cost when our minds wander.

Davidoff and Johnson (1964) investigated 36 patients with epilepsy in which the patient was not known to be otherwise neurologically abnormal (i.e. organic factors were not suspected). All subjects had an EEG with clearly definable bursts of bilateral, synchronous waves which disappeared quickly, with essentially normal activity in between the bursts. Nineteen of the subjects had *grand mal* epilepsy, and 8 *petit mal*. No relation could be found between performance on a battery of tests and the particular kind of EEG activity, there being a wide variety of idiosyncratic responses. However, discharges of long duration and discharges clearly of a 'clinical' type were significantly more likely to be associated with a depression of concentration and learning ability than short or 'sub-clinical' bursts.

Grissell *et al.* (1964) found that in six epileptic patients there was a consistent lengthening in auditory reaction time associated with paroxysmal EEG activity.

Guey *et al.* (1967) studied 25 children with *petit mal* epilepsy who had been treated with the anticonvulsant drug ethosuximide ('Zarontin'). W.I.S.C. testing before and after the administration of the drug showed a significant decline in test results. In 60 per cent of the cases there was also a lowered score on Bender's visual retention test. The authors suggest that this decline in performance may be due to the effects of the drug.

Cognitive functioning and brain damage and the hyperkinetic syndrome

A common accompaniment of brain damage in children is impairment of intellect. Kushlick (1964), reviewing literature on the causes of mental deficiency suggests that pathological changes in the brain account for about 40 per cent of cases of mental deficiency.

McFie (1961) showed how, in 40 children admitted to the National Hospital with cerebral lesions beginning after the age of one, these lesions affected intellect. The greatest impairment seemed to be in children with parietal lobe tumours (mean IQ 77·8) and the least in children with temporal lobe tumours (mean IQ 90·1).

The largest bulk of literature in this field refers to the cognitive effects of the hyperactive, hyperkinetic, or minimal brain damage syndrome.

Bradley and Bowen (1941) described the hyperkinetic children as having a short span of attention and an erratic school performance which accompanied their impulsive, explosive behaviour. This syndrome, the authors suggested, apparently disappeared with the maturation of the C.N.S. Similar observations about the learning and school difficulties for the epileptic child have been made by Bradley (1951) in a paper indicated above.

Ounsted and Smith (1955) reported the interesting finding that in children with minimal brain damage due to tuberculosis meningitis, and in whom basic intelligence was unimpaired, the increased energy and drive which the children seemed to have was accompanied by over-achievement. However, in about 20 per cent of cases, children surviving tuberculosis meningitis had gross brain damage with idiocy or low IQ and convulsions.

Ingram (1956), reporting on the overactive syndrome in 25 brain-damaged children (13 of whom were epileptic) found that the overall intelligence in these cases was well below average. All cases had histories suggestive of brain injury.

Ounsted (1955) described 70 epileptic children who were hyperkinetic. The cases displayed the 'common brain-injured features' of distractability, short span of attention, and wide scatter on the IQ sub-tests. The range of intelligence was from idiotic to high normal, so that low intelliegnce cannot be said to be *sine qua non* of hyperactivity in epileptic children. However, in a later study of 100 children with temporal lobe epilepsy (Ounsted *et al.*, 1966) it was found that the 26 hyperkinetic cases had a significantly lower IQ than the non-hyperkinetic cases. In fact, only two of the hyperkinetic cases had an IQ above the median score (90) for the series. In 22 of the 26 hyperkinetic cases the behaviour of the children became intolerable to the teachers in normal school classes, from which the children were consequently excluded.

Hutt and Hutt (1964) studied 16 brain-damaged, hyperkinetic children, 14 of whom had epilepsy, compared with non-hyperkinetic controls. On a battery of learning tests the hyperkinetic children had a much quicker learning process, with less variability in learning time than non-hyperkinetic but brain-damaged, epileptic controls˙ These latter controls themselves learned more quickly and efficiently on the tests than normal subjects. The hyperkinetic children, suggest the authors, plunge over-readily into the problem they are faced with in a manner which likens them to the extreme extravert, whose test performance they resemble.

Generalizing from this study and that of Ounsted and Smith (1955) hyperactive children might be expected to do well in some learning situations, despite (or perhaps because of) their short attention-span, distractability and readiness to attack a new problem.

The study by Stevens *et al.* (1967) of 26 children with minimal brain damage and matched controls found that hyperactive children had lower W.I.S.C. scores on arithmetic and number tests. They also found that the minimal brain-damaged children were slower to respond and less able to follow verbal instructions.

Pond (1963) commenting on the finding of a number of authors that hyperkinesis disappears as the patient matures, suggested that epileptics who have been hyperkinetic in childhood may become apathetic in later life, with a withdrawal of interest in motivation as a basic personality pattern. Animal evidence is cited of rhinencephalic lesions causing such a withdrawal of motivation.

However, Levy (1966) has reported the syndrome of hyperactivity occurring in adolescent children.[1]

Intelligence, learning and behaviour disorder in non-epileptic children

The epileptic child is viewed, from a conceptual point of view, as a *child* who has *epilepsy*, and who is sometimes *brain-damaged.* It is for this reason that the literature on psychiatric disturbance apart from brain damage and disorders of learning and intellect is taken into consideration. What have been the trends in the literature about the relationship of psychiatric disturbance in non-epileptic, non-brain-damaged children to intellect and learning?

An interesting controversy was raised by Davis and Kent (1955) and Lynn (1955), who reported, in apparently contradictory studies, firstly, that anxiety in children was not associated with learning disorder (Davis and Kent), and, secondly, that it was (Lynn). Lynn showed that children who scored highly on a questionnaire about worries and fears also had a higher reading attainment than their verbal mental age would lead one to expect. This apparent contradiction was solved by Castaneda (1956), who showed that an intervening variable was the level of task difficulty. On the less difficult tasks the highly anxious children did better than those without

[1] Over half of the 25 hyperactive children in the present series (*vide supra*, p. 182) were aged 12 or over.

anxiety. But at the highest level of difficulty they did *less* well than those children without anxiety. This finding suggests that the anxious child has high motivation to succeed, and may apply himself with great assiduity to learning tasks; but at the higher levels of difficulty the anxiety which motivates the child also interferes with his performance.

Later writers have suggested an association between anxious or neurotic pictures in children and above average intelligence. Davidson *et al.* (1957) found that children with a linear body build did better on verbal intelligence tests and showed more anxiety, emotional unrest, terrors, etc., than the children with a high amount of muscle and bone, who tended to be low on anxiety symptoms and do less well on the verbal tests.

Burns (1959) found that a high proportion of grammar school children referred to a child guidance clinic displayed neurotic symptoms. Eysenck (1960) in a factor analysis of the symptoms and attributes of children referred to a child guidance clinic found that being 'intelligent' correlated with a cluster of psychoneurotic symptoms, no such correlation appearing with the cluster of aggressive symptoms. Eysenck and Rachman (1965) have suggested that these two basic clusters of symptoms arise because of the intervening variable of the previous personality—introverted or extraverted—of the child, so that in the face of stress the introverted children may show anxious, neurotic symptoms and the extraverted children aggressive, outgoing symptoms. This finding is in keeping with that of Davidson *et al.*, outlined above (p. 94), since Eysenck has also shown (*vide supra*, p. 95) that a lean body build is associated with introversion, and a muscular one with extraversion.

It is interesting to compare these findings with those of writers on the hyperactive child, which Hutt and Hutt (*vide supra*, p. 87) have conceptualized as an extreme extravert. The hyperactive child in some studies appears to have gained from his 'aggressive' attack on learning problems, but on other occasions is handicapped by inappropriately aggressive behaviour.

Nicholls (1962) reviewed research on the causes of retarded reading, and noted the following causes: (1) Ocular abnormalities in the child. (2) Auditory abnormalities. (3) Neurological abnormalities, especially in the pariotemporal area. (4) Emotional factors, e.g. parental discord. (5) Poor teaching methods. The fourth kind of factor was identified by Tuckman (1963) in a study of children with retarded reading ability.

Much of the earlier literature on intelligence and childhood psychiatric disorder has been reviewed by Rutter (1964), who shows that a number of contradictory findings have been presented: high intelligence in some studies has been associated with over-inhibited behaviour, and low intelligence with delinquency, but that in other studies these relationships did not emerge. He criticizes these studies for their frequent lack of rigour and the failure to consider referral policies as artefacts in determinants of intellectual level in the children studied. Rutter studied the intelligence of 306 children with psychiatric disorder (a study briefly referred to above, since this number contained an unstated number of epileptic children). He was unable to show any significant variation in the intelligence of the psychiatric diagnostic groups within this population.

It should be noted that Rutter did not test the difference of the mean IQ for the different diagnostic groups (he does not, in fact, give this figure in his paper) and only examines the total *distribution* of intelligence over all the diagnostic groups by the χ^2 test. However, it is possible to calculate the means for the diagnostic groups from the data given by Rutter. The results of this exercise are presented in Table 28. It will be seen that there is in fact a significant difference between the intelligence of the children with conduct disorders and those with neurotic illness (rather than neurotic behaviour disorder).

Table 28 Mean IQ in child psychiatric disorder

IQ	*Conduct behaviour disorder*	*Neurotic behaviour disorder*	*Neurotic illness*	*Mixed behaviour disorder*
Mean	95·8	96·3	102·6	96·43
S.D.	15·9	17·75	16·2	14·0
N.	107	113	37	49

Data derived from Rutter (1964).

Significant Difference: Conduct behaviour disorder of neurotic illness, $T = 2{\cdot}23$, P less than 0·05, greater than 0·02. (The normality of the two distributions was established by G. Fisher's test, 1965.)

Rutter's criteria for 'neurotic behaviour disorder' were: 'Symptoms . . . mainly in the fields of primary or secondary habit disorder, motor disorder, somatic disorder of functional origin, psychic disorder, or allergic disorder.' The 'conduct behaviour disorder' symptoms were 'predominantly those of socially disapproved conduct (including delinquency)'. Cases in which neither of these two pictures predominated over the other were termed 'mixed behaviour disorder'. Syndromes approximating to those found in adults (anxiety state, obsessional neurosis, hysteria, depressive illness, etc.) were classified separately as 'neurotic illness'.

Since Rutter's distinction between 'conduct behaviour disorder' and 'neurotic illness' approximates to the categories in the present study of 'aggressive' and 'anxious', it will be of interest to see if the factor of intelligence differentiates these categories in the present study.

Neuman and Krug (1964) report their impressions that it is in arithmetic rather than reading that the 'emotionally disabled child' most frequently fails at school. They suggest that insecure children may resent the absoluteness of their mistakes in this subject.

Wolf (1965) studied 80 neurotic children, using a normal sibling as control for each child. By means of longitudinal study, the pairs were age-matched. Standardized tests of reading could not discriminate between the subjects and controls, leading Wolf to conclude that reading retardation was not a deficiency displayed by neurotic children.

Schwebel (1966) found a correlation between impulsiveness and lower intelligence in children, a finding which may suggest a link between the apparent association of lower intelligence, aggressiveness and extraversion.

Maguire (1966), in a study of 335 children of normal intelligence, found that subjects showing high anxiety (according to the Castaneda questionnaire) did better than other subjects on a rote learning test (memorizing Latin words and their meanings).

Rushton (1966) found that extraversion had a positive relationship with verbal reasoning in a sample of English children from 14 schools, and anxiety a negative relation. (Anxiety and extraversion were measured by Cattell's children's personality questionnaire.) Rushton found that the most academically successful child was the stable extravert. These results do not necessarily contradict those which have found a possible link between aggression, extraversion and lower intelligence, and between introversion, anxiety and higher intelligence, since the higher attainment in Rushton's study was achieved by *normal* subjects. These results do show, however, how complex and multi-dimensional the problem of relating emotional disorder to intelligence and learning is.

Child (1966) compared extraversion-introversion (from the J.M.P.I.) and social class in 395 subjects in four schools. It was found that children who achieved rapid 'promotion' between forms and streams because of their examination performance were significantly more introverted and of higher social status than the rest of the sample. Since there is a link between high social status and higher intelligence (Rutter, 1964), these results also tend to show a link between introversion and higher intelligence.

McLaughlin and Eysenck (1967) studied the relationship of extraversion and anxiety to the speed of learning lists of nonsense words. Two lists were used, one easy, the other difficult. The extraverts, as predicted, learned both lists faster than introverted subjects. A moderate level of anxiety was found to facilitate the learning of the easy list of words; however, when it came to the difficult list, subjects who were *low* on anxiety did best. These results confirm Casteneda's study (*vide supra*, p. 207) of the relation to task difficulty to the learning performance of anxious subjects. The findings with regard to extraverts tend to support the impression that subjects who attack a learning problem without any 'inner' reflection or anxiety about the task in hand may have an advantage in some kinds of learning situation. Frost (1968) has confirmed the complexity of the phenomenon under discussion, suggesting that there is a complex interrelationship of types of anxiety, types of achievement, and sex of subject.

Epilepsy, behaviour disorder and cognition handicap: discussion and conclusions

With regard to the connections of epilepsy and its correlates (EEG type, behaviour abnormality, aetiology, etc.) with intellectual factors the literature reviewed suggests the following conclusions:

1 Brain damage, which may also be accompanied by epilepsy, is an important cause of low intelligence in children.

2 Given this fact, it is not surprising that a number of studies have shown epileptic populations to have a lower intelligence than the normal population. However, the average intelligence of epileptic populations studied does not seem to be markedly below normal. Relationships have been found between lower intelligence, brain damage, early onset of epilepsy, fits occurring over a long period of time and resistant to control by drugs; which of these factors is primary and which is secondary is not clear. Brain damage has not in fact been implicated as a totally unequivocal cause of low intelligence. The fits themselves or the disturbed EEG which underlies them may be of equal or greater importance in retarding intellectual capacity.

3 One writer has suggested that epileptics may have a particular difficulty with mathematics as a school subject. No test of this hypothesis with a series of epileptic children seems to have been made.

4 Studies relating intellectual performance to abnormalities on the EEG have been in agreement in finding that periods of a clinically abnormal EEG are accompanied by a decreased capacity for concentration or speed of thought. Children with generalized abnormalities on the EEG seem most handicapped in this respect.

5 There is some evidence that damage to the temporal lobes can impair intellectual functioning—in particular, affecting visual learn-

ing and retention. Studies of temporal lobe epileptics, however, have been equivocal. Some studies (reviewed in an earlier section on temporal lobe epilepsy (pp. 53–70)) have associated this condition with low intelligence, but studies comparing psychomotor or temporal lobe cases with other kinds of epilepsy have not indicated particular incapacities in learning in epilepsy originating in the temporal lobes. In fact, the reverse has been the case in a number of recent studies.

6 The evidence on the connection of *petit mal* is, like that on temporal lobe epilepsy, equivocal with respect to intellectual functioning. Some studies have shown *petit mal* cases to have the highest IQ of all epileptics. But other studies of the effect of 3 per second spike-and-wave on the EEG (the *petit mal* pattern) have shown that this kind of discharge particularly handicaps learning, causing retrograde and anterograde amnesia. In addition, this kind of discharge seems to reduce alertness.

7 There is some evidence that anticonvulsants may have an adverse effect on learning behaviour and measured intelligence.

8 The evidence on the relationship of behaviour disorder and intellectual capacity in epileptics is equivocal. Some writers have found a relationship between aggression and low intelligence, but this finding has not been consistently made. In Nuffield's study, in which organic factors were shown to be important in epileptic behaviour disorder, there were no significant associations between diagnosis (aggressive or neurotic) and intellectual level, although a trend towards an association of lower intelligence and aggression was observed. Rutter's study of intelligence and childhood psychiatric disorder included an unstated number of epileptics; this study was unable to find any relationship between the distribution of intelligence and diagnosis. However, a re-analysis of this data in the present study suggests that children with conduct behaviour disorder have a significantly lower intelligence than children with neurotic illness.

9 The hyperactive syndrome, which is probably the result of minimal brain damage, occurs in about 10 per cent of epileptics. Hyperactive epileptics seem to have an IQ which is well below the mean for the normal population. Hyperactive children (both epileptic and non-epileptic) suffer from short attention-span in learning situations, high distractability, and show a high scatter on IQ subtests. Their over-active behaviour in the classroom may adversely affect the attitude of teachers and other children towards them, thus causing further barriers to effective learning. However, there is also some evidence that the extreme willingness of these children to attack new situations (a characteristic of their extreme extraversion) may be beneficial in some learning situations.

With regard to the recent literature on the relationship of psychiatric disturbance to intelligence and learning activity, it may be said, first of all, that the amount of literature on this interesting subject relevant for the present study seems rather small. The controversy surrounding the relationship of anxiety to learning activity seems to have been satisfactorily solved by the discovery of the importance of the intervening variable of task difficulty, so that anxiety is functional for learning performance only at lower levels of difficulty.

There appears to be little recent literature on the relationship of aggression to learning disorder in children. A number of studies, however, have related this kind of disorder to lower intelligence, while other studies have associated anxiety with higher intelligence. Rutter's study (1964) may be counted among these, despite the formal conclusions of the author.

Eysenck's work provides an interesting link between learning, personality, and psychiatric disturbance, since it seems that extraverted children under stress tend to become aggressive and introverted children to become anxious or neurotic. Extraverted children have some advantages in learning situations which require an immediate 'attack' on the situation, and in which pausing for reflection would be dysfunctional. The similarities with the hyperactive child whose extreme extraversion (Hutt and Hutt) has an organic origin are interesting. A recent study (Rushton, 1966) has suggested that the child who does best academically is the stable extravert.

However another recent study (Child, 1966) has suggested that introverted children (who may have strongly internalized parental values about striving and doing well at school) do better than other children. Here the factor of social class may be an intervening variable.

Retardation in reading has been related in one recent study (Tuckman, 1963) to emotional factors in the home; but another study (Wolf, 1965) could find no relationship between neurosis in children and reading disability. One impressionistic study has suggested that the relationship between arithmetic retardation and emotional disturbance is stronger than that between reading retardation and emotional disturbance. This hypothesis remains to be investigated.

The controversies which have arisen in this field are interesting. This is an obvious field for further research. Future studies will have to carefully separate out the factors to be studied: intellectual level (IQ); performance on particular sub-tests making up the IQ test and on related types of tests; retardation in English and arithmetic on tests with standardized norms, retardation being measured by the gap between the child's potential, as indicated by his IQ, and his achievement, as indicated by the attainment test (e.g. Vernon or Schonell); the existence of extraversion or introversion; the existence of carefully defined and measured behavioural abnormality; the existence of emotional discords in the home; an assessment of the school situation itself, and the attitude of peers (including sociometric status); social class.

Further possible constraints on intellectual, learning, and attainment capacity are organic factors, including epilepsy. For the epileptic we will need to know whether early brain damage by itself can be associated with low intelligence; whether early onset of fits (associated, perhaps, with brain damage) is the crucial variable; and the part played in this process by the frequency of fits. The influence on the kinds of brain damage, and the kinds of epileptic discharge in the EEG will also have to be elucidated. The actual relationship of I.Q. to psychiatric diagnosis and of retardation (as defined above) must be investigated.

The effect of the epileptic child on the school and of the school on the epileptic child

The influence of the school on the behaviour of the epileptic child as well as on the course of his epilepsy has been described by two early writers (Bridge, 1934; Cobb, 1940). Bridge showed how an emotionally disturbing situation, such as rejection by schoolmates, and in some cases by teachers, could make both the behaviour of the epileptic and the epilepsy itself worse. Cobb showed how placement in a special school in which the needs and behaviour of the epileptic child were understood reduced the number of fits as well as the child's anxiety about his fits.

Carter (1947) in a study of the attitudes of epileptic children toward their illness, described a group of children who expressed resentment at the fact that teachers prevented them from taking part in the activities of other children; some were even excluded from playing with other children because they might have fits.

Price (1950), in a study of 50 American children, described the improvement of behaviour which resulted when school authorities received counselling about the problems of the epileptic child. When the teacher provided a 'matter-of-fact' environment for the child having a fit, the children in the class accepted the fit in this way as well. This process '. . . has been most helpful in preventing anxiety, tensions, and fear of the seizures'.

The *Lancet*, in an annotation (1953), commented that:

> The doctor who has to do with epileptics soon discovers that ostracism is often responsible for character traits sometimes attributed to the disease. School teachers commonly show a surprising eagerness to eliminate affected children from

school, and even people with a medical training may show a disproportionate emotion when trying to persuade a mother to send her epileptic child to a colony or home.

Henderson (1953) studied a stratified random sample of 365 children in normal schools in England and Wales. According to teachers' descriptions, about 12 per cent of these children displayed serious emotional disturbance in school. It is of interest that only 9 per cent of the children actually had fits whilst at school. Teachers apparently find hyperkinesis and overactivity in the epileptic child (and presumably in other hyperkinetic children without epilepsy) most difficult to tolerate. Ounsted *et al.* (1966) describing 100 children with temporal lobe epilepsy, found that in every case where the child was hyperkinetic and also suffered from 'catastrophic rages' the child was excluded from normal schooling. The authors comment:

> The mythology surrounding epilepsy appears to have been the most potent factor in determining teachers' attitudes. Teachers would often tolerate bad behaviour of an anti-social type, but reject a child who had quite a small number of psychomotor seizures at school. This reaction was an important factor in the lives of many of our patients. It resulted in undue changes of school and of class which reinforced the insecurity that these children experienced, and hence, in a circular manner, reinforced their disorders of behaviour and perhaps also their propensity to seizures.

Some of the studies of interaction (described in an earlier section) illustrate this 'circular' process described by Ounsted and his colleagues. Patterson *et al.* (1965), for example, in a controlled situation, showed how the environment of a hyperactive child (without epilepsy) could be manipulated to provide reinforcement for *good* behaviour. In an uncontrolled situation, it is easy to imagine how reinforcement from the children's peers could provide reinforcement for disturbed behaviour.

Lacey (1966) has provided an interesting picture of this 'circular' process in a sociological case study of the interactions between teachers and children in a grammar school, in which the system of streaming served to justify the teacher's perceptions of the children placed in the bottom stream, since the fact of being placed in this stream disposed the child to act in a way which merely confirmed the teacher's original judgment. Lacey mentions the case of a child with epilepsy which was apparently aggravated by the anxiety of keeping up with a stream in which he was placed and worry about being down-graded.

Conclusions

It seems clear from these studies that an adverse school environment (teachers who reject the epileptic child or exclude him from the company or activities of other children, and a school peer group which rejects the epileptic child) can make both the behaviour and the fits of the child worse. There is some rather disturbing evidence that teachers react in a hostile or over-anxious way to children with epilepsy. It is evident, too, that the teacher can have much influence on the adjustment of the epileptic child by providing an environment in the classroom which is understanding and non-alarmist about his fits, and provides a structured situation which reinforces his good behaviour in the case of hyperactive, epileptic children.

The lack of any literature on the subject of epilepsy in British education textbooks and journals may be a factor which hampers the teacher's understanding of this illness.

Intellectual factors in the present series of epileptic children

The distribution of scores on the W.I.S.C. test for the epileptic children in the present series is given in Table 29.[1]

It will be seen that the mean IQ of the 116 epileptic children considered (scores not being available in two cases) was 99·85, which is very close to the mean for the normal population of 100. However, the intelligence scores are not distributed normally, there being more cases with low intelligence than would be expected, so that the curve for intelligence is skewed to the left.

Since upper social classes are over-represented in the present series, the mean IQ for the social class groups has been calculated (Table 30). The higher scores for social classes I and II and the lower scores for classes IV and V are in keeping with earlier work (e.g. Rutter, 1964), which has shown a relationship between social class and intelligence.

A *hypothetical* mean has been calculated (Table 30) for a population having a distribution of social classes similar to the population at large from the data given by the Registrar General for the 1961 Census. This correction does not appreciably reduce the IQ of this epileptic population, the mean IQ 'corrected' for social class distribution, being 98·71.

These data suggest that the present series—a population of epileptic children in the general community, but selected on the basis of

[1] In a small number of cases, a Stanford-Binet score was converted to its W.I.S.C. equivalent, using the formula given by Weider *et al.* (1951). The same procedure was carried out for the control subjects, where the I.Q. score was based on the Stanford-Binet rather than the W.I.S.C. test.

Table 29 The distribution of IQ scores in 116 epileptic children

IQ score	*Number*
Less than 50	2
50–9	4
60–9	7
70–9	8
80–9	13
90–9	19
100–9	22
110–19	20
120–9	14
130–9	7
Total	116

Distribution significantly different from normal at the 0·01 level by G. Fisher's test (1965).
Mean IQ 99·85.

attendance at a neurological hospital—has a mean IQ that is similar to that of the normal population. This mean, however, is not distributed normally.

IQ and psychiatric diagnosis

There has been some suggestion in earlier literature that aggressive behaviour in both epileptic and non-epileptic children has been associated with lower intelligence and anxious behaviour with higher intelligence. This finding has not, however, been made consistently,

Table 30 Social class and IQ in 116 epileptic children

Social class	*No. of epileptic children*	*Actual mean IQ*	*No. in social class groups in 116 children in the normal population*
I and II	30	104·8	21
III	67	99·3	61
IV and V	19	93·9	34

Mean IQ of 116 children with social class distribution as in the normal population for the catchment area and an average IQ score by social class as in the present epileptic population = 98·71.

Table 31 IQ scores and behavioural category in 116 epileptic children

IQ score	*Normal*		*Anxious*		*Aggressive*		*Mixed*		*Totals*
	n	*cum. p.*	*n*	*cum. p.*	*n*	*cum. p.*	*n*	*cum. p.*	
Less than 80	6	0·17	2	0·08	9	0·3	4	0·16	21
80–9	3	0·26	3	0·19	3	0·4	4	0·32	13
90–9	3	0·34	4	0·35	8	0·7	4	0·48	19
100–9	8	0·57	6	0·58	3	0·77	5	0·68	22
110–19	8	0·8	3	0·69	5	0·93	4	0·84	20
120 or more	7	1·0	8	1·0	2	1·0	4	1·0	21
Totals	35		26		30		25		116
Means (ungrouped data)	102·11		105·03		90·56		99·0		

Note: IQ data not available in two cases.
Significance: Kolmogorov-Smirnov one-tailed test:

Comparison	χ^2 *(2 d.f.)*	*Probability level*
Normal-anxious	0·01	Greater than 0·5
Normal-aggressive	8·37	Less than 0·02, greater than 0·01
Normal-mixed	1·68	Greater than 0·5
Anxious-aggressive	6·81	Less than 0·05, greater than 0·02

and Rutter's paper (1964) discussed above (p. 209), illustrates the controversy which surrounds this area.

The IQ scores of the 116 epileptic children are examined in Table 31 according to the distribution about the median of the whole series for each of the four behavioural categories.

The aggressive children have significantly more IQ scores in the lower categories than both the normal and the anxious children. The children in the mixed group occupy an intermediate position. The difference in mean IQ is particularly marked for the anxious children (mean, 105·03) and the aggressive children (mean, 90·56).

What factors underlie low intelligence in the epileptic children in the present series? The distribution of IQ scores according the likelihood of brain damage is given in Table 32. Surprisingly, the relationship between brain damage and low IQ fails to reach the 5 per cent level of significance. In the range below 80 there are markedly more cases with brain damage than without. However, in the upper ranges of intelligence, and especially in the range 120 plus, there are as many cases with brain damage as there are without. In the previous chapter it was noted that hyperactivity was significantly associated with low intelligence in this series of epileptic children. These data suggest that when brain damage is associated with low intelligence it is also associated with hyperkinesis, and this relationship in turn accounts for the association of low IQ with aggressive behaviour disorder.

The IQ distribution according to the existence or absence of minor fits with motor involvement (which in this series are good predictors of an aggressive or mixed behaviour disorder) is given in Table 33. There is no relationship between such fits and low intelligence, even though low intelligence itself is a good predictor of aggressive behaviour.

Table 32 Brain damage and IQ in 116 epileptic children

IQ score	*Brain damage unlikely*		*Brain damage likely*	
	n	*cum. p.*	*n*	*cum. p.*
Less than 80	4	0·07	17	0·27
80–9	6	0·18	7	0·39
90–9	9	0·35	10	0·55
100–9	14	0·61	8	0·68
110–19	11	0·81	9	0·82
120 or more	10	1·0	11	1·0
Totals	54		62	

Significance: Kolmogorov-Smirnov one-tailed test—X^2 (2 d.f.) = 4·71
P less than 0·1, greater than 0·05

The IQ distribution according to the time that has occurred since the first fit is given in Table 34. There is a positive association between the time that has elapsed since the first fit and low intelligence. Whether this was due to a trauma of the C.N.S. caused by fits when the child was young (since this is an age-homogeneous sample, there is a close relationship between early onset of fits and the time that has elapsed since their onset) or whether to the accumulated effect of the fits over the years is difficult to say. It seems unlikely that brain damage precedes both the early onset of fits and low intelligence, since there is only a slight relationship in the present series between brain damage and low intelligence.

The IQ distribution according to the E.E.G. categories is given in Table 35. The most marked difference is that between the 'generalized brain damage' category, which has the lowest IQ of all, and the 'temporal lobe focus' category, which has the highest IQ of all the groups. Since the temporal lobe group is itself a brain-damaged category, this explains why there is no relationship between brain damage as such and low IQ. This relationship only holds good for cases with damage to the brain *other* than in the temporal lobes.[1]

Table 33 Minor motor fits and IQ in 116 epileptic children

IQ score	*Other types of fits*		*Minor motor fits*	
	n	*cum. p.*	*n*	*cum. p.*
Less than 80	8	0·15	13	0·21
80–9	4	0·22	9	0·35
90–9	9	0·38	10	0·52
100–9	13	0·63	9	0·66
110–19	10	0·8	10	0·82
120 or more	10	1·0	11	1·0
Totals	54		62	

Significance: Kolmogorov-Smirnov one-tailed test:
X^2 (2 d.f.) = 2·01
P less than 0·5, greater than 0·3

The IQ distribution for the three diagnostic groups of non-epileptic children from a child guidance clinic used as controls for the epileptic children (*vide supra*, p. 152) is given in Table 36. Although the clinic children were matched for sex and age and social class group, as well

[1] It follows, and is the case in fact, that those cases with a temporal lobe focus who have low intelligence are the most likely of the temporal lobe cases to be hyperkinetic, since there is a relationship between hyperactivity and low intelligence (*vide supra* p. 182) and a random association with type of brain damage.

Table 34 Time since first fit and IQ of 116 epileptic children

IQ score	*Time equal to, or less than median (0–4 years)*		*Time greater than median (5+ years)*	
	n	*cum. p.*	*n*	*cum. p.*
Less than 80	6	0·1	15	0·27
80–9	4	0·16	9	0·44
90–9	11	0·34	8	0·58
100–9	11	0·52	11	0·78
110–19	16	0·79	4	0·85
120 or more	13	1·0	8	1·0
Totals	61		55	

Significance: Kolmogorov-Smirnov one-tailed test:
X^2 (2 d.f.) = 8·62
P less than 0·01, greater than 0·005

as diagnosis, IQ was not used as a matching factor, since it was assumed at the time of the matching, from Rutter's paper (1964), that IQ level was not connected with psychiatric disorder. It will be seen that the rank order of IQ level is the same as that for the epileptic children (1st, anxious children; 2nd, mixed; 3rd, aggressive) although the differences of the mean IQ between the diagnostic groups of clinic children are not as great as in the epileptic children, and are not significant. The fact that the clinic sample contains no brain-damaged children may account for the higher IQ of the clinic aggressive children when compared with the aggressive epileptic children.

It is interesting to note that the IQ level of the anxious and the aggressive clinic children is similar to the mean IQ for the 'conduct behaviour disorder' and 'neurotic behaviour disorder' groups reported by Rutter (1964). If the present sample had been the same size as Rutter's, and the mean IQ for the aggressive and the anxious groups remained the same, the result, like that in Rutter's study, would have been significant at the 5 per cent level.

Discussion

In the review of literature on intelligence and psychiatric disorder above it was noted that a number of workers had found a relationship between anxiety and high intelligence and aggression and lower intelligence, independently of brain damage. This relationship occurs in the present series of epileptic children. There is no relationship of

Table 35 EEG category and IQ in 114 epileptic children

IQ score	*Normal*		*Epileptic*		*Petit mal*		*Immature*		*Generalized brain damage*		*Temporal lobe focus*	
	n	*cum. p.*	*n*	*cum. p.*	*n*	*cum.p.*	*n*	*cum. p.*	*n*	*cum. p.*	*n*	*cum. p.*
Less than 80	4	0·13	0	0·0	1	0·09	2	0·33	11	0·37	2	0·08
80–9	3	0·23	1	0·08	2	0·27	0	0·33	4	0·5	2	0·16
90–9	6	0·43	2	0·25	1	0·36	0	0·33	8	0·77	2	0·24
100–9	5	0·6	4	0·58	5	0·82	1	0·5	2	0·83	5	0·44
110–19	6	0·8	2	0·75	1	0·9	2	0·83	1	0·87	8	0·76
120 or more	6	1·0	3	1·0	1	1·0	1	1·0	4	1·0	6	1·0
Totals	30		12		11		6		30		25	

Note: IQ data not available in two cases; EEG data not available in two cases.
Significance: The distribution of IQ scores for each EEG category has been tested against that for each other category. Only results attaining the 5 per cent level of significance or beyond are presented. (Kolmogorov-Smirnov one-tailed test.)

Comparison	χ^2 *(2 d.f.)*	*Probability Level*
Generalized B.D.; cf. Temporal lobe focus	15·2	Less than 0.001
Generalized B.D.; cf. Epileptic	9·13	Less than 0·02, greater than 0·01
Generalized B.D.; cf. Normal	6·65	Less than 0·05, greater than 0·02
Generalized B.D.; cf. *Petit mal*	6·11	Less than 0·05, greater than 0·02

Table 36 IQ and psychiatric diagnosis in 79 non-epileptic children

IQ score	*Anxious*		*Aggressive*		*Mixed*	
	n	*cum. p.*	*n*	*cum. p.*	*n*	*cum. p.*
Less than 80	4	0·14	5	0·18	3	0·13
80–9	4	0·28	6	0·39	4	0·3
90–9	6	0·5	5	0·57	7	0·61
100–9	6	0·71	8	0·86	5	0·83
110–19	4	0·86	1	0·89	2	0·91
120 or more	4	1·0	3	1·0	2	1·0
Totals	28		28		23	
Mean score (ungrouped data)	101·4		95·2		98·4	

Note: Data not available in four cases.

Significance: Kolmogorov-Smirnov one-tailed test: no difference between any of the groups reaches the 5 per cent level of significance.

intelligence with brain damage as such, although there is a relationship between lower intelligence and a certain type of brain damage (generalized brain damage, not involving the temporal lobes). However, no significant relationship exists (*vide supra*, pp. 179–80) between generalized brain damage and disturbed behaviour, although there is a significant, positive relationship between all types of brain damage combined and aggressive behaviour. Thus the relationship of lower intelligence and aggressive behaviour cannot be accounted for solely by the association of generalized brain damage and low intelligence, since the temporal lobe cases, who have in fact the highest IQ of all, also have a tendency to aggression.

The position is complex, but the evidence seems to suggest that two factors underlie the association of lower intelligence and disturbed behaviour: perhaps generalized brain damage, and perhaps the factor which tends to make children of lower intelligence over-represented in populations of non-brain-damaged, aggressive children.

It is important to note that there are *two* factors of an 'organic' nature—minor motor fits and lower intelligence—which are independent of one another, but both predicting aggressive behaviour in the children. It seems likely that higher aggression scores will occur in those cases who have both low intelligence and minor motor fits. Two other predictors of disturbed behaviour have been identified—disturbed parental attitudes and behaviour, and environmental hazards. All four factors are largely independent of one another. It seems probable that the highest yield of disturbed behaviour will be in those cases in which all four adverse factors combine—in the children with low intelligence, a history of minor motor fits, disturbed attitudes in the parents, and a high number of environmental hazards. This hypothesis will be tested in a subsequent chapter.

Reading and arithmetic age retardation

Reading retardation is defined as the negative discrepancy between the child's reading age, as measured by the Schonell Reading Test, and the Verbal Mental Age from the Wechsler Intelligence Scale for Children. The sub-tests making up the verbal scale are: vocabulary; comprehension; arithmetic; similarities; and digit span. Arithmetic retardation is defined as the negative discrepancy between the child's arithmetic age on the Schonell Arithmetic Test and the Verbal Mental Age on the W.I.S.C. (which includes sub-tests on arithmetical items).

The child's academic potential in reading and arithmetic can be taken to be the equivalent of his mental age from the IQ test (Kornrich, 1965). In some cases the child's attainment age may exceed his mental age, because of such factors as extra tuition in the subject or parental stimulation. In other cases the child may not be working up to his full potential in reading and arithmetic, because of such factors as poor teaching, absence from school, or emotional disorder. The exact relationship of emotional disorder to academic retardation is not entirely clear, as the literature reviewed above shows. No studies seem to have been carried out on this kind of retardation in epileptic children, apart from Bradley's early report (1951), that epileptic children experience 'a specific difficulty with maths as a school subject'. Bradley gave no figures relating to this difficulty, but suggested that it only occurred in some epileptic children.

In making the estimates of reading and arithmetic retardation for the present series of epileptic children, it should be pointed out that the figures presented in the following two tables are likely to underestimate the amount of retardation. This is because, first of all, the Schonell Reading Age has been standardized on a population with an age range of 5 to 15 years, so that norms for children older than 15 are not known. A majority of the epileptic children are aged between 12 and 14, and approximately half of these children have verbal IQs over 100, so that over a quarter of the children in the series have verbal mental ages *greater than* 15. For example, a 14-year-old child with a verbal mental age of 16 and a reading age at the test ceiling of 15 years cannot be said to be retarded on the evidence available, because the reading test norms do not extend to his actual verbal mental age; in this case the retardation is assumed to be zero, although in actual fact, if a test with 16-year-old norms were available, it *might* be shown that the child was 12 months retarded in reading ability.

The degree of underestimation of retardation is likely to be more marked in the case of arithmetic age, since the Schonell Test of Arithmetic has been standardized on a population aged 7 to 14½ years. It would be possible in this case for a 14-year-old boy with a verbal mental age of 17½ to be up to 3 years retarded in arithmetic, without this being indicated by comparing the maximum possible arithmetic age and the verbal mental age.

The results of comparing verbal mental age with arithmetic and reading ages on standardized tests, are given in Tables 37 and 38. Because the distributions of retardation for the various groups approximate to a normal distribution, the data have been analysed, using means, standard deviations and the *t*-test.

All groups considered have mean reading and arithmetic ages

Table 37 Reading age retardation in 107 epileptic children and controls

Category	*Mean retardation in months*	*Standard deviation*	*N*
Epileptic:			
Normal	− 4·8 months	12·0	33
Anxious	−15·8 months	12·2	24
Aggressive	−11·9 months	10·6	27
Mixed	−11·2 months	10·4	23
Non-epileptic controls:			
Anxious	−14·0 months	9·3	22
Aggressive	−16·4 months	10·2	24
Mixed	−15·1 months	8·9	20

Note: Data not available for eleven epileptic cases and for seventeen controls. The mean rates take into account both negative and positive discrepancies of Schonell Reading Age from W.I.S.C. Verbal Mental Age.

Significance (epileptic and control subjects compared by Sandler's adaption of the *t*-test for matched pairs). Only results exceeding the 5 per cent level are presented.

Comparison epileptic groups	*Value of t*	*Probability level*
Normal-anxious	3·91	Less than 0·002, greater than 0·001
Normal-aggressive	2·88	Less than 0·05, greater than 0·02
Normal-mixed	3·96	Less than 0·002, greater than 0·001
Epileptic cf. controls	No difference significant	

Table 38 Arithmetic age retardation in 99 epileptic children and controls

Category	*Mean retardation in months*	*Standard deviation*	*N*
Epileptic:			
Normal	−23·1 months	15·1	31
Anxious	− 8·0 months	13·9	23
Aggressive	−30·48 months	19·6	25
Mixed	−24.0 months	16·3	20
Non-epileptic controls:			
Anxious	−10·3 months	11·4	22
Aggressive	−18·0 months	12·2	23
Mixed	−15·4 months	13·1	20

Note: Data not available for 19 epileptic cases, and for 18 epileptic controls. The mean rates take into account both negative and positive discrepancies of Schonell Arithmetic Age from W.I.S.C. Verbal Mental Age.

Significance (epileptic and control subjects compared by Sandler's adaption of the t-test for matched pairs). Only results exceeding the 5 per cent level are presented.

Comparison Epileptic groups	*Value of t*	*Probability Level*
Normal-anxious	3·81	Less than 0·001
Anxious-aggressive	4·61	Less than 0·001
Anxious-mixed	3·42	Less than 0·002, greater than 0·001
Epileptic cf. Controls		
Aggressive-non-epileptic aggressive	2·61	Less than 0·02, greater than 0·01

which are less than their potential as indicated by verbal mental age. However, in respect of reading age, the retardation of the behaviourally normal epileptics is significantly less than that for the other three behavioural groups. The highest degree of retardation is found in the anxious epileptics. No difference in reading retardation can be found between the disturbed epileptics and their controls, suggesting that the same factors which underlie this retardation in the disturbed non-epileptic children may underlie this retardation in the disturbed epileptic children.

Although showing some significant differences, the results for arithmetic retardation are in marked contrast to the results for reading age. The behaviourally *normal* epileptics have an arithmetic retardation much greater than that for any of the *disturbed* non-epileptic groups, suggesting that difficulty with arithmetic is associated with epilepsy, rather than with behaviour disorder. The highest amount of retardation occurs in the aggressive children, whose average retardation is —30·48 months. This is a very high degree of retardation, and in fact eleven children on the right-hand side of the curve have a retardation in arithmetic of 3 years or more. These figures must be considered, too, against the fact that this estimate of retardation is likely to be an underestimate.

Although the anxious epileptics had the highest degree of reading retardation, they have the lowest amount of arithmetic retardation in comparison with the aggressive epileptics, who have the highest amount of arithmetic retardation. In this respect, the rank order for the three disturbed groups is the same in the epileptics as in the controls.

These data would be consistent with the following hypothesis: Previous work has shown the level of task difficulty to be an intervening variable affecting the result of tests carried out by anxious and aggressive subjects, so that in some kinds of test (relatively easy) anxious subjects do better than aggressive subjects, while in others (relatively difficult) it is the aggressive subjects who do best. The two approaches might be conceptualized (from the previous studies) as (*a*) inhibition and reflection, (*b*) an 'attack' on the intellectual task by the aggressive subjects. These two types of approach seem to be functional for different types of intellectual task. In the present study, anxiety may be dysfunctional for reading ability, or tests of reading ability, in comparison with the performance of aggressive subjects. However, the reverse seems to be true with regard to arithmetic tests, where it is the aggressive subjects (both epileptic and non-epileptic) who do worst, relative to the anxious subjects. Thus the anxious epileptics have much less arithmetic retardation than both the behaviourally normal epileptics and the other disturbed epileptics. There appears to be a specific factor associated with epilepsy which causes an arithmetic retardation in epileptic subjects to be much higher than in non-epileptic subjects. The nature of this factor requires further investigation.

It is not immediately explicable what this factor might be, since any test of relationship between the hypothetical factor and arithmetic retardation must take into account that, since arithmetic retardation does not distinguish the normal from the aggressive and the mixed cases, the factor is unlikely to be one of those which has been shown to discriminate between normal and aggressive cases. The anxious cases, which have a markedly lower amount of arithmetic retardation than the other cases, are distinguished from the other three behavioural groups to a greater or lesser degree by the two factors of intelligence (high in the anxious cases) and time since first fit (tending to be less in the anxious cases). These two factors have been examined, but no relationship appears between the amount of arithmetic retardation and the time since first fit or the level of intelligence. No particular EEG group can be implicated, although there is a trend, just reaching the 10 per cent level of significance, for brain damage to be associated with arithmetic retardation.

A fuller exploration of hypothetical factors which underlie arithmetic retardation in these epileptic children would be possible, given the data available, but this exercise would extend beyond the scope of the present study, which is principally concerned with behaviour and its ramifications, rather than with intellect itself.

The present series: conclusion

1 The epileptic children under consideration, 116 referrals for the neurological investigation of epilepsy, have a mean IQ of 99·85. However, the intelligence scores are not distributed normally, there being a longer left-hand tail than a standard normal distribution. An adjustment for social class distribution does not appreciably affect this mean IQ.

2 Both the behaviourally normal and the anxious children have a significantly higher IQ than the aggressive children.

3 No relationship between brain damage or between minor motor fits (two factors which are known to differentiate the anxious and the normal subjects from the aggressive subjects) and low IQ can be found. These findings suggest that low IQ is a relatively independent factor differentiating aggressive children with epilepsy.

4 A significant relationship between low IQ and the time that has elapsed since the first fit has been found.

5 The EEG category of generalized brain damage has a significantly higher proportion of low IQ scores than the EEG categories, '*petit mal*', 'normal,' 'epileptic', and 'temporal lobe focus', the latter group having the highest IQ of all.

6 Behaviourally normal epileptic children have significantly less reading retardation than mixed, aggressive and anxious epileptic children, this last group having the greatest amount of retardation in reading age. There is no difference in the level of reading retardation between disturbed epileptics and matched, non-epileptic controls with similar types of psychiatric disturbance.

7 Retardation of performance in arithmetic is particularly marked in the epileptic children. However, anxious epileptic children have significantly less arithmetic retardation than normal, mixed and

aggressive epileptics. This last group has the highest amount of arithmetic retardation, with an average of a 2½ year discrepancy between mental age and arithmetic age. The aggressive epileptic children have significantly more arithmetic retardation than their non-epileptic, aggressive controls.

8 It is suggested that reading retardation in the epileptic children is related principally to the type of psychiatric disorder rather than epilepsy, while arithmetic retardation in the epileptic children is related principally to a specific epileptic factor rather than to psychiatric disorder. However, it has not been possible to isolate any factor connected with epilepsy which underlies arithmetic retardation. This factor requires further investigation.

24 The integration of medical, social and educational agencies in the treatment of the epileptic child

There is general agreement among social administrators that the fragmentation of services concerned with particular aspects of the same social problem is not in the best interests of the client or patient, since the decisions of some agencies may actually conflict with those of others. This phenomenon has been commented on by Robb (1961), and Balbernie (1966) writing about the decision whether or not to place a child in residential care (a decision that may have to be taken with the epileptic child), stated:

> The various agencies concerned, each of whom had various overlapping powers and responsibilities, could each act independently and pull in different directions. Each had different but ill-defined official functions in relation to the boy and powers of decision-making that were unrelated to those actually in roles in ɪelation to the boy and whose views, in fact, were at times ignored *because* they were in key roles. Those involved were the school health service, the educational authority, the children's department of the referring area and also the local one, the employer, the child guidance clinic, the school, and John's mother. . . .

This lack of integration of the work of the school, the school health service, and the health authorities (the hospital) seems manifest in the treatment of the 118 epileptic children in the present series. Although good channels of communication existed between the hospital and the disablement resettlement officer, the lines of communication between the hospital and the school and the school health service were extremely unclear. There were no formal processes by which the school health service and the child's teacher could be informed that the child had epilepsy, a condition which the previous chapter has shown has important educational implications.

Lord Cohen, in a report on the medical care of epileptics (1956), recommended that diagnostic clinics under the direction of Regional Hospital Boards should be set up for the special investigation and treatment of epilepsy. Lord Cohen's report advocates the closest links between those responsible for the schooling of the epileptic child and those carrying out medical investigations of epilepsy. Lord Cohen advocates strong efforts to keep the epileptic child in the normal school whenever possible.

Pond (1965) describing the advanced services for epileptics in the Netherlands, pointed out that the important recommendations of the Cohen Report had not been adopted. At the time of writing (1970) these recommendations have still not been implemented.

Social class and the treatment of epilepsy

In the present series it has been found that the parents of the epileptic children have a significantly higher distribution of individuals in the upper social classes than would be expected in a sample representing the population at large. This can either be explained by some factor by which epilepsy is connected with upper social classes; or by the selection mechanism in operation, which prevents lower-class patients receiving the best treatment available.

The evidence relating to social class and epilepsy seems sparse, but *a priori* reasoning points to the association of epilepsy with *low* economic status. The Lennoxes (1960) suggest that

> Probably epilepsy is more common among those with low incomes . . . in previous decades the poor received inadequate obstetric attention, had poor living conditions, and experienced excessive infections; but at the present these discrepancies have lessened. The incidence of congenital defects and of epileptic relatives of high and low-income groups deserves attention (p. 498).

Winston and Chilman (1964), writing, like the Lennoxes, about America, said that

> While there is no available evidence to indicate that epilepsy is more common among low-income groups, logic would suggest that rates may be higher for disadvantaged populations because one of the chief causes of epilepsy and related disorders appears to be associated with inadequate obstetric and pediatric care . . . the possible association of epilepsy with poverty will remain in the speculative realm until adequate epidemiological studies can be made.

In Britain the general practice surveys of epilepsy carried out by Pond, Bidwell and Stein (1960) and Pond and Bidwell (1960) found that epileptic patients were more likely to receive a full investigation of their illness if they lived nearer to a teaching hospital. Cooper (1965), describing epilepsy in a national sample of schoolchildren, found that of the 107 children having fits under the age of 2 years, 75 had fits unaccompanied by any other illness. The author reports a slight *excess* from the upper social groups in the children with fits without illness.[1] However, examination of the ratings for standard of material care and housing showed that, in spite of this, more of these children without an obvious direct cause (i.e. febrile illness, such as measles, meningitis, etc.) for their fits came from homes rated poorly for the standard of care.

Rutter *et al.* (1966), reporting the results of a survey of 9 to 12-year-old schoolchildren in the Isle of Wight, reported that 'The social class distribution for children with psychiatric disorder, epilepsy, or a neurological condition was similar to that in the general population'.

Although these findings are slightly equivocal about the possible excess of patients from low social class families, there is certainly no evidence to suggest that the excess of upper classes in the London sample is due to an association of higher social class with factors likely to be associated with epilepsy.

What other factors can account for this association? One explanation would be that, akin to the finding in the general practice studies, upper-class patients are prepared to travel further to a teaching hospital to obtain advice about their children, so that the hospital will cater for two groups of patients—those in the geographically adjacent catchment area with a social class distribution similar to that for the general population in this area, *plus* a population of children whose parents come from upper social classes who have the time, the funds, and the motivation to travel long distances to the hospital.

An interesting finding, analogous to the above hypothesis, has been made by Walker (1967) in a comparative study of English and West Indian children attending the Psychiatric Out-patients Department of the Paddington Children's Hospital. This hospital has an 'open' clinic which sees patients in the evening without a referral note from the general practitioner. Walker studied a sample of West Indian children and English control children attending this clinic, and found marked differences between the two groups in respect of areas of residence. The English children came from a fairly wide area of London, whilst the West Indian children without exception lived

[1] Cf. the distribution by class of epilepsy in patients of all ages in Watts' study (1962) of general practice records in England and Wales. This study gave class rates as follows: Class 1, 4·1/1,000; Class 2, 2·8; Class 3, 3·4; Class 4, 4·0; Class 5, 5·5.

in the Paddington area; the large majority of these West Indian children lived, too, close to the no. 18 bus route, which terminated at the hospital. Walker suggested that the availability of transport to a hospital which was also nearby was a significant factor in selecting West Indian patients for this clinic. The implication of this finding is that parents with only a partial awareness of services or knowledge of transport facilities or the available time to travel may well not be attending the hospital; however, the need for a medical service can be assumed to apply equally to West Indians who do not use the hospital services because of the time, knowledge and distance factors.

These findings are analogous to the suggestion that low social classes do not use, to the fullest extent, hospital services for epileptic children because of lack of knowledge of the services available, and the difficulties of time and expense in travelling long distances which these classes experience relative to upper classes, just as West Indian immigrants experience such difficulties relatively to the indigenous population.

This hypothesis has been examined (Table 39) by comparing the distance of the patient's home from the hospital, according to social class distribution. The hypothesis is supported, since there is a significant difference between the high and low social class groups in respect of distance from the hospital of the patient's home in the expected direction.[1] Distance from home to hospital was measured 'as the crow flies', using a map with a scale of 2½ inches to 1 mile.

The teacher and the epileptic child

To what extent are the teachers of the children in the present series aware that the child has epilepsy? A questionnaire was sent to the child's teacher asking a number of questions about his school progress, health and behaviour. Hospital etiquette forbade that the neurologist's diagnosis should be communicated to the school, and the teacher was merely informed that the child was attending the hospital for treatment. Two questions were asked which were aimed to elicit the teacher's knowledge about epilepsy in the child: 'Please state: The nature of school problem (if any) and any known physical disabilities . . . ' A section was also included for 'Additional comments'.

The questionnaire was completed for 109 of the 118 children; in the remaining nine cases the child had either left school or the school did not return the form, or the parents refused permission for the form to be sent to the school.

[1] A recent study by Collver *et al.* (1967) of the use of maternal health services in Detroit has shown that a significant factor influencing the use of these services by low-income mothers was distance of residence from hospital.

Table 39 Distance of patient's home from hospital and social class in 118 epileptic children

Distance	*Social class group of Registrar General*					
	I and II professional		*III skilled and clerical*		*IV and V semi- and unskilled*	
	n	*cum. p.*	*n*	*cum. p.*	*n*	*cum. p.*
Less than 1 mile	8	0·11	23	0·34	10	0·53
1 to 3 miles	9	0·55	25	0·71	5	0·79
4 miles or more	14	1·0	20	1·0	4	1·0
Totals	31		68		19	

Significance: Kolmogorov-Smirnov one-tailed test:

Comparison	χ^2 *(2 d.f.)*	*Probability level*
I and II: cf. IV and V	8·32	Less than 0·02, greater than 0·01

Only 43 of the teachers appeared to be aware that the child had epilepsy. The remaining 66 teachers gave no indication that they were aware of the existence of epilepsy, although many of these teachers volunteered detailed information about the child's health and behaviour.

The ignorance of the teachers in this respect seems to be due to the reluctance of parents to communicate the information that their child has epilepsy, and the formal system whereby the hospital diagnosis is not passed to the school medical officer or the school itself.

If epilepsy had no other implications than those surrounding the fits, this lack of knowledge might not be detrimental to the relationship of teacher and child. However, as we have seen in the two previous chapters, epileptic children may be hyperactive, a condition which requires special understanding and treatment, and which may not be understood by the teacher unless he knows much more fully the clinical background and history of the child he is teaching; and secondly, epilepsy seems to have ramifications in the field of learning, either through maladjustment or directly from some neurological factor.[1] In particular, the epileptic child is particularly likely to be handicapped with arithmetic, and to require special assistance from the teacher with this subject.

In the questionnaire, teachers were asked to give an estimate of the child's *intelligence* (as well as of his ability in particular school subjects). The comparison of the teachers' estimates and the W.I.S.C. results is given in Table 40. The cases below the dotted line are those in which it is considered that the teachers have underestimated the child's academic potential in terms of his basic ability as indicated by an IQ test. Although in the majority of cases in the 90–109 range the teacher's assessment is compatible with the IQ score (e.g. 'below average' or 'average' for children with an IQ in the 90–9 range, and 'average' or 'above average' for children with an IQ in the 100–9 range), in 25 cases in which the child's IQ on the W.I.S.C. is above 90 the teacher's underestimate of his intelligence might have serious implications from the point of view of the child's academic progress.

Brief case histories of the twenty-five children are given below.

1 A 13-year-old boy with an aggressive behaviour disorder and an IQ of 94. The teacher did not know he had epilepsy, and described

[1] Cf. Rutter *et al.* (1966): '. . . one child in ten in the general population [of the Isle of Wight] suffered from severe reading backwardness, maladjustment, epilepsy or a neurological disorder. From a service point of view the most striking finding, apart from the size of the problem, was the very considerable degree of overlap between the three handicapped conditions. In particular, severe reading retardation was common among anti social children and among those with epilepsy or a neurological disorder.'

Table 40 A comparison of teachers' estimates of intelligence and W.I.S.C. results in 99 epileptic children

W.I.S.C. intelligence quotient	*Teacher's estimate of child's intelligence*					
	Well below average	*Below average*	*Average*	*Above average*	*Well above average*	*Totals*
Less than 80	7	8	2	0	0	17
80– 9	2	3	1	1	0	6
90– 9	1	9	9	0	0	19
100– 9	0	7	10	4	0	21
110–19	0	6	5	4	1	16
120 or more	0	1	8	8	3	20
Totals	10	34	35	16	4	99

Note: Teachers' estimates of intelligence not available in seventeen cases, and IQ test data in two cases. Cases below broken line are those in whom it is considered that the teacher underestimates the child's basic academic ability.

him as of 'well below average' in intelligence. The Schonell tests were not carried out at the hospital for this boy.

2 A 15-year-old boy, behaviourally normal and with an IQ of 104, was described by his teacher as of 'below average' intelligence. The teacher did not know about the epilepsy. The child was 62 months retarded in reading ability and working up to the level of his W.I.S.C. verbal mental age in arithmetic. This child had brain damage located in the temporal lobe area, and was thought to be dyslexic. This was unknown to his teacher.

3 A 15-year-old boy, behaviourally normal, with an IQ of 106, was described by his school as of 'below average' intelligence. The child had *petit mal* attacks (with an underlying 3 per cent spike-and-wave formation) at the rate of one or two a day. These were unknown to his teacher, who wrote a detailed report about him. He was 13 months retarded in arithmetic (according to the Schonell tests given at the hospital). His teacher (in the 'B' stream of a secondary modern school) wrote: 'He has below average achievement because of lack of concentration. He could do better if he tried.' It seems unlikely that the teacher would have written this if he had been aware of the child's underlying neurological condition.

4 An 11-year-old boy with an IQ of 105 and an anxious behaviour disorder was assessed by his teacher as of 'below average' intelligence. He was 51 months retarded in reading and 71 months retarded in arithmetic. In this case the teacher knew of the child's epilepsy.

5 A 15-year-old girl with an aggressive behaviour disorder and an IQ of 103 was described by her teacher as of 'below average' intelligence. Her reading was up to the level of her verbal mental age, but she was 27 months retarded in arithmetic. The teacher was unaware of the child's epilepsy.

6 A 13-year-old boy with an IQ of 117 was described by his school as of 'below average' intelligence. He was working up to the expected level in reading, but was 54 months retarded in arithmetic. The teacher described periods of 'blankness' during school lessons, and complained of the child's slowness without apparently appreciating the significance of the attacks.[1]

7 A 14-year-old boy, behaviourally normal, with an IQ of 117 was described by his teacher as of 'below average' intelligence. He was 30 months retarded in reading and 36 months retarded in arithmetic. This child was in the 'D' stream of a secondary modern school, and was described by his teacher as 'quiet and rather slow'. The teacher was unaware that the boy had epilepsy.

8 A 14-year-old girl with an IQ of 117, behaviourally normal, was described by her teacher as of 'below normal' intelligence. She

[1] In this case the teacher is included among those who reported knowledge of the child's epilepsy.

was working up to expectation in reading, but was 12 months retarded in arithmetic. The teacher appeared unaware of the epilepsy.

9 A 14-year-old boy, IQ 116 and an anxious behaviour disorder, was described by his teacher as of 'below average' intelligence. He was 8 months retarded in reading; the Schonell arithmetic test was not given when the child visited the hospital. The teacher knew about the epilepsy.

10 An 11-year-old boy with an aggressive behaviour disorder and an IQ of 114 was assessed by his teacher as of 'below normal' intelligence. He was 39 months retarded in reading and 31 months retarded in arithmetic. In this case the teacher estimated the child's IQ to be 85. The teacher did not know about the epilepsy.

11 A 15-year-old boy was described by his teacher as of 'below average' intelligence. He had an IQ of 107, but was 60 months retarded in reading and 46 months retarded in arithmetic. He had an anxious behaviour disorder. The teacher did not know of the child's epilepsy.

12 An 8-year-old girl with an anxious behaviour disorder and an IQ of 123 was described by her teacher as of 'below average' intelligence. She was 10 months retarded in reading and 23 months retarded in arithmetic. The school was unaware of the child's epilepsy.

13 A 12-year-old boy, IQ 109, behaviourally normal, was said to be of 'below average' intelligence. He was 4 months retarded in reading and 14 months retarded in arithmetic. The teacher was unaware of the epilepsy.

14 An 8-year-old boy with a mixed behaviour disorder and an IQ of 114 was described as being of 'average' intelligence. He was 43 months retarded in reading and 37 months retarded in arithmetic. The teacher did not know about the epilepsy.

15 A 10-year-old boy with an IQ of 112 and an anxious behaviour disorder was said to be of 'average' intelligence. He was 33 months retarded in reading and 24 months retarded in arithmetic. The teacher was unaware of the epilepsy.

16 A boy aged 15, behaviourally normal, with an IQ of 113 was said by his teacher to be of 'average' intelligence. He was 4 months retarded in reading, and 24 months retarded in arithmetic. The teacher did not know about the epilepsy.

17 A 14-year-old boy, IQ 114, was said to be of 'average' intelligence. He was 23 months retarded in reading and 27 months retarded in arithmetic. The teacher did not know the child was epileptic. This child was behaviourally normal.

18 A 9-year-old boy with an aggressive behaviour disorder, IQ 116, was said by his teacher to be of 'average' intelligence. He was 31

months retarded in reading and 46 months retarded in arithmetic. The school did not report the child's epilepsy.

19 A behaviourally normal boy of 14 with an IQ of 127 was said to be of 'average' intelligence. He was working up to the expected level in reading, but was 15 months retarded in arithmetic. The school knew about the epilepsy. Despite his IQ, this boy was at a secondary modern school, having failed his 11+. His parents expressed surprise at this, since his non-epileptic sister, who seemed to them to be less bright, had in fact passed the 11+ and was attending a grammar school.

20 A 12-year-old boy, IQ 121, was described as being of 'average' intelligence. The boy, behaviourally normal, was not retarded in reading, but was 36 months retarded in arithmetic. The school knew about the epilepsy.

21 A 13-year-old girl with an anxious behaviour disorder had an IQ of 120. Her intelligence was said by her teacher to be 'average', and she was in fact in the 'D' stream of a secondary modern school. She was 18 months retarded in reading and 19 months retarded in arithmetic. The school was unaware of the epilepsy.

22 A 13-year-old boy with an IQ of 125 was said to be of 'average' intelligence by his teacher. The boy had an anxious behaviour disorder, and was 21 months retarded in reading and 42 months retarded in arithmetic. The school was unaware of the epilepsy.

23 A 13-year-old boy with an anxious behaviour disorder and an IQ of 120 was said to be of 'average' intelligence. He was 26 months retarded in reading and 15 months retarded in arithmetic. The school knew about his epilepsy.

24 A 15-year-old boy with an aggressive behaviour disorder and an IQ of 124 was described by his grammar school headmaster as of 'fair average' intelligence. The boy was working up to expectation in reading, but was 27 months retarded in arithmetic. This boy was later expelled from school on the grounds of 'laziness, poor school work, and cheekiness'. The school was unaware of the boy's epilepsy.

25 A behaviourally normal boy of 15 with an IQ of 113 was described by his grammar school of being 'only of average intelligence'. The school, which was unaware of the boy's epilepsy, complained that he was lazy, and could not or would not concentrate. He was working up to the expected level in reading, but was 18 months retarded in arithmetic.

26 A 12-year-old boy with an anxious behaviour disorder and an IQ of 133 was said by his teacher in a secondary modern school (he had failed the 11+) to be 'average or slightly below' in intelligence. He was described by the teacher (who knew about the epilepsy) as 'slow but sure'. He was 22 months retarded in reading and 21 months retarded in arithmetic.

No control subjects are available for this aspect of the investigation into the epileptic child's classroom experience; but this does not mitigate the seriousness of the findings, for in all the cases cited above it appears that the teacher is unaware of the child's true academic potential. The implications for the child's future are serious; many educational sociologists (e.g. Lacey, 1966) have shown how the teacher's perception of a child's academic ability can be self-confirming, so that the child comes to regard his current academic achievement as his maximum potential, when in fact, under different teaching conditions, his academic achievement could be brought up to the level indicated by his mental age revealed by intelligence testing.

What the teachers of these 28 children seem to have been doing is assuming that the child's current academic achievement is the *equivalent* of his basic IQ.[1] To what extent teachers make this assumption about non-epileptic children is unknown, but the problem is serious enough to bear further investigation.[2]

The following four case histories of children other than those reported above may illustrate aspects of the school's relationship with the epileptic child:

27 A 13-year-old boy with a mixed behaviour disorder was extremely anxious about his school situation, and was given psychotherapy by the hospital child psychiatrist on this account. He had an IQ of 96, and was regarded (realistically) as of 'average' intelligence by his secondary modern school. He was 57 months retarded in reading and 95 months retarded in arithmetic. The teacher's report on this boy was framed in somewhat hostile terms. Commenting on his achievement, the teacher said: 'He is well below the lowest grade in the school'. The teacher gave no reasons for this, although the fact that he had 'black-outs' was mentioned. His behaviour was described by the school as 'Ingratiating, lying, cowardly, disobedient'. The boy had no friends in school, and was himself victimized and bullied by other children.

The family lived in very poor circumstances. The boy shared a bed with his two brothers in the same room occupied by his parents and

[1] Cf. Ingram and Mason (1965): '. . . there are too many children in each class and reliable assessments of intelligence are seldom available, so that the position is reversed—teachers tend to judge the intelligence of a pupil by his progress in reading. Thus special learning difficulties may escape recognition for years.'

[2] It is the writer's experience that current practice in colleges of education is to instruct student teachers in the use of group intelligence tests and standardized achievement tests for use at the beginning of each school year for the class of which he is form-master, and to give remedial teaching to retarded children, as well as investigating the possible causes of this retardation, passing on a report at the end of the school year to the next form-teacher.

a small baby. The parents were extremely depressed by these circumstances. Efforts by the social worker to have the family rehoused by the local authority were unsuccessful.

28 A 14-year-old girl, IQ of 107, was described (fairly realistically) by her school to be of 'average' intelligence. She was behaviourally normal, and was 10 months retarded in reading and 30 months retarded in arithmetic. The case is of interest for the attitudes of the teachers at this all-girls secondary modern school. The girl had 'minor major' attacks, falling down and being unconscious for five minutes, but without motor involvement. On one occasion when this happened at school the teacher poured a bowl of cold water over the girl, and she arrived home soaking wet. On other occasions the teacher made her run round the playground after an attack. Neither of these strategies could be regarded as realistic behaviour in the face of an attack. The girl was particularly hurt when the teachers prevented her from attending the school prize-giving, fearing that she might have an attack.

29 This 14-year-old boy, IQ of 94, with a mixed behaviour disorder, was described by his teacher (realistically) as of 'average' intelligence and, was 2 months retarded in reading and 26 months retarded in arithmetic. The headmaster contacted the hospital, after learning that the child was receiving treatment, and requested more information about him. Permission being obtained from the consultant in charge of the case and the boy's parents, the results of psychometric testing were sent to the head master, with recommendations for special tuition in mathematics. On receipt of these reports this extra tuition was arranged.

30 A 10-year-old girl with an IQ of 129 and an anxious behaviour disorder was described by her headmaster as being of 'well above average intelligence'. This headmaster contacted the hospital for further information about the child, saying that of the panel of teachers which made recommendations for transfer to a grammar or a secondary modern school, only he felt that her intelligence (which had not previously been tested) warranted her transfer to a grammar school. The other teachers felt that her standard of work justified her transfer to a secondary modern school (she was 22 months retarded in arithmetic, but working up to the expected level in reading). If it had not been for the fact that the hospital contacted the school for a report at this time, the majority recommendation (secondary modern) would have been carried out. However, after permission was gained from consultant and parents, the IQ test results and recommendations were sent to the girl's headmaster. As a result of this, she was in fact transferred to a grammar school. It is interesting to note in this case that this important decision was being made by teachers without access to objective information about the child's ability.

It is possible that the teachers may have been influenced by the child's appearance and home background. She came from an extremely poor home. For most of her life the girl had lived in overcrowded rooms with her mother and four siblings in circumstances of poverty. Occasionally the father would live with the family, on his release from prison, during which another pregnancy would be initiated. The family had been taken into care several times when the family had been evicted, and the girl had attended several primary schools because of the family's frequent changes of accommodation. The longest separation from her mother followed the mother's suicide attempt after the child's father received a further prison sentence.

It may be that, knowing the child's home circumstances, the child's teachers did not perceive her as a child likely to be of high intelligence or as one who would do well at a grammar school.

The last two case histories offer some evidence that if the hospital which has carried out a full range of diagnostic testing can counsel the school about the best educational treatment for the child, and the implications of the child's epilepsy, the result is very much in the child's interest.

Discussion

The above tables and case histories have been presented in support of the contention that the treatment of the epileptic child, from both an educational and a clinical point of view, could be improved. Enough of the diagnostic centres of the kind recommended by Lord Cohen are necessary to ensure that children in all areas, and regardless of social class, obtain adequate investigation and treatment of their epilepsy.

The establishment of channels of communication between school and hospital (and between school and diagnostic centre) might have many beneficial results. The teacher would be aware of the implications of factors associated with epilepsy for the child's behaviour, of the child's academic potential, and the areas in which to give special tuition.[1] What seems to be needed are formal channels of communication whereby a synopsis of the relevant clinical and psychometric details about the child should be automatically sent to the child's head teacher, and advice given on the handling of behaviour disorder and on the handling of epileptic fits. The present system too easily

[1] The situation in France is certainly no better than in Britain. Jacquet (1968) estimated that only 3,572 of France's 60,000 children estimated to have epilepsy were known to the school medical service. This is attributed to a 'conspiracy of silence' between families of the children, and G.P.s. Fifty per cent of the epileptic children known to the school had 'serious scholastic difficulties'.

assists the parents' desire to keep the knowledge of their child's epilepsy from as many people as possible.

The conclusions of a *Lancet* annotation of 4 February 1967 still have very great relevance:

> . . . that report on the welfare services for these patients was produced in 1953, and it was followed in 1956 by the Cohen Report on the medical care of epileptics (the continued interest in this report led to its being reprinted in 1965). It was a careful analysis of the help available, and ended with 23 recommendations. Many of these suggestions were concerned with the need for co-operation between the various services and with the establishment of regional diagnostic and treatment clinics and long-stay treatment and rehabilitation centres. These changes would have cost money, but they did not need complex legislation. The first thing a patient needs is a full medical and social assessment before the best treatment and social advice can be given. Among doctors, co-ordination is not always close enough between the neurologist, paediatrician, psychiatrist, and general practitioner. Similarly, communications may be poor between those educating the patients and those who will help them find jobs and employ them. . . . The regional centres, as suggested by the Cohen Report, would promote more efficient co-operation between all those concerned with the care of these patients. . . . After so much painstaking work, these recommendations have produced little change. The capital cost of implementing them will continue to rise, legislation will not become easier, and the services are not yet available. Another review of all the services is being carried out, and further advice and recommendations will be produced. To seek advice, and even to make recommendations, is relatively easy. What is required is action on the suggestions that have already been made.

Conclusions

1 The excess of children with parents from the upper social classes in the present series may reflect the distance, time and expense which a parent is willing to travel and to sacrifice in order to take the child to a teaching hospital for consultation. There is a significant relationship between the distance of the patient's home from the hospital and the social class of the child's parent.

2 A questionnaire was completed by teachers for 109 of the epileptic children. Sixty-six of these teachers gave no indication that they were aware that the child had epilepsy. This fact probably reflects the lack of formal communication between hospital and school.

3 In 28 cases the teachers appeared to underestimate the basic academic potential of the epileptic child. It appears that the teachers are basing their estimates of the child's intelligence on his level of attainment. In the epileptic child, as the previous chapter showed, this attainment is often depressed in relation to the child's ability as revealed by his IQ.

4 Thirty case histories have been presented in support of the contention that the education and the welfare of the children could be aided by establishing formal links between the hospital and the school.

25 A genetic hypothesis

In the review of literature above, it was concluded that in a number of studies there had appeared an association between a history of epilepsy in family members of the epileptic, and a history of a number of abnormal behaviour conditions, such as neurosis, psychosis, alcoholism, etc. This finding has been repeated in the present study.

Some writers have tried to account for such findings by positing a general constitutional weakness in the epileptic and his family, allied to the concept of the epileptic personality (e.g. Bleuler, 1960). However, the notion of 'constitutional weakness' seems vague and difficult to examine systematically.

A possible alternative explanation may be advanced, based on a number of known facts about epilepsy. First of all, there is evidence (reviewed above, p. 108) that the epileptic is subject to prejudice and social rejection. This has been true in historical times, in simple societies, and in modern society. It would follow that as a result of this social rejection the epileptic would find difficulty in finding partners for marriage.[1] There is evidence, in fact, that marriage rates of epileptics are less than those in the normal population. A crucial hypothesis is that in order to fulfil his normal sexual and social needs, the epileptic is forced to take as marriage partners those who were themselves rejected by society—the physically and emotionally disabled. Given that some of these conditions have a

[1] Supportive evidence for this proposition is provided by Watts' study of epilepsy in general practice in England and Wales (1962). He found that epilepsy was twice as common in unskilled, single female workers as in male unskilled workers. He attributes the large number of single women with epilepsy to the fact that 'the marriage market for epileptic women is not a good one'.

genetic basis,[1] the familial association of epilepsy and abnormal behavioural (and perhaps physical conditions) becomes explained.[2]

In the anthropologist's term, this is a final cause theory, since it suggests the origin of present phenomena by events in history, so that an empirical examination of the hypothesis is not possible. The hypothesis must be accepted or rejected on grounds of plausibility. If it is rejected, the question must be answered: How *else* can the familial association of epilepsy and abnormal behaviour be accounted for?

This familial association has some important implications for the study of behaviour disorder. In the present study we have found a significant association between the number of hazards in the environment of the epileptic child (poverty, overcrowding, disturbing relatives, breaks and changes of environment, etc.) and a history of epilepsy in the family members of the epileptic child. There are grounds for supposing that the abnormal behaviour in family members may underlie these environmental hazards. In addition, a significantly inverse relationship was found between a history of brain damage and the number of environmental hazards.

It thus seems, so far as environmental hazards are concerned, that the child whose epilepsy seems to be the result of brain damage is likely to be relatively free of these environmental hazards. This may explain why some writers (notably Bridge, 1949, and the Lennoxes, 1960) have found an apparently inverse or random relationship between brain damage and adverse behaviour. However, in the present study brain damage itself appears to be an important precipitant of behaviour disorder, so that in those cases in which the child is both brain-damaged and there are a high number of hazards in the environment, the child will be particularly at risk for behaviour disorder.

Brain damage and heredity are not *absolutely* inverse conditions as factors in the aetiology of epilepsy. Rodin and Gonzales (1966), for example, in a study of EEG in the family members of epileptic patients and of control subjects, found that abnormal EEGs in the family members of patients with psychomotor seizures were more common than in the families of the control subjects. Ounsted and his colleagues (1966) found, in a study of 100 children with temporal lobe epilepsy, that the sibling risk of convulsive disorder was 15 per cent, much higher than that in children in the general population. These

[1] Cf. the theory of Sir Julian Huxley *et al.* (1964) on the historical survival of the schizophrenic gene. Cf. similar 'historical' genetic theories on albinism (Wade, 1969), and shortsightedness (Douglas *et al.*, 1968).

[2] Alström (1950) in a Swedish study, could not demonstrate an association of epilepsy and disturbed behaviour in families; but in Sweden epileptics were forbidden by law, from 1760 to 1920, from marrying.

results are at first puzzling, since psychomotor and temporal lobe epilepsy by definition involve an injury to the brain. A possible explanation comes from the data of Ounsted *et al.*: the highest sibling risk was found in those children in whom the aetiology of the temporal lobe damage seemed to be *status epilepticus* occurring early in the child's life. The writers suggest that in these cases the child is genetically disposed to febrile convulsions. The convulsions, when they occur, chance to be severe or continuous, and in the course of them Ammon's horn is damaged. Sclerosis follows, and an epileptogenic lesion arises.

In this way the paradoxical findings of some writers (summarized by W.H.O., 1957) of an association of temporal lobe epilepsy and abnormal behaviour in family members, might be explained.

Conclusion

A persistent finding in studies of epileptics has been the familial association of epilepsy and behaviour disorders. A hypothesis that epileptics, because of prejudice, are forced to choose behaviourally abnormal individuals as marriage partners, has been advanced to account for this phenomenon.

26 Residual areas

A 'residual area' is that area of a problem which the research in question[1] has not been able to illuminate. Parsons has stressed that these areas must be specified so that the value of those findings about which full information is available, and which have been more or less accurately measured, may be considered in the light of the extent of the problem as a whole.

There are at least five such areas in the present study, involving variables which may have an important relation to behaviour disorder in epileptic children, but for which there are insufficient data or data are in an insufficiently systematic form, or for which an appropriate analysis has not yet been undertaken because of technical difficulties. These five areas are: delinquency; the effect of anticonvulsant drugs; body build factors; the pre-morbid personality of the child; and the long-term adjustment of these children.

Some perspectives and preliminary findings for these areas are given below.

Delinquency

The previous literature on this subject (*vide supra*, p. 78), like much of the literature on epileptic children and adolescents, is equivocal. The general conclusion from this literature is that heinous crimes, such as murder or sexual assault, do not appear to be any more prevalent than in the population at large; but there is some evidence that minor crimes, probably due to inadequacy or frustration, may be more prevalent in some epileptic populations.

In the present series, lying and stealing and aggressive symptoms occurred with some frequency in 30 children categorized as 'aggres-

[1] See Talcott Parsons: *The Structure of Social Action* for an expansion of this idea.

sive' and in 25 children categorized as 'mixed'. However, it is only very rarely that these symptoms seem to have involved the children in trouble with the police. Six of the 118 children were known to have been found guilty (over a period of about one year before interview) at a juvenile court for an offence—in all cases involving theft. This rate of 5·1 per cent is somewhat higher than the yearly rate for London in the early 1960s of about 1 per cent of children in the age range 8 to 17 (Bagley, 1965). However, there was a cluster of epileptic children in the age range 12 to 15, and a predominance of boys in excess of the number of boys expected in the general population, so that a direct comparison of the two percentages is not realistic. In addition, delinquency is known to have great variations between neighbourhoods, so that a few streets can provide 50 per cent of the delinquents in a much larger administrative area (Bagley, 1965). It is impossible to know how the delinquency rate of the epileptic children compares with that of the children in their immediate neighbourhood, since control subjects matched for this variable were not studied.

One case is of interest in this respect. A 13-year-old boy with a mixed behaviour disorder was said to be solitary and unpopular at school at the time the study was undertaken, and was known through a follow-up study to have made a relatively good behavioural adjustment. Concomitant with this, he was accepted by his neighbourhood sub-culture and engaged in the delinquent pastimes of this group. His subsequent appearance in juvenile court in fact appeared to be an index of his behavioural *adjustment*.

A further case is of interest. This 14-year-old boy was subject to violently aggressive outbursts in which he sometimes physically-attacked members of his family. Despite the fact of having a generalized brain damage situated in the left hemisphere, the boy was highly intelligent, with a W.I.S.C. IQ of 135. He was a solitary boy, and very sensitive and self-conscious. He had experienced 'catastrophic rage outbursts' since the age of 3. Parental attitudes and behaviour towards this boy were extremely disturbed, and the environment was also extremely unstable. Two years later the boy was placed on remand after an arrest for 'suspected loitering with intent to commit a felony'. In the remand home he was extremely recalcitrant, his behaviour being diagnosed as 'aggressive psychopathy', and he was subsequently committed to an institution for the criminally insane. However, his adjustment in this institution was so good that he was eventually released. Though we run the risk of the *post hoc ergo propter hoc* fallacy, it is interesting to speculate whether the removal of this boy from a highly disturbing home environment was connected with his eventual good adjustment.

Anticonvulsant medication

There are grounds for believing, from the work of Reynolds and his colleagues (*vide supra*, p. 85), that prolonged anticonvulsant medication may be a cause of mental disturbance in epileptics by causing folic acid deficiency in the patient. In the present series only a fairly small number of children were taking anticonvulsants at the time they were investigated psychiatrically. No relationship can be established between taking anticonvulsants, and disturbed behaviour. However, this analysis did not take into account the amount of the dosage, the type of anticonvulsant, nor the length of time that the child had been taking the anticonvulsants.

Anthropometric factors

In the review of literature above it was concluded that anthropometry had never been systematically undertaken with epileptic children, although the balance of opinion from clinical impressions seemed to suggest that aggressive children were likely to be stocky and muscular.[1] This relationship has been systematically demonstrated with non-epileptic children.

In the present series a number of body measurements are available for the children. However, the range of measurements is not complete enough for any of the conventional anthropometric profiles to be constructed. It is eventually hoped to compare the available body measurements with the means of the national population, when these

Table 41 Linearity scores in anxious and aggressive epileptic children

Per cent of linearity score of a child of similar age and sex in the normal population	*Anxious*		*Aggressive*	
	n	*cum. p.*	*n*	*cum. p.*
−15 to −19	1	0·04	0	—
−10 to −14	1	0·07	0	—
− 5 to −9	4	0·22	4	0·14
− 1 to −4	15	0·78	9	0·45
+ 0 to +4	6	1·0	16	1·0
Totals	27		29	

Note: Data not available in two cases.
Significance: Kolmogorov-Smirnov one-tailed test:
Anxious cf. Aggressive, X^2 (2 d.f.) =6·09
less than 0·05, greater than 0·02

[1] But note that Rey *et al.* (1949) found the reverse to hold.

are available. At the time of the study, only national means for height and weight are available (Tanner, 1958).

It has been possible to construct an index of linearity (height divided by the cube root of weight) for the children. This is not a complete anthropometric profile, but is in effect one third of it (Parnell *et al.*, 1962), two other measures—of the amount of fat and of the amount of muscle—going to make up the full profile. However, as Sheldon *et al.* (1940, p. 140) point out, an individual who has a high linearity score will tend to have a dearth of fat and muscle in relation to height, i.e. will tend to have an asthenic body build.

The linearity scores of the two most contrasted behavioural groups, the anxious and the aggressive have been compared. The linearity scores distinguish the anxious and the aggressive epileptic children at the 2 per cent level, but *not* in the expected direction. The anxious children, in fact, seem to have much more fat and muscle in relation to their height than the aggressive children. In order to correct for the effect of age and sex (which cause slight variations in linearity), the linearity scores of the two disturbed groups of epileptic children have been expressed as percentages of the linearity score of a child in the normal population of similar age and sex, using the national means of height and weight given by Tanner (1958). The results remain significant at the 5 per cent level.

Pre-morbid personality

According to interaction theory, one of the variables affecting the final behavioural outcome in epilepsy in children will be the personality of the child before the onset of epilepsy. No measure of this (e.g. extraversion-introversion) is available for the present series; indeed such information would only be available if a large population of children were studied from birth, the data on pre-morbid personality of the epileptic being considered if and when epilepsy had its onset.

According to some previous studies, body build may correlate with personality orientation. In the present study, what evidence there is on body build shows an atypical trend—for anxious children to be less linear than aggressive children—so that it is difficult to hypothesize that epileptic children who become anxious were lean and introverted before the onset of epilepsy, and the aggressive child muscular and extraverted.

Only one clue to the pre-morbid personality of the children exists for the present series—an onset of behaviour disorder *before* the onset of epilepsy. In 23 of the epileptic children sufficient information was available to say that the behaviour disorder preceded the epilepsy, sometimes by many years. These cases are randomly distributed by the brain-damaged/not brain-damaged categories, so that brain damage cannot be implicated as a factor in the early onset of behaviour disorder. If, as we have suggested, behavioural pathology of family members of the epileptic underlies the existence of environmental hazards, there is no reason why some of these environmental factors should not have been in operation *before* the onset of epilepsy, when they might in themselves cause behaviour disorder. A similar suggestion has been made by Pond (1961).

Long-term prognosis

Robins (1966), in a follow-up study of child guidance clinic referrals and control children which investigated the subjects up to thirty years after the original referral, found that the children referred for anti-social problems ('aggressive children' in our present terms) very often became sociopathic personalities in adult life, in contrast with both the neurotic children and the normal controls, whose adjustment in adult life was largely normal. As adults, the anti-social children were much more likely to appear before the courts, to have unstable marriages, to be alcoholic, to be often unemployed, to wander around the country (the United States), to be dishonourably discharged from the Army, and not to rise in the social scale.

A deductive generalization from this study would suggest that the aggressive epileptic children may show this pattern of adjustment in later life. Systematic follow-up studies may investigate this, but at the present time, three to five years after the original investigation of the children, systematic details about their present adaption are not known, except in a few cases.

One such case has already been mentioned in the section on delinquency above (p. 249), in which a highly aggressive boy was committed to an institution for the criminally insane, and was subsequently discharged. One girl developed a psychotic state in her mid-'teens. This girl's previous behaviour had been exemplary, and there were no grounds from her previous history to suggest this outcome. One boy developed Giles de la Tourette's syndrome, with compulsive coprophilia, and in his late 'teens was institutionalized in a mental hospital. This boy died during an attack of *status epilepticus.* One girl whose parents had refused permission for her to be included in the research series developed a psychotic state in her mid-'teens, and it is probable that this girl had been a behaviour problem for some years.

Conclusion

For the five 'residual areas' specified, the following conclusions can be made:

1 The data do not suggest any marked differences between the delinquency rate of the epileptic children and children in the general population, although an accurate comparison cannot be made with the present data.

2 No firm conclusions can be drawn about the effect of anticonvulsant medication on the children's behaviour.

3 A comparison of the linearity scores for the anxious and the aggressive epileptic children produced results contrary to theoretical expectation, the anxious children being *less* linear than the aggressive. There is some indication that children who are more physically robust (i.e. the anxious children) also have higher intelligence than the less intelligent children, who tend to be less physically robust and to have an aggressive behaviour disorder. These relationships are hypothetical, and require further investigation.

Maturity, measured by bone-age photography, does not appear to be related to the behaviour disorder.

4 No accurate indicators of the pre-morbid personality of the epileptic children are known. In 23 children the behaviour disorder had its onset before the occurrence of epilepsy. Brain damage cannot be implicated as a factor in this early onset of behaviour disorder.

5 Two cases are known to have become psychotic in their later 'teens. One of these cases died during *status epilepticus*.

27 An interaction hypothesis

In the review section of this study (*vide supra*, pp. 114–25) a number of studies were mentioned which appear to show, or to suggest, that a number of factors may *interact* together to produce particular kinds of behavioural outcome. There seems to be no logical reason why this kind of interaction of particular constraints on behaviour should not take place among the factors which bear on the behaviour of epileptic children, and a number of writers (e.g. Gudmundsson, 1966) have made the hypothesis that this interaction does in fact take place. Indeed, the hypothesis of interaction, that many different factors have a partial influence on the final behavioural outcome in epilepsy, may help to explain some of the apparently contradictory findings (e.g. brain damage versus social environment) which have emerged in some studies.

The interaction of constraints on aggressive behaviour

In the present study, four relatively independent factors discriminating normal from aggressive cases have been identified: minor motor fits (and to a lesser extent the brain damage which probably underlies these fits); a high number of environmental hazards; a high number of adverse parental attitudes and behaviours; and low intelligence. Parental attitudes and environmental hazards do have an association at the 5 per cent level of significance, although a substantial number of cases have a high adverse parental attitude *or* a large number of environmental hazards, so that these two factors may be said to be relatively independent.

The hypothesis that will be tested below is that the highest behavioural yield in terms of aggressive behaviour (i.e. the highest number of cases with an aggression score greater than the median for the series) will occur in those cases in which all four of the hypothetical constraints are combined; the lightest yield will be in those cases in which none of these constraints is present; those cases in which only some constraints are present will occupy an intermediate position, more cases being aggressive when two rather than one constraint is present, and more still when three constraints are present.

A further hypothesis to be tested is that each of these four factors significantly adds to the aggressive behavioural yield when the effect of the other three factors is held constant.

The data and the test of these hypotheses are given in Tables 42, 43 and 44.

The principle underlying the interaction table (Table 42) is the dichotomization of each variable in terms of each other variable. In the discussion of such tables, in the chapters on interaction and parental attitudes and behaviour (*vide supra*, p. 114–25 and 184–99) it was pointed out that a variety of treatments of the results of the interaction table (i.e. of the proportion of cases in each cell having the particular outcome in question) is possible, including the full range of factorial treatments.[1] In the present study, the relatively simple analysis of comparing the cells by the χ^2 technique is used.

The final outcome examined in the interaction table (Table 42) is the proportion of cases which have an aggression score above the median aggression score for the whole series. This means, in effect, considering the proportion of cases which have been classified as aggressive and mixed behaviour disorders.

All of the interaction hypotheses are confirmed (Tables 43 and 44). Each of the four constraints on aggressive behaviour significantly adds to the load of aggressive behaviour when its interaction with the three other factors is considered. The two most potent factors in this respect are seen to be parental attitudes and minor motor fits, each of which adds to the behavioural yield at a very high level of significance. Environmental hazards have the lowest significance in this respect; this reflects the fact that this constraint also appears to be a factor in precipitating anxiety in the present series of epileptic children, so that its significance in the interaction table rests on its power to discriminate between the normal and the aggressive and the mixed cases, (but not between the anxious and the aggressive and mixed cases).

It is interesting to note that low intelligence *by itself* is in no case associated with aggressive behaviour disorder. Children of low intelligence tend to be aggressive only when some other factor is present, which probably provides stress to which such a child is particularly susceptible.

Table 44 shows that the more constraints there are in combination,

[1] Cf. the somewhat similar tables for the calculation of the analysis of variance and covariance given by Moroney (1956), pp. 396–7.

Table 42 The interaction of parental attitudes, fits, environment and intelligence as constraints on aggressive behaviour in 118 epileptic children

Parental attitudes	− 58								+ 60							
Environmental hazards	− 38				+ 20				− 23				+ 37			
Intelligence	− 24		+ 14		− 8		+ 12		− 10		+ 13		− 14		+ 23	
Fits	− 16	+ 8	− 5	+ 9	− 4	+ 4	− 4	+ 8	− 4	+ 6	− 7	+ 6	− 7	+ 7	− 8	+ 15
Normal	11	2	5	5	3	1	0	0	1	1	2	0	1	1	1	1
Anxious	4	4	0	1	1	1	3	1	2	0	1	0	2	3	3	2
Aggressive	0	1	0	0	0	0	0	4	1	3	2	5	0	1	4	9
Mixed	1	1	0	3	0	2	1	3	0	2	2	1	4	2	0	3
Aggression below median	15	6	5	6	4	2	3	1	3	1	3	0	3	4	4	3
Aggression above median	1	2	0	3	0	2	1	7	1	5	4	6	4	3	4	12
Constraints	0	F	I	IF	E	EF	EI	EIF	P	PF	PI	PIF	PE	PEF	PEI	PEIF

Note: For parental attitudes, data divided as near to the median as possible, — indicating a score below the median and + a score above it. The number of environmental hazards has been similarly divided, '—' indicating a score below the median.

Intelligence quotients have also been divided at the median, but in this case '—' indicates high intelligence (above the median) and '+' low intelligence.

For fits, '—' indicates fits other than the minor motor types; '+' indicates minor motor fits.

In two cases the IQ was not known, and these cases were allocated randomly to the high and low categories.[1]

The 'constraint' cells at the bottom of the table indicate the combinations of hypothetical factors influencing aggressive behaviour. Thus EIF, for example, indicates that the cases in this category have a high number of environmental hazards, minor motor fits, and low intelligence.

[1] Both of these cases have an anxious behaviour disorder. In the case randomly allocated to the 'low intelligence' group, the teacher described the child's intelligence as 'average'. In the case randomly allocated to the 'high intelligence' group the teacher described the child's intelligence as 'well above average'.

Table 43 A test of the independence of the constraints on aggressive behaviour

(*Data from Table 1*)

(*a*) *Parental Attitudes*

	P not a constraint (−)	P a constraint (+)	
Aggression low	42	21	63
Aggression high	16	39	55
	58	60	118

χ^2 (1 d.f.)=15·9
P less than 0·001

(*b*) *Environmental Hazards*

	E not a constraint (−)	E a constraint (+)	
Aggression low	39	24	63
Aggression high	22	33	55
	61	57	118

χ^2 (1 d.f.)=5·63
P less than 0·02, greater than 0·01

(*c*) *Low Intelligence*

	I not a constraint (−)	I a constraint (+)	
Aggression low	38	25	63
Aggression high	18	37	55
	56	62	118

χ^2 (1 d.f.) =8·96
P less than 0·005, greater than 0·001

(*d*) *Minor Motor Fits*

	F not a constraint (−)	F a constraint (+)	
Aggression low	40	23	63
Aggression high	15	40	55
	55	63	118

χ^2 (1 d.f.)=14·87
P less than 0·001

Note: 'F not a constraint' (for example) combines the cells in Table 42, 0, I, E, EI, P, PI, PE, and PEI. 'F a constraint' combines the cells F, IF, EF, EIF, PF, PIF, PEF and PEIF.

Table 44 The number of constraints and the proportion of cases who have high aggression scores

Number of constraints	*Low aggression score*		*High aggression score*		*Proportion with high aggression*
	n	*cum. p.*	*n*	*cum. p.*	*score*
0	15	0·24	1	0·02	0·06
1 (F, I, P)	18	0·52	3	0·07	0·14
2 (IF, EF, EI PF, PI, PE)	18	0·81	19	0·42	0·52
3 (EIF, PIF, PEF, PEI)	9	0·95	20	0·78	0·69
4 (PEIF)	3	1·0	12	1·0	0·8
Totals	63		55		

Significance: Kolmogoroc-Smirnov one-tailed test:
Distribution of constraints between low aggression scorers, and high aggression categories, X^2 (2 d.f.)=23·78, P less than 0·001.
Data from Table 42.

the more likely it is that there will be a high number of cases with high aggression scores. When there are no constraints (cell 0 in Table 42) only one of the sixteen cases has a high aggression score. When there are four constraints (cell PEIF in Table 42) twelve of the fifteen cases have high aggression scores. There is a highly significant difference in the distribution of the number of constraints when the cases with low aggression scores, and high aggression scores are compared.

The interaction of constraints on anxious behaviour

There has been marked tendency for the data in the present study to distinguish the behavioural groups of epileptic children in the following way, (1) normal, (2) anxious, (3) mixed, (4) aggressive, so that the greatest difference is found between the normal and the aggressive cases, with the anxious cases often having a rather similar incidence of the variable in question to the normal cases, with the mixed cases more often having an incidence of the variable in question that resembles the aggressive rather than the anxious cases. The similarity of the aggressive and the mixed cases is reflected in Table 42 (above, p. 256) so that when these two behavioural groups are combined to form a group with high aggression scores, the difference in incidence of the four variables in question between the low and high aggression cases is very marked.

When factors which distinguish the low anxiety from the high anxiety cases are considered, it is more difficult to find variables which should, by hypothesis, distinguish the two groups of cases at a high level of significance, since the mixed cases, by virtue of having high anxiety as well as high aggression scores, must be grouped with the anxious cases (which they have not, in the chapters above, resembled in terms of the incidence of the variables examined).

One variable does, however, have a rather similar incidence in the anxious and the mixed cases, distinguishing them from the normal and the aggressive cases—the incidence of girls. In the 118 children, there is a higher proportion of boys than girls—74/118, or 63·0 per cent. Rather similar sex ratios have been observed in series of epileptic patients by Lennox (1960) and Ounsted (1955). The exact reason for this higher incidence of boys in epileptic populations is not known, although there is some suggestion in the data presented by Gudmundsson (1966) that girls are less likely to be brain-damaged than boys. The present series is too small to test this hypothesis, although there is a relationship, significant at the 10 per cent level only, between being male and being brain-damaged, and a relationship at a similar level of significance between being female and having a middle sibship. There is an inverse relationship, significant at the 5 per cent level, between sibship in the first or last ordinal position and having epilepsy, when the epileptic children are compared with the ordinal position of their 211 siblings. This comparison is based on 99 epileptic children, since 19 of the series were only children. The relationship of birth order and the incidence of epilepsy has been the subject of some controversy (Bridge, 1949; Brain, 1956; Collver and Kerridge, 1962; Metrakos and Metrakos, 1963), a relationship between being first-born and being epileptic occurring in some studies, but not in others. The present data suggest that both the first and the last ordinal positions carry a greater risk of epilepsy. The hypothetical cause of this greater risk of developing epilepsy is that first-born children, and children born to older mothers, carry a greater risk of trauma to the central nervous system.

The number of girls does not distinguish any one behavioural group from any other; nor does it distinguish the high and low aggressive cases. It does, however, distinguish the high and low anxiety cases at a significant level: 19 of the 65 cases with low anxiety scores (i.e. normal plus aggressive cases) are female, compared with 25 of the 53 cases with high anxiety scores (i.e. anxious plus mixed cases). This difference is significant at the 5 per cent level (χ^2 1 d.f.= 4·02). The most marked difference in sex incidence between any of the four behavioural groups is between the aggressive cases (6/30 girls, or 20·0 per cent) and the mixed cases (15/25 girls, or 60·0 per cent).

Two factors have been indentified in previous chapters which distinguish the normal from the anxious cases at a significant level—the number of environmental hazards and the number of cases with major motor or *grand mal* fits. The variable of intelligence has distinguished the anxious from the aggressive cases, with both the normal and mixed cases occupying an intermediate position. Hypothetically, the variables of environmental hazards, major motor fits, and high intelligence will distinguish the low and high anxiety groups at a moderate level of significance, while the factor of sex should distinguish the two groups at a stronger level of significance when these four variables are considered in interaction with one another.

In terms of interaction theory, the highest yield of anxious behaviour should be in those cases who are girls with high intelligence, major motor fits, and who experience a high number of environmental hazards.

The test of these hypotheses is presented in Tables 45, 46 and 47. It will be seen that all results are at a lower level of significance than the levels obtained in the test of constraints on aggressive behaviour. Only environmental hazards and female sex attain the 5 per cent level of significance when their interaction with other factors is considered as constraints on anxious behaviour. The variable of major fits does not quite reach the 5 per cent level, and the variable of high intelligence is clearly not a significant constraint on anxious behaviour when the anxious and the mixed cases are considered together.

It will be seen from Table 47 that there is a significant relationship between a high number of constraints and a high anxiety score.

Discussion and conclusion

These data support the picture of an interaction of constraints on the behaviour of the epileptic child. This interaction is highly complex, and it is not possible to tell from the data whether the interaction is additive or whether there are any catalytic effects. Children with brain injury or minor motor fits and low intelligence, seem particularly susceptible to both stresses in their environment and adverse behaviour on the part of their parents. Neither minor motor fits nor intelligence seem to be *by themselves* marked discriminants of aggressive behaviour. Only in combination with the other two variables (environment or parental behaviour) does the existence of these constraints lead to behaviour disorder.

It is more difficult to find powerful discriminants of anxious behaviour. The two principal reasons for this are that parental behaviour and attitudes which strongly discriminate the aggressive and the mixed cases do not discriminate the anxious cases from the

Table 45 The interaction of environment, high intelligence, major fits, and female sex as constraints on anxious behaviour in 118 epileptic children

Environmental hazards	— 61								+ 57							
Intelligence	— 28				+ 33				— 34				+ 23			
Major Fits	— 22		+ 6		— 24		+ 9		— 28		+ 6		— 18		+ 5	
Sex	— 10	+ 12	— 5	+ 1	— 18	+ 6	— 7	+ 2	— 19	+ 9	— 3	+ 3	— 12	+ 6	— 0	+ 5
Normal	6	4	2	0	8	4	3	0	1	2	0	1	2	1	0	1
Anxious	1	1	0	0	4	0	4	2	3	2	2	2	4	1	0	2
Aggressive	3	3	2	0	4	0	0	0	10	3	1	0	4	0	0	0
Mixed	0	4	1	1	2	2	0	0	5	2	0	0	2	4	0	2
Anxiety below median	9	7	4	0	12	4	3	0	11	5	1	1	6	1	0	1
Anxiety above median	1	5	1	1	6	2	4	2	8	4	2	2	6	5	0	4
Constraints	0	S	M	MS	I	IS	IM	IMS	E	ES	EM	EMS	EI	EIS	EIM	EIMS

Note: The 'Constraint' cells at the bottom of the table indicate the combinations of hypothetical factors influencing aggressive behaviour. Thus IMS, for example, indicates that the cases in this category have high intelligence, major fits, and are female. '+' indicates female sex in the fourth row of horizontal cells, high intelligence in the second row, and major fits in the third row.

Table 46 A test of the independence of the constraints on anxious behaviour

(*Data from Table 45*)

(*a*) *Environment Hazards*

	E not a constraint (−)	E a constraint (+)	
Anxiety low	39	26	65
Anxiety high	22	31	53
	61	57	118

χ^2 (1 d.f.)=4·03
P less than 0·05, greater than 0·02

(*b*) *High Intelligence*

	I not a constraint (−)	I a constraint (+)	
Anxiety low	38	27	65
Anxiety high	24	29	53
	62	56	118

χ^2 (1 d.f.)=2·01
P less than 0·2, greater than 0·1

(*c*) *Major Fits*

	M not a constraint (−)	M a constraint (+)	
Anxiety low	55	10	65
Anxiety high	37	16	53
	92	26	118

χ^2 (1 d.f.)=3·72
P less than 0·1, greater than 0·05

(*d*) *Female Sex*

	S not a constraint (−)	S a constraint (+)	
Anxiety low	46	19	65
Anxiety high	28	25	53
	74	44	118

χ^2 (1 d.f.)=4·02
P less than 0·05, greater than 0·02

Table 47 The number of constraints and the proportion of cases who have high anxiety scores

No. of constraints	*Low anxiety score*		*High anxiety score*		*Proportion with high anxiety score*
	n	*cum. p.*	*n*	*cum. p.*	
0	9	0·14	1	0·02	0·1
1 (S, M, I, E)	34	0·66	20	0·04	0·37
2 (MS, IS, IM, ES, EM, EI)	19	0·95	19	0·75	0·5
3 (IMS, EMS, EIS, EIN)	2	0·98	9	0·92	0·82
4 (EIMS)	1	1·0	4	1·0	0·8
Totals	65		53		

Significance: Kolmogorov-Smirnov one-tailed test: Distribution of constraints between low anxiety and high anxiety categories:
χ^2 (2 d.f.)$=7{\cdot}89$
P less than 0·02, greater than 0·01
Data from Table 45

normal; and the tendency, in several areas, for the mixed cases to resemble the aggressive cases more closely than the normal ones. Only two variables discriminate both the anxious and the mixed cases from normal at a significant level—environmental hazards and female sex.

What these tables have not demonstrated is whether particular combinations of variables form significant factors in the statistical sense of the term. We have attempted such an analysis, making (perhaps unwarrantedly) parametric and equal interval assumptions for the data, in Ch. 28. This analysis does in fact also confirm the interaction hypothesis.

28 A parametric study of the data

In Ch. 2, pp. 6–12, in a discussion of the methods used in the analysis of data, we concluded that in the present study the most appropriate statistics were non-parametric ones, which did not make assumptions of normal distribution or equal interval measures. But we also noted that some writers (e.g. Labowitz, 1967) have argued that parametric statistics could be used with such data because the error involved in so doing was small and the increase in the refinement and speed of analysis was very great.

As a conclusion to the empirical study of the interaction of social, psychological and biological factors leading to behaviour disorder in epileptic children, we have undertaken a parametric analysis of the data, using the method of product moment correlations and factor analysis by the principal components method. The analysis required that data should be complete for each case, and in order to achieve this we have omitted from the analysis data about verbal-performance discrepancy, reading and arithmetic ages, and heredity of epilepsy. In addition, six cases for which data were missing on other variables have been omitted, giving an N for this analysis of 112.

The method of principal components analysis extracts 'factors' from a matrix of associations for the data. A factor represents a group of variables which occur together with high frequency. These factors then become variables in their own right. The methods and assumptions of such an analysis are explained by Hope (1968). The programme used in the present analysis is that written by White and Hendrickson[1] for the I.B.M. 70–90 computer of Imperial College, London. This uses the technique of promax rotation in calculating principal components. An example of the use of this programme with non-parametric data is the study by Eysenck and Eysenck (1968),

[1] See Hendrickson and White (1964) for a theoretical discussion of the properties of this programme.

which extracted principal components representing 'neuroticism', 'extraversion' and 'psychotism' from responses to a questionnaire. Answers to questions such as 'Are there people who keep trying to avoid you?' were used to calculate product moment correlations for the resulting factor analysis. The answers to these questions are not normally distributed, but are in most cases 'J' shaped (i.e. the large majority of respondents will answer 'Not at all' to a question such as this), and no assumption about equal intervals can be made about numbers assigned to verbal responses to questions such as this. Despite these probably mild theoretical objections to their method, the authors concluded that their data ' . . . support the notion of a psychoticism factor as one of the major dimensions of personality'.

Methods

The methods used were to correlate the four kinds of behaviour derived from the cluster analysis (Ch. 16)—normal, anxious, aggressive, and mixed; the eighteen items of parental attitudes and behaviour; data on IQ., brain injury, EEG, fit pattern, fit frequency, fit rank, years since first fit, age, sex, linearity and ordinal position. Then the first twelve principal components were calculated. The twelve principal components were then subjected to a further factor analysis and reduced to five components. The process was repeated to reduce the number of components to two, and then one.

Next, the four components with the highest loadings on the four kinds of behaviour—normal, anxious, aggressive and mixed—were located. These components are set out in Tables 48 to 51.

The first twelve components extracted account for 55 per cent of the variance. Behaviour categorized as 'normal' in terms of the cluster analysis technique of Ch. 16 has its highest loading on the final, single component (Table 48). This component, being derived from all of the twelve components extracted, accounts for 55 per cent of the variance.

The 'normal' component

On this component the two highest loadings are 'normal' (—0·68) and 'father's non-support' (0·70). Thirteen of the eighteen items of parental attitudes and behaviour have fairly high loadings on this component indicating as our analysis in Ch. 22 suggested, that there is a generally high and positive intercorrelation among these items.[1]

[1] Fifteen of the eighteen items of parental behaviour have significant, positive associations with one another. The three items which have negative associations with the other items are: mother's over-ambition; mother's non-understanding; and father controlling.

Table 48 The 'normal' component

Variable	*Loading on 'normal' component*
'Normal'	−0·68
'Aggressive'	0·37
'Mixed'	0·33
Mother's anxiety	0·48
Mother's coping	0·51
Mother depressed	0·27
Mother critical	0·51
Mother's sibling preference	0·33
Parental conflict	0·57
Father punishing	0·36
Father controlling	0·22
Father critical	0·53
Mother's guilt	0·36
Mother's non-support	0·42
Mother's over-emphasis	0·24
Father's non-support	0·70
Mother's guilt (cause)	0·22
Environment hazards	0·26
Brain injury	0·30
IQ (low to high)	−0·44
Immature EEG	−0·42
Epileptic EEG	−0·33
Petit mal EEG	−0·23
Petit mal fits	−0·55
Major fits	−0·21
Minor fits	0·41
Linearity (less to more)	0·34

Note: Insignificant factor loadings, below 0·20, have been omitted.

Environmental hazards, and brain injury are positively correlated with this component. IQ, as our previous analysis suggests is negatively correlated—i.e. normal behaviour and high IQ go together in being negatively correlated with this component. Five neurological variables (immature, epileptic and *petit mal* EEGs, and *petit mal* and major fits) are negatively correlated with this component—i.e. are associated with normal behaviour. But minor fits, as in our earlier analysis are inversely related to normal behaviour. The interesting variable of linearity also has a positive loading on this component. This means that *high* linearity is associated with abnormal behaviour, a finding reported in the non-parametric analysis in Chapter 26. In terms of previous work this finding is paradoxical and extremely interesting.

One point which should be stressed is that the technique we are using calculates the correlation of items with the component *after* accounting for the correlation of the items with each other. Thus, for example, both *petit mal* fits and *petit mal* EEG are both negatively associated with this component. In fact in the product moment correlation matrix these two variables have a correlation of 0·25; they are significantly and positively correlated with one another (although the correlation, in terms of the amount of variance it accounts for, is small). The correlation of the two variables with the component 'holds constant' the association of these two variables with one another. From the point of view of our interaction hypothesis, the items identified as correlated with a component of behaviour are correlated with that component independently of one another.

Table 49 The 'anxious' component

Variable	*Loading on 'anxious' component*
'Anxious'	−0·51
'Normal'	0·37
Mother's anxiety	−0·49
Mother's coping	−0·40
Mother depressed	−0·52
Mother critical	−0·24
Mother's over-ambition	0·21
Mother's irritation	−0·59
Father controlling	0·33
Father critical	−0·29
Mother's guilt	−0·46
Mother's non-understanding	0·20
Mother's over-emphasis	−0·28
Father's non-support	−0·26
Mother's guilt (cause)	−0·34
Age (younger to older)	0·29
Sex (male)	0·36
Environmental hazards	−0·33
IQ (low to high)	−0·52
Immature EEG	−0·49
Epileptic EEG	−0·26
Major fits	−0·31
Fit rank	−0·30
Social class (high to low)	0·21

Note: Insignificant factor loadings, below 0·20, have been omitted.

Table 50 The 'aggressive' component

Variable	*Loading on 'aggressive' component*
'Aggressive'	−0·73
'Normal'	0·32
'Anxious'	0·28
Mother's anxiety	−0·21
Mother's coping	−0·52
Mother depressed	−0·22
Mother critical	−0·72
Mother's sibling preference	−0·65
Mother's irritation	−0·58
Parental conflict	−0·38
Father punishing	−0·21
Father controlling	−0·22
Father critical	−0·47
Mother's non-support	−0·50
Mother's non-understanding	−0·29
Father's non-support	−0·64
Brain injury	−0·28
Temporal lobe EEG	−0·20
Generalized EEG	−0·53
Normal EEG	0·42
Minor major fits	0·27
Major fits	0·26
Minor fits	−0·42
Fit rank	−0·25
Years since 1st fit	−0·30
1st or last born	−0·33

Note: Insignificant factor loadings, below 0·20, have been omitted.

The 'anxious' component

The component on which 'anxious' behaviour has its highest loading is the seventh of the twelve first-order components, and accounts for 6·5 per cent of the variance (Table 49). The highest loadings are on mother's irritation (−0·59), mother's depression (−0·52), and 'anxiety' (−0·51). It is interesting to note that on three of the parental attitudes—mother's over-ambition, mother's non-understanding, and father controlling—there are positive loadings, i.e. these items are inversely related to anxiety in the children.

The age and sex loadings suggest that children who are anxious tend to be young and female. Both environmental hazards and I.Q. have negative loadings (i.e. are associated with anxiety) as would be predicted from the non-parametric analysis. Three interesting neurological correlations of anxiety are immature EEG, epileptic EEG and major fits. This last variable emerged as a correlate of anxiety in the non-parametric analysis above, but the association of the epileptic and the immature EEGs is an interesting new finding. The association of fit rank (i.e. of the outward manifestations of the the fit) with anxiety was shown in Table 10 in Ch. 18.

The 'aggressive' component

The 'aggressive' component is the second of the first-order factors, and accounts for 12·7 per cent of the variance. Its highest loadings are 'aggression' (—0·73), mother's sibling preference (—0·65), and father's non-support (—0·64). The neurological factor with the highest loading is generalized EEG (—0·53). This is in keeping with our previous findings. Minor fits too are correlated with the component in the expected direction, but an interesting and unexpected finding is the loading of —0·20 of temporal lobe EEG. Being first or last born (loading —0·33) is another possible index of brain damage.

The 'mixed' component

This component is the third of the first-order components, and accounts for 7 per cent of the variance. Its highest loadings are

Table 51 The 'mixed' component

Variable	*Loading on 'mixed' component*
'Mixed'	—0·63
'Normal'	0·47
'Anxious'	—0·30
'Aggressive'	—0·26
Parental conflict	—0·38
Father punishing	—0·25
Mother's non-understanding	0·25
Mother's over-emphasis	—0·21
Petit mal EEG	0·28
Petit mal fits	0·22
Minor major fits	0·27
Minor fits	—0·30
Mental illness in child's relatives	—0·20

Note: Insignificant factor loadings, below 0·20, have been omitted.

'mixed' (—0·63), 'normal' (0·47), and parental conflict (—0·38). As expected, the 'anxious' and 'aggressive' types of behaviour have moderate but significant correlations with the component in the same direction as 'mixed' behaviour disorder. The highest neurological correlate is minor fits (—0·30) but *petit mal* EEG is related to the component in the opposite direction (0·28). The correlation of 'mental illness in the child's relatives' with this component of 'mixed' behaviour disorder is interesting, and deserves further study.

Conclusions

The results of the principal components analysis are encouraging, since the results show a good concordance with the results of the non-parametric analysis.[1] The results support, too, our hypothesis that behaviour disorder in epileptic children is the result of the *interaction* of a number of factors. This is shown most clearly in the 'normal' component, which summarizes the whole of the principal components analysis. Parental attitudes, environmental hazards, brain injury, IQ minor fits and linearity are all associated with this component in the opposite direction of normality, and associated independently of any association they have with one another. The potential usefulness of this parametric technique is illustrated by its apparent sensitiveness in locating some inverse correlates of disturbed behaviour—immature, epileptic, and *petit mal* EEG and *petit mal* fits—which had been largely unnoticed in the non-parametric analysis. While we cannot be exactly sure of the degree of error involved in the parametric analysis, its usefulness with categorical and ordinal data is clearly demonstrated by this analysis.

Used with care, and with proper regard for the possibility of error in its method, the technique can be used with 'soft' data, not least because of the extreme rapidity with which high-speed computers can perform such tasks. In undertaking further studies of this kind, we would first carry out a standard parametric analysis, which would illustrate the main trends in the data and suggest specific hypotheses. These would then be examined in detail, using the more statistically correct non-parametric methods. One disadvantage of the principal components method is that it is based on an *R*-matrix of characteristics, rather than a *Q*-matrix of individuals. The cluster analysis reported in Ch. 16 analysed the characteristics of individuals; but in the analysis in the present chapter we have lost sight of individuals. When we are dealing with hospital patients for whom we wish to derive optimum *individual* strategies, this is a serious drawback.

[1] A principal components analysis has been carried out on the thirty-nine items of child behaviour, and this categorization has an excellent concordance with the results of the cluster analysis employed in the study.

29 Conclusion: the integration of sociology, psychology and biology

We have led the reader through what must, at times have seemed a bewildering complexity of neurological, social and psychological data. It is not customary for a single work to range over several disciplines in this way, but we undertook the study with a specific theoretical perspective outlined in detail in an earlier study (Bagley, 1967): that of providing some base lines and experimentation in the difficult and interesting area of the integration of sociology, biology and psychology.[1]

A number of writers have offered valuable perspectives on the possibilities of integrating disciplines concerned with individual man (e.g. psychology) and those concerned with social man (e.g. sociology): Georg Simmel on the 'inner unity' of an individual who is faced dialectically with a range of group interests (Levine, 1965); George H. Mead (1956) on the interaction between the individual and the social world; Gardner Murphy (1947) on the interaction of genetics, physiology and psychology (including perception of the social world); Spiro (1951) on how the individual, possessing a psychobiological constitution, learns social system behaviour through his interaction with others; Parsons and Shils (1951) on individuals with 'need dispositions' interacting with others to form an agreed structure of values, norms and symbols guiding behaviour; Parsons (1964) on the similarity of Durkheim and Freud on the internalization of the moral rules of society; Sullivan (1965) on the basic similarity of psychiatry and social science, stressing that abnormality of behaviour only has meaning within the context of interaction with others; Kluckhohn and Murray (1964) on personality in nature, society and culture; Morris (1956) on the interaction of social, psychological

[1] We also have an obvious clinical or empirical interest in using this integrated approach to show as exactly as possible what factors underlie behaviour disorder in epileptic children.

and biological factors in determining values in six cultures.

We argued (Bagley, 1967) that none of these writers, with the exception perhaps of Morris, has developed a clear conceptual scheme allowing due weight to the *three* determinants of personality—social, psychological and biological. Many lay stress on only two ignoring relevant work in, say, the biological field. Moreover, few of these models are based on empirical studies.

Our own solution to the problem of integrating the sciences of human behaviour—individual and social—is implicit in the present study of behaviour disorder in epileptic children. The writer is by training a sociologist, but has been influenced, working in the fields of education and medicine, by psychological and biological perspectives of behaviour. His conception of sociology is similar to that of Sir John Bucknill, who was first editor of the *Journal of Mental Science*. This journal changed its title in 1963 to the *British Journal of Psychiatry*, and the editor, Dr Eliot Slater, quoted Bucknill's editorial to the very first number. Bucknill wrote that he intended to deal with 'mental science in its practical, that is in its *sociological* point of view', and to cover 'mental physiology and pathology, with their vast range of inquiry into insanity, education, crime and all things which tend to preserve mental health or to cause mental disease'. (Italics added.)

This is probably one of the most explicit statements of the Comtean notion of sociology as a generalized science of social and mental life, with a final rationale in the understanding of individual behaviour.[1]

Our argument for the unification of the sciences of human behaviour is as follows: the individual is endowed at birth with potentialities for action. These potentialities are acquired through heredity, and through organic trauma before and during birth. Personality is formed by the way in which other people (notably the child's parents) interact with the child. The responses to the behaviour of others are influenced both by the nature of that behaviour and the child's innate response tendencies.

As the child grows older, he internalizes moral norms from his parents, peers and teachers, and is assigned an increasing complexity of roles to perform. How he performs these roles will depend on his personality—his chronic style of action. It is perfectly legitimate to study just one aspect of human behaviour, such as the influence of

[1] Cf. Fletcher (1966) on *Auguste Comte and the Making of Sociology*:
'He is surely right in maintaining that the *social* framework of reference is essential for the psychological study of the human individual, and that sociology and psychology should work in the closest combination. One of the tragedies—one might almost say one of the inanities—of the present-day situation is that, in so many of our universities, psychology and sociology have come to be not only separated from each other, but in a state of enmity with each other: a fantastic situation!'

body type, or parental behaviour, or peer group pressure, or rapid social change, on the way individuals behave. But it is inadmissible for any one discipline to claim that these are the only factors influencing the behaviour in question.

Disciplines working in isolation and in enmity with one another, but on essentially the same problem may produce diametrically opposed solutions to the same problem. Stott (1964), for example, writing about delinquency has pointed out that

> . . . our present disagreements about delinquency constitute an epistemologically intolerable situation. We have two disciplines—sociology and psychology—each, in their extreme wings, offering theories about causation and denigrating those of the other discipline.[1]

The behavioural scientist is driven by a categorical imperative to seek for truth in his study of behaviour. He may not ritualistically defend the status of his own department or discipline at the expense of scientific study. In the final analysis the social scientist *must* take account of the work of psychologists and physiologists whose work has a bearing on the subject he is studying, such as deviant behaviour.

In the field of behaviour disorders in epileptic children we have noted that various writers have offered apparently conflicting explanations of deviant behaviour in the children. But we have shown that none of the various factors implicated—social, psychological, biological—can by themselves fully explain this behaviour.

The behaviour of children is easier to study than that of adults, because the number of roles a child has to perform is much less than for an adult. The child has three chief roles—as a son or daughter, as a pupil and as a member of one or more peer groups. In this study we have only dealt in any systematic way with the first role, which involves the behaviour of the parent towards the child, and the child's behaviour in relation to his parent. The determinants of role behaviour are first of all, the normative rules governing such behaviour. If there are conflicting normative standards (e.g. parental disagreement on behaviour appropriate in the child, or peer group pressure to behave differently from parental norms of behaviour), 'deviance' or disorganized behaviour may result.

The self-perception that a person has of his own worth can fundamentally influence his role behaviour. This self-concept is derived from his interaction with others and the perception that others have of him. The symbolic interactionist theorists have provided evidence that individuals tend to internalize the concept of

[1] Cf. our attempts to formulate integrated theories of suicide (Bagley, 1968), incest behaviour and taboo (Bagley, 1969) and schizophrenia (Davison and Bagley, 1970).

themselves given to them by others (e.g. Rose 1962; Meadow, 1969), a self-concept which in turn profoundly influences an individual's behaviour.

The individual's performance of roles in the social system is influenced, too, by his psychobiological predisposition towards action (e.g. extraversion-introversion), and this predisposition can also be influenced by organic factors, such as hyperactivity due to organic brain damage.

The epileptic child is open to a number of influences upon his behaviour in the role of son or daughter. The way the parents perceive him and behave towards him is of fundamental importance for his own behaviour. How he reacts to his parents' behaviour is in turn influenced by his innate psychological disposition to action, his cognitive state (e.g. the ability to process and organize information from significant others), the structural constraints on behaviour (e.g. poverty, overcrowding), type of epileptic fit and location of brain damage.

All of these factors are largely independent of one another, and interact in a complex way to influence the degree of, and kind of, disturbed role behaviour ('child psychiatric disorder') in the child.

Sociology, psychology and biology merge in describing constraints on *role behaviour*.[1] All of these factors have a profound influence on such behaviour, and in the interests of scientific inquiry all of them should be considered in offering explanations of behaviour. The purpose of sociology *is* to offer explanations of behaviour of man the social animal behaving in a social world. Our ultimate purpose is to explain, for example, why *this man* committed suicide, and to know how people facing similar stresses may be helped.

A variety of studies may have contributed to such knowledge: Durkheim, and Gibbs and Martin on the stability and clarity of norms governing behaviour; studies on the relationship of parental loss and later suicide and attempted suicide; studies of amine deficiency in the brains of suicides; and studies of body build and endocrine factors. These factors (reviewed by the writer, 1968) have all been validly and independently identified as being associated with suicide. It is the *combination* of these factors which influences any individual in the direction of suicide. At any one time the number of people in a state of profound *anomie* (normative confusion about role behaviour) may be very great, and much greater than the score or so of individuals per 100,000 population who kill themselves each year. The determinant of suicide is not *anomie* as such, but the coincidence of states of social structure with individuals whose psychological experience and psychobiological constitution dispose

[1] Cf. proposals for integrating different kinds of study of human behaviour proposed by Emmett (1960) and Inkeles (1963).

them to negative self-evaluation and self-destructive behaviour.

The theory applies equally to behaviour disorders in epileptic children. These are influenced (Ch. 27) by the variety of factors we have identified. The degree and type of the behaviour disorder is influenced by the *particular combinations* of these constraints in any one individual. In the final analysis we have to consider the uniqueness of each individual in our matrix. Our social matrix is a matrix of individuals interacting with one other, and in so doing forming agreement on the kinds of roles which are to make up a social system, and how these roles are to be performed. Describing the social system (e.g. as in organization theory) is a necessary precursor to understanding role behaviour. But role behaviour *in the final analysis* can only be adequately explained by reference to individuals occupying those roles.[1]

Our position, in sum, is that sociology, psychology and biology can merge in describing constraints on *role behaviour*. Sociology has the task, too, of describing how roles develop within social systems, and how roles are related to one another. It is the task of social scientists to integrate studies of the various constraints upon role behaviour.

[1] Cf. Popper (1961), p.136: '. . . the task of social theory is to construct and to analyse our sociological models carefully in descriptive or nominalist terms, that is to say, *in terms of individuals*, of their attitudes, expectations, relations, etc.—a postulate which may be called "methodological individualism".' (Italics in original.) Cf. also Homans (1964): ' . . . the same set of general propositions . . . are needed for explaining the phenomena of both personality and society'.

Bibliography

AALL-JILEK, L. (1965), 'Epilepsy in the Wapagora Tribe in Tanganyika' *Acta Psychiat. Scand.*, *61*, (57–86).

ACHENBACH, T. (1966), 'The Classification of Children's Psychiatric Symptoms', *Psychol. Monograph*, *80*, No. 7.

ADEY, W. R. (1959) 'Recent Studies of the Rhinencephalon in Relation to Temporal Lobe Epilepsy and Behaviour Disorders', *Internat. Rev. Neurobiol.*, *1*, (1–47).

AIRD, R. (1959), 'Modern Concepts on the Value of E.E.G. in Epilepsy', *Int. J. Neurol.*, *1*, (66–75).

AIRD, R. and TSUBAKI, T. (1958), 'Common Sources of Error in the Diagnosis and Treatment of Convulsive Disorders, *J. Nerv. Ment. Dis.*, *127*, (400–6).

AIRD, R. VENTURINI, A., and SPIELMAN, P. (1967), 'Antecedents of Temporal Lobe Epilepsy', *Arch. Neurol.*, *16*, (67–73).

ALSTRÖM, C. H. (1950), 'Epilepsy in Its Clinical, Social and Genetic Aspects', *Acta Psychiat. Neurol. Scand. Suppl.*, *63*.

ALTABLE, J. P. (1947), 'Rorschach Psychodiagnosis in a Group of Epileptic Children', *Nervous Child*, *6*, (22–33).

AMYOT, R. (1957), 'Des Faites nouveaux en Sclerose en Plaques et Schizophrenie', *Union Med. du Canada*, *86*, (781–4).

BAER, P. E. (1961), 'Problems in the Differential Diagnosis of Brain Damage and Childhood Schizophrenia', *Am. J. Orthopsychiat.*, *31*, (728–38).

BAGLEY, C. (1965), 'Juvenile Delinquency in Exeter: and Ecological and Comparative Study', *Urban Studies*, *2*, (33–50).

BAGLEY, C. (1966), 'Does candidates' Position on the Ballot Paper influence Voters' Choice? A Study of the 1959 and 1964 British General Elections', *Parl. Affairs*, *59*, (162–74).

BAGLEY, C. (1967), 'On the Integration of Sociology, Psychology and Biology', Part III of 'Studies in the Scope of Social Administration', unpublished M.A. thesis, University of Essex.

BAGLEY, C. (1968), 'The Evaluation of a Suicide Prevention Scheme by an Ecological Method, *Soc. Sci. and Med.*, *2*, (1–14).

BAGLEY, C. (1969), 'Incest Behaviour and Incest Taboo', *Social Problems*, *16*, (505–19).

BAGLEY, C. (1970), 'The Educational Performance of Children with Epilepsy', *Brit. J. Ed. Psychol.*, *40*, (82–3).

BAGLEY, C. and EVAN-WONG, L. (1970), 'Psychiatric Disorder and Adult and Peer Group Rejection of the Child's Name', *J. Child Psychol. Psychiat.*, *11*, (19–27).

BAKER, H. and TRAPHAGEN, V. (1936), *The Diagnosis and Treatment of Behavior Problem Children*, New York: Macmillan.

BALBERNIE, R. (1966), *Residential Work with Children*, Oxford: Pergamon Press.

BANAY, R. (1961), 'Criminal Genesis and the Degrees of Responsibility in Epilepsies', *Am. J. Psychiat.*, *117*, (873–6).

BANISTER, H. and RAUDEN, M. (1944), 'The Problem Child and His Environment, *Brit. J. Psychol.*, *34*, (60–5).

BARTHEIMER, L. (1942), 'Some Observations on Convulsive Disorders in Children', *Amer. J. Orthopsychiat.*, *2*, (260–7).

BEARD, A. W. (1963), 'The Schizophrenia-like Psychoses of Epilepsy: (ii) Physical Aspects', *Brit. J. Psychiat.*, *109*, (458).

BECK, H. S. (1959), 'Comparison of Convulsive Organic, Non-convulsive Organic, and Non-organic Public School Children', *Amer. J. Ment. Defic.*, *63* (866–75).

BECKER, W. C. and KRUG, R. S. (1965), 'The Parent Attitude Research Instrument: a Research Review', *Child Develop.*, *36* (329–65).

BELLAK, L. (1958), *Schizophrenia*, New York: Logos Press.

BENDER, L. (1961), 'Childhood Schizophrenia and Convulsive States', in Wortis, J. (ed.), *Recent Advances in Biological Psychiatry*, New York: Grune and Stratton.

BENNETT, A. E. (1962), 'Psychiatric Aspects of Psychomotor Epilepsy', *Calif. Med.*, *97*, (346–49).

BENNETT, A. E. (1965), 'Mental Disorders Associated with Temporal Lobe Epilepsy', *Dis. Nerv. Syst.*, *26*, (275–80).

BENNETT, C. A. and FRANKLIN, N. L. (1954), *Statistical Analysis in Chemistry and the Chemical Industry*, New York: John Wiley.

BENNETT, I. (1960), *Delinquent and Neurotic Children*, London: Tavistock.

BINGEL, A. (1967), 'Misinterpretation of Encephalographic Findings', *Int. J. Neuropsychiat.*, *3*, (29–39).

BIRCH, H. (ed.) (1965), *Brain Damage in Children: Biological and Social Aspects*, London: Ballière.

BIRCH, H., THOMAS, A. and CHESS, S. (1964), 'Behavioural Development in Brain-damaged Children', *Arch. Gen. Psychiat.*, *11*, (596–603).

BLAU, A. (1937), 'Mental Changes following Head Trauma to Children', *Arch. Neurol. Psychiat.*, *35*, (723–69).

BLEULER, E. (1960), *Textbook of Psychiatry*, London: Allen and Unwin.

BLUM, H. (1954), 'A Note on the Reliability of Electro-encephalographic Judgments', *Neurology*, *4*, (143–6).

BLUMER, D. and WALKER, A. (1967), 'Sexual Behaviour in Temporal Lobe Epilepsy', *Arch. Neurol.*, *16* (37–43).

BOTTOMS, A. E. (1967), 'Delinquency amongst Immigrants', *Race*, *8*, (357–83).

BOWSHER, D. (1961), *Introductory to Neuroanatomy*, Oxford: Blackwell.

BOZZO, M. and GIUGANINO, B. (1965), 'A Study of the Correlations between the E.E.G. Findings and the Results of the Wechsler Intelligence Scale for Children', *Arch. Psicol. Neurol. Psichiat.*, *26*, (401–11).

BRADLEY, C. (1947), 'Treatment of the Convulsive Child in a Children's Psychiatric Hospital', *Nerv. Child.*, *6* (76–85).

BRADLEY, C. (1951), 'Behavior Disturbances in Epileptic Children', *J. Am. Med. Ass.*, *146*, (436–41).

BRADLEY, C. and BOWEN, M. (1941), 'Amphetamine Therapy of Children's Behavior Disorder', *Am. J. Orthopsychiat.*, *11*, (92).

BRADY, J. P. (1964), 'Epilepsy and Disturbed Behaviour', *J. Nerv. Ment. Dis.*, *138*, (468–73).

BRAIN, W. (1926), 'The Inheritance of Epilepsy', *Quart. J. Med.*, (299–309).

BRAIN, LORD (1956), *Diseases of the Nervous System* (5th ed.), Oxford University Press.

BRAZIER, M. (1961), *Computer Techniques in E.E.G. Analysis*, Amsterdam: Elsevier.

BREWIS, H., POSKARIZER, D., HOLLAND, C. and MILLER, H. (1966), 'Neurological Disease in an English City', *Acta Neurol. Scand. Suppl.*, *24*.

BRIDGE, E. (1934), 'Mental State of the Epileptic Patient', *Arch. Neurol. Psychiat.*, *32*, (723–36).

BRIDGE, E. (1949), *Epilepsy and Convulsive Disorders in Children*, New York: McGraw Hill.

BRIKMAYER, W. and LENZ, H. (1938), 'Mitteilung eines Falles von Friedrichscher Ataxia und Schizophrenia', *Wien. Klin. Wochenschr.*, *52*, (667–9).

BROMBERG, W. (1966), *Crime and the Mind*, New York: Collier-Macmillan.

BROME, V. (1966), *The World of Luke Simpson*, London: Heinemann.

BROWN, G. W. and RUTTER, M. (1966), 'The Measurement of Family Activities and Relationships', *Hum. Relat.*, *19*, (241–63).

BURNS, C. L. C. (1959), 'Maladjusted Children in Grammar Schools', *Brit. J. Ed. Psychol.*, *29*, (198–206).

BURT, C. (1952), 'The Nature and Causes of Maladjustment among Children of School Age', *Brit. J. Psychol. Stat. Section*, *5*, (39–57).

BURTON, L. (1965), 'The Child in the Road Accident', *New Society*, 6 May, (10–12).

CAIRNS, H. (1950), 'Mental Disorders with Tumours of the Pons', *Folia Psychiat. Neurol. Neurochir. Neerl.*, *53*, (193–203).

CARTER, J. D. (1947), 'Children's Expressed Attitudes toward Their Epilepsy', *Nerv. Child.*, *6*, (34–7).

CASTANEDA, A. (1956), 'Complex Learning and Performance of Anxiety in Children and Task Difficulty', *Child. Devel.*, *27*, (327–32).

CAVENESS, W. F., MERRITT, H. H., GALLUP, G. H. and RUBY, E. H. (1965), 'A Survey of Public Attitudes toward Epilepsy in 1964', *Epilepsia*, *6*, (75–86).

CAZZULLO, Q. C. (1959), 'Psychiatric Aspects of Epilepsy', *Int. J. Neurol.*, *1*, (53–65).

CHAMPION, D. (1968), 'Some Observations on Measurement and Statistics: Comment', *Social Forces*, *46*, (541).

CHAUNDRY, M. and POND, D. (1961), 'Mental Deterioration in Epileptic Children', *J. Neurol. Neurosurg. Psychiat.*, *24*, (213–19).

CHEN, C. and HIGGINS, C. (1966), 'Children's Behaviour Disorders and E.E.G. Patterns', *Dis. Nerv. Syst.*, *27*, (52–6).

CHESS, S. and BIRCH, H. (1963), 'Interaction of Temperament and Environment in the Production of Behavioral Disturbances in Children', *Am. J. Psychiat. 120*, (142–7).

CHESSICK, R. and BOLIN, R. (1962), 'Psychiatric Study of Patients with Psychomotor Seizures', *J. Nerv. Ment. Dis.*, *134*, (72–9).

CHILD, D. (1966), 'Personality and Social Status', *Brit. J. Soc. Clin. Psychol.*, *5*, (196–9).

CHRISTIAN, W. (1957), 'E.E.G.—Befund bei einem Fall von Epileptischer Halluzinose', *Dtsch. Z. Nervenheilk.*, *176*, (693–700).

CHRISTIAN, W. (1962), 'E.E.G.—Verandergungen bei der Psychomotorischen Epilepsie', *Dtsch. Z. Nervenheilk.*, *183*, (218–44).

CLARK, L. P. (1917), *Clinical Studies in Epilepsy*, Utica: State Hospital Press.

CLARK, L. P. (1927), 'A Critical Discussion of the Constitutional Anomalies of Epileptics', *Psychiat. Quart.*, *1*, (26–43).

COBB, S. (1940), 'Psychiatric Approach to the Treatment of Epilepsy', *Am. J. Psychiat.*, *96*, (1,009–22).

COHEN, J. (1969), 'Multiple Regression as a General Data-analytic System', *Psychological Bulletin*, *70* (426–43).

COHEN, LORD (1956), *Medical Care of Epileptics*, London: H.M.S.O. (Central Health Services Council).

COHEN, LORD (1958), 'Epilepsy as a Social Problem', *Brit. Med. J.*, i, (672–5).

COLEMAN, J. (1964), *Introduction to Mathematical Sociology*, New York: Free Press.

COLLINS, L. F., MAXWELL, A. E. and CAMERON, K. (1962), 'A Factor Analysis of Some Child Psychiatric Clinic Data', *J. Ment. Sci.*, *108*, (274–85).

COLLINS, L. F., MAXWELL, A. E. and CAMERON, K. (1963), 'An Analysis of the Case Material of the Younger Maladjusted Child', *Brit. J. Psychiat.*, *109*, (758–65).

COLLVER, A., HARE, R. and SPREARE, M. (1967), 'Factors Influencing the Use of Maternal Health Services', *Soc. Sci. and Med.*, *1*, (293–308).

COLLVER, T. and KERRIDGE, O. F. (1962), 'Birth Order in Epileptic Children', *J. Neurol. Neurosurg. Psychiat.*, *25*, (59–62).

COMFORT, A. (1967), *The Anxiety Makers*, London: Nelson.

CONNERS, C. and GREENFIELD, D. (1966), 'Habituation of Motor Startle in Anxious and Restless Children', *J. Child Psychol. Psychiat.*, *7*, (125–32).

CONRAD, K. (1937), 'Heredity in Epilepsy, IV: a Study of the Child of Epileptic Parents', *Zeitschr. f.d.ges. Neurol. Psychiat.*, *159*, (521–40).

COOPER, J. E. (1965), 'Epilepsy in a Longitudinal Survey of 5,000 Children', *Brit. Med. J.*, i, (1,020–2).

CRASKE, S., ELITHORN, A. and BAGLEY, C., 'Psychiatric Symptoms as Side-effects of Anti-convulsants', unpublished paper.

CREAK, M. (1961), 'Schizophrenic Syndrome in Children', *Brit. Med. J.*, ii, (889–90).

CREAK, E. M. (1963), 'Childhood Psychosis: a Review of 100 Cases', *Brit. J. Psychiat.*, *109*, (84–9).

CRUICKSHANK, W. (ed.) (1966), *The Teacher of Brain-injured Children*, Syracuse University Press.

CURRIER, R., KOOI, K. and SAIDMAN, L. (1963), 'Prognosis of "Pure" *Petit Mal*', *Neurology*, *13*, (959–67).

DAUBROS, S. and DANIELS, G. (1966), 'An Experimental Approach to the Reduction of Overactive Behaviour', *Behav. Res. Therap.*, *4*, (251–8).

DAVIDOFF, E. (1947), 'The Treatment of Institutionalized Epileptic Children', *Neur. Child.*, *6*, (57–75).

DAVIDOFF, R. and JOHNSON, L. (1964), 'Paroxysmal E.E.G. Activity and Cognitive-motor Performance', *Electroenceph. Clin. Neurophysiol.*, *16*, (343–54).

DAVIDSON, M., MCINNES, R. and PARNELL, R. (1957), 'The Distribution of Personality Traits in Seven-year-old Children: a Combined Psychological, Psychiatric and Somatotype Study', *Brit. J. Ed. Psychol.*, *27*, (48–61).

DAVIES, B. and MORGANSTERN, F. (1960), 'A Case of Cysticercosis, Temporal Lobe Epilepsy and Transvestism', *J. Neurol. Neurosurg. Psychiat.*, *23*, (247–9).

DAVIES-EYSENCK, M. (1952), 'Cognitive Factors in Epilepsy', *J. Neurol. Neurosurg. Psychiat.*, *15*, (39–44.)

DAVIS, D. R. and KENT, M. (1955), 'Psychological Factors in Educational Disability', *Proc. Roy. Soc. Med.*, *48*, (993).

DAVIS, R. (1959), 'Explosive or Episodic Behaviour Disorders in Children as Epileptic Equivalents', *Med. J. Aust.*, *2*, (474–81).

DAVISON, K. and BAGLEY, C. (1970), *Schizophrenia-Like Psychoses Associated with Organic Disorders of the Central Nervous System*, London: Royal Medico Psychological Association.

DAWSON, S. and CONN, J. (1929), 'The Intelligence of Epileptic Children', *Arch. Dis. Chil.*, *4*, (142–51).

DELAY, J., PICHOT, P., LEMPÉRIERE, T. and PERSE, J. (1955), *Le Test de Rorschach et la Personnalité Épileptique*, Paris: Presses Universitaires de France.

DENHOFF, E. and HOLDEN, R. (1954), 'Family Influence on Successful School Adjustment of Cerebral Palsied Children', *Except. Child*, *20*, (5–8).

DENNERILL, R., RODIN, E., GONZALEZ, S., SCHWARTZ, M. and LIN, Y. (1966), 'Neurological and Psychological Factors related to Employability of Persons with Epilepsy', *Epilepsy*, *7*, (318–29).

DEUTSCH, C. (1953), 'Differences among Epileptics and between Epileptics and Non-epileptics in Terms of Some Memory and Learning Variables', *Arch. Neurol. Psychiat.*, *70*, (474–82).

DEUTSCH, L., and WIENER, L. (1948), 'Children with Epilepsy: Emotional Problems and Treatment', *Amer. J. Orthopsychiat.*, *18*, (65–72).

DIETHELM, O. (1934), 'Epileptic Convulsions and the Personality Setting', *Arch. Neurol. Psychiat.*, *31*, (755–67).

DIETHELM, O. (1948), 'Differential Diagnosis of Epilepsy', *in* Hoch, P. and Knight, R. (eds.), *Epilepsy*, London: Heinemann.

DITFURTH, H. V. (1953), 'Zur Problematik der Modernen Epilepsiebehandlung, Zugleich ein Kasuistischer Beitrag Zur Frage der sog. Epilepsiepsychosen', *Nervenarzt 24*, (348–9).

DOUBROS, S. and DANIELS, G. (1966), 'An Experimental Approach to the Reduction of Overactive Behaviour', *Behav. Res. Therap.*, *4*, (251–8).

DOUGLAS, J. and ROSS, J. (1964), 'Age of Puberty related to Educational Ability, Attainment and School Leaving Age', *J. Child Psychol. Psychiat.*, *5*, (185–96).

DOUGLAS, J. ROSS, J. and SIMPSON, H. (1965), 'The Relation between Height and Measured Educational Ability in School Children of the Same Class, Family Size and Stage of Sexual Development', *Human Biol.*, *37*, (178–86).

DOUGLAS, J., ROSS, J. and SIMPSON, H. (1968), 'The Myopic *Élite*', *New Society*, 3 October, (483–4).

DUTRA, V. (1963), 'Behavioural Disorders in Epileptic Children', *J. Brasileiro de Psiquiatria*, *12*, (473–93).

EARL, C. L. (1936), 'The Affective Psychology of Imbecile Children', *Brit. J. Med. Psychol.*, *15*, (266–78).

ECLAND, B. (1967), 'Genetics and Sociology: a Reconsideration', *Am. Soc. Rev.*, *32*, (173–93).

EISENBERG, L. (1957), 'Psychiatric Implications of Brain Damage in Children', *Psychiat. Quart.*, *31*, (77–92).

EISENBERG, L. (1964), 'Behavioral Manifestations of Cerebral Damage in Childhood', *in* Birch, H. (ed.), *Brain Damage in Children*, Baltimore: Williams and Wilkins.

ELLINGSON, R. J. (1966), 'Relationship between E.E.G. and Test Intelligence: a Commentary', *Psychol. Bull.*, *65*, (91–8).

EMMETT, D. (1960), 'How far can Structural Studies take Account of Individuals?', *J. Roy. Anthrop. Inst.*, *90*, (191–200).

EPPS, P. and PARNELL, R. W. (1952), 'Physique and Temperament of Women Delinquents compared with Women Undergraduates', *Brit. J. Med. Psychol.*, *52* (249–55).

EPSTEIN, A. W. (1961), 'Relationship of Fetishism and Transvestism to Brain and particularly to Temporal Lobe Dysfunction', *J. Nerv. Ment. Dis.*, *133*, (247–53).

ERVIN, F., EPSTEIN, A. and KING, H. (1955), 'Behaviour of Epileptic and Non-Epileptic Patients with "Temporal Spikes" ', *Arch. Neurol. Psychiat.*, *74*, (488–97).

EYSENCK, H. and RACHMAN, S. (1965), *The Causes and Cures of Neurosis*, London: Routledge.

EYSENCK, H. J. (1957), *The Dynamics of Anxiety and Hysteria*, London: Routledge & Kegan Paul.

EYSENCK, H. J. (1959), 'The Rees-Eysenck Body Index and Sheldon's Somatype System', *J. Ment. Sci.*, *105*, (1,053–8).

EYSENCK, H. J. (1960), *The Structure of Human Personality*, London: Methuen.

EYSENCK, H. J. and EYSENCK, S. B. G. (1970), *Personality Structure and Measurement*, London: Routledge & Kegan Paul.

EYSENCK, M. D. (1950), 'Neurotic Tendencies in Epilepsy', *J. Neur. Neurosurg. Psychiat.*, *13*, (237–40).

EYSENCK, S. and H. (1968), 'The Measurement of Psychoticism: a Study of Factor Stability and Reliability', *Brit. J. Clin. Soc. Psychol. 7*, (284–94).

FALCONER, M. A. (1965), 'Some Functions of the Temporal Lobes, with Special Regard to Affective Behaviour in Epileptic Seizures', *J. Psychosom. Res.*, *9*, (25–8).

FALCONER, M. and POND, D. (1953), 'Temporal Lobe Epilepsy with Personality and Behaviour Disorders caused by an Unusual Calcifying Lesion', *J. Neurol. Neurosurg. Psychiat.*, *16*, (234–44).

FENICHEL, O. (1945), *Psychoanalytic Theory of Neurosis*, New York: Norton.

FIELD, E. (1967), *Types of Delinquency and Home Background*, London: Home Office Research Unit.

FISCHER, M., KORSAKJAER, G. and PEDERSEU, E. (1965): 'Psychotic Episodes in Zarontin Treatment', *Epilepsia*, *6* (325–33).

FISHER, G. (1965), *The New Form Statistical Tables*, University of London Press.

FLETCHER, R. (1966), *Auguste Comte and the Making of Sociology*, University of London: The Athlone Press.

FOXE, A. (1948), *The Antisocial Aspects of Epilepsy*, London: Heinemann.

FRANKE, G. (1937), 'Erbbiologische Untersuchingen an Kindern von Epileptikern', *Zeitschr.f.d.ges. Neurol. Psychiat.*, *160*, (381–401).

FREMONT-SMITH, F. (1933), 'Influence of Emotion in Precipitating Convulsions', *Arch. Neurol. Psychiat.*, *30*, (234–6).

FROST, B. (1968), 'Anxiety and Educational Achievement', *Brit. J. Ed. Psychol.*, *38*, (293–301).

FUSTER, B., CASTELLS, C. and ETCHVERRY, M. (1954), 'Epileptic Sleep Terrors', *Neurology*, *4*, (531–40).

GASTAUT, H. (1964), 'Proposed International Classification of Epileptic Seizures', *Epilepsia*, 5, (297–306).

GASTAUT, H. *et al.* (1969), 'Epilepsy and Heredity', *Epilepsia*, *10*, (3–96).

GEIST, H. (1962), *The Etiology of Idiopathic Epilepsy*, New York: Exposition Press.

GIBBENS, J. C. N. (1965), 'The Inadequate Recidivist', *Proc. Roy. Soc. Med.*, *58*, (705–6).

GIBBERD, F. B. (1966), 'The Clinical Features of Petit Mal', *Acta Neurol. Scand.*, *42*, (176–90).

GIBBS, F. (1951), 'Ictal and Non-ictal Psychiatric Disorders in Temporal Lobe Epilepsy', *J. Nerv. Ment. Dis.*, *113*, (522–8).

GIBBS, F. (1959), *Epilepsy Handbook*, Oxford: Blackwell.

GIBBS, F. and GIBBS, E. (1952), *Atlas of Electroencephalography*, Vol. II, Cambridge, U.S.A.: Addison-Wesley.

GIBBS, F. and GIBBS, E. (1963), 'Fourteen and Six Per Second Positive Spikes', *EEG Clin. Neurophysiol.*, *15*, (553–8).

GIBBS, F. and STAMPS, F. (1958), *Epilepsy Handbook*, Springfield, Ill.: Thomas.

GIBSON, H. (1968), 'The Measurement of Parental Attitudes and Their Relation to Boys' Behaviour,' *Brit. J. Ed. Psychol.*, *38*, (233–9).

GIEL, R. (1968), 'The Epileptic Outcast', *E. African Med. J.*, *45* (27–31).

GINSBURG, B. (1966), 'All Mice are not created Equal: Recent Findings on Genes and Behaviour', *Social Service Review*, *40*, (121–34).

GLASER, G. and DIXON, M. (1956), 'Psychomotor Seizures in Childhood', *Neurology*, *6*, (646–55).

GLASER, G., NEWMAN, R. and SCHAFER, R. (1963), 'Interictal Psychosis in Psychomotor Temporal Lobe Epilepsy', *in* Glaser, G. (ed.), *E.E.G. and Behaviour*, New York: Basic Books.

GLASER, G. H. (1963), 'The Normal E.E.G. and Its Reactivity', *in* Glaser, G. (ed.), *E.E.G. and Behaviour*, New York: Basic Books.

GLUECK, S. and GLUECK, E. (1950), *Unravelling Juvenile Delinquency*, New York: Commonwealth Fund.

GOLD, S. and NEUFELD, I. (1967), 'Symptom Complexes in Childhood Psychosis', *Aust. N.Z. J. Psychiat.*, *1*, (30–4).

GOLDENSOHN, E. (1963), 'E.E.G. and Ictal and Postictal Behavior', *in* Glaser, G. (ed.), *E.E.G. and Behaviour*, New York: Basic Books.

GOLTSCHALK, L. A. (1953), 'Effects of Intensive Psychotherapy on Epileptic Children: Report on Three Cases with Idiopathic Epilepsy', *Arch. Neurol. Psychiat.*, *70*, (361–84).

GORDON, N. and RUSSELL, S. (1958), 'The Problem of Unemployment among Epileptics', *J. Ment. Sci.*, *104*, (103–14).

GOWER, J. C. (1966), 'Some Distance Properties of Latent Root and Vector Methods used in Multivariate Analysis', *Biometrika*, *53*, (325–38).

GOWER, J. C. (1967), 'A Comparison of Some Methods of Cluster Analysis', *Biometrics*, *23*, (623–37).

GOWERS, W. (1881), *Epilepsy and Other Chronic Convulsive Diseases*, London: Churchill.

GRAHAM, P. and RUTTER, M. (1968), 'Organic Brain Dysfunction and Child Psychiatric Disorder', *Brit. Med. J.*, iii, (695–98).

GREEN, J.B. (1961), 'Association of Behaviour Disorder with an E.E.G. Focus in Children without Seizure', *Neurology*, *11*, (337–44).

GRISSELL, J. L., LEVIN, S. M., COHEN, B. and RODIN, E. (1964), 'Effects of Subclinical Seizure Activity on Overt Behaviour', *Neurology*, *14*, (135–45).

GROSS, M. D. and WILSON, W. C. (1964), 'Behaviour Disorders of Children with Cerebral Dysrhythmias', *Arch. Gen. Psychiat.*, *11*, (610–19).

GRUNBERG, F. and POND, D. (1957), 'Conduct Disorders in Epileptic Children', *J. Neurol. Neurosurg. Psychiat.*, *20*, (66–8).

GUDMUNDSSON, G. (1966), 'Epilepsy in Iceland', *Acta Neurol. Scand. Suppl.*, *25*, (43).

GUERRANT, J., ANDERSON, W., FISCHER, A., WEINSTEIN, M., JAROS, R and DESKINS, A. (1962), *Personality in Epilepsy*, Springfield, Ill.: Thomas.

GUEY, J., CHANES, C., COQUERY, C., ROGER, J. and SALAYROL, R. (1967), 'Study of Psychological Effects of Ethosuximide (Zarontin) on 25 Children suffering from Petit Mal Epilepsy', *Epilepsia*, *8*, (129–41).

GUINENA, Y. (1953), 'The Unitary Conception of the Epilepsies and Psychoses or the Irritative Encephalopathic Syndrome', *J. Roy. Egypt. Med. Ass.*, *36*, (116–42).

GUNN, J. (1969), 'The Prevalence of Epilepsy in Prisoners', *Proc. Roy. Soc. Med.*, *62*, (60–3); and M.D. Thesis, University of Birmingham.

HACHIYA, H. (1960), 'Epileptic Psychosis with Schizophrenic-like Manifestations', *Psychiat. Neurol. Jap.*, *62*, (992–1011).

HALBERSTADT, G. (1962), 'Le Demence Précoce Infantile', *Rev. Neurol.*, *2*, (209–19).

HALSTEAD, H. (1957), 'Abilities and Behaviour of Epileptic Children', *J. Ment. Sci.*, *103*, (28–47.)

HALTON, D. A. (1966), 'The Child with Minimal Cerebral Dysfunction', *Develop. Med. Child. Neurol.*, *8*, (71–8).

HARE, E. and SHAW, G. (1965), *Mental Health on a New Housing Estate*, London: Oxford University Press.

HASS, A. L. de (1959), 'Rehabilitation of Adult Epileptics in the Netherlands', *Sem. Med. Prof. Med. Soc.*, *35*, (477–9).

HAUCK, G. (1968), 'The Attitude towards Epilepsy of the General Population of Germany and the U.S.A.', *Nervenarzt*, *39*, (181–3).

HAUCK, G. (1969), 'Soziale Ursachen und Folgen von kindlicher Epilepsie', *Social Psychiatry*, *4*, (32–42).

HEIMLER, E. (1967), *Mental Illness and Social Work*, London: Pelican.

HELGASON, T. (1964), 'Epidemiology of Mental Disorders in Iceland', *Acta. Psychiat. Scand. Suppl.*, *173*.

HEMMING, J. (1966), 'Interaction as a Model of the Educational Process', *Bull. Brit. Psychol. Soc.*, *19*, (73–4).

HENDERSON, P. (1953), 'Epilepsy in School Children', *Brit. J. Prev. Soc. Med.*, *7*, (9–13).

HENDRICKSON, A. and WHITE, P. O. (1964), 'Promax: a Quick Method for Rotation to Oblique Simple Structure', *Brit. J. Statist. Psychol.*, *17*, (65–70).

HENRY, C. (1963), 'Positive Spike Discharges in the E.E.G. and Behaviour Abnormality', *in* Glaser, G. (ed.), *E.E.G.* and *Behavior*, New York: Basic Books.

HERSOV, L. (1963), 'Emotional Factors in Cerebral Palsy', *Develop. Med. Child. Neurol.*, *5*, (504–11).

HERTZIG, M., BORTNER, M. and BIRCH, H. (1969), 'Neurologic Findings in Children Educationally Designated as "Brain-damaged" ', *Amer. J. Orthopsychiat.*, *39*, (436–46).

HERZ, E. (1928), 'Über Heredogenerative und Symptomatische Schizophrenien', *Psychiat. Neurol. Monatschrift*, *68*, (265–319).

HEWITT, L. and JENKINS, R. (1946), *Fundamental Patterns of Maladjustment: the Dynamics of their Origin*, State of Illinois.

HILL, C. (1965), *How Colour Prejudiced is Britain?*, London: Gollancz.

HILL, D. (1948), 'The Relationship between Epilepsy and Schizophrenia: E.E.G. Studies', *Folia Psychiat. Neerl.*, *51*, (95–111).

HILL, D. (1952), 'E.E.G. in Episodic Psychotic and Psychopathic Behaviour', *E.E.G. Clin. Neurophysiol.*, *4*, (419–42).

HILL, D. (1953), 'Psychiatric Disorders of Epilepsy', *Med. Press.*, *229*, (473–5).

HILL, D. (1956), 'Clinical Applications of E.E.G. in Psychiatry', *J. Ment. Sci.*, *102*, (264–71).

HILL, D. (1958), 'Value of the E.E.G. in Diagnosis in Epilepsy', *Brit. Med. J.*, i, (663–6).

HILL, D. (1959), 'The Difficult Epileptic and His Social Environment', *Trans. Ass. Industr. Med. Offrs.*, *9*, (46–50).

HILL, D. and POND, D. (1952), 'Reflections on One Hundred Capital Cases submitted to Electroencephalography', *J. Ment. Sci.*, *98*, (23–43).

HOCH, P. and KNIGHT, R. (eds.) (1948), *Epilepsy—Psychiatric Aspects of Convulsive Disorders*, London: Heinemann.

HOCHAPFEL, L. (1938), 'Ueber Gleichzeitiges Vorkommen von Schizophrenie und Progressiver Muskeldystrophie', *Allg. Zeit. Psychiat.*, *109*, (16–31).

HODGE, R., WALTER, V. and WALTER, W. (1953), 'Juvenile Delinquency: an Electrophysiological, Psychological and Social Study', *Brit. J. Del.* (155–72).

HOENIG, J. and LEIBERMAN, D. M. (1953), 'The Epileptic Threshold in Schizophrenia', *J. Neurol. Neurosurg. Psychiat.*, *16*, (30–4).

HOLLINGSHEAD, A. and REDLICH, F. (1958), *Social Class and Mental Illness: A Community Study*, New York: John Wiley; London; Chapman & Hall.

HOLMES, S. S. (1936), *Human Genetics and Its Social Import*, New York: McGraw Hill.

HOMANS, G. C. (1964), 'Bringing Men Back In', *Amer. Sociol. Rev.*, *29*, (809–18).

HOPE, K. (1968), *Methods of Multivariate Analysis*, University of London Press.

HUESSY, H. (1967), 'Study of the Prevalence and Therapy of the Choreatiform Syndrome or Hyperkinesis in Rural Vermont', *Acta Paedopsychiatrica*, *34*, (130–5).

HUTT, S., JACKSON, P. and BELSHAM, A. (1968), 'Perceptual-motor Behavior in Relation to Blood Phenobarbitone Level: a Preliminary Report', *Develop. Med. Child. Neurol.*, *10*, (626–32).

HUTT, S. and HUTT, C. (1964), 'Hyperactivity in a Group of Epileptic (and Some Non-epileptic) Brain-damaged Children', *Epilepsia*, *5*, (344–52).

HUTT, S., LEE, D. and OUNSTED, C. (1963), 'Digit Memory—Evoked Discharges in Four Light-sensitive Children', *Develop. Med. Child. Neurol.*, *5*, (559–71).

HUXLEY, SIR J., MAYR, E., OSMOND, H. and HOFFER, A. (1964), 'Schizophrenia as a Genetic Morphism', *Nature*, *204*, (220–1).

INGRAM, T. T. S. (1956), 'A Characteristic Form of Overactive Behaviour in Brain-damaged Children', *J. Ment. Sci.*, *102*, (550–8).

INGRAM, T. T. S. and MASON, A. W. (1965), 'Reading and Writing Difficulties in Childhood', *Brit. Med. J.*, ii, (463–5).

INKELES, A. (1963), 'Sociology and Psychology', in *Psychology: a Study of a Science*, *6*, ed. S. Hoch, New York: McGraw-Hill.

JACKSON, J. H. (1931), *Selected Writings*, *1*, London: Hodder and Stoughton.

JACQUET, M. (1968), 'The Education of Epileptics', *Rev. Hyg. Med. Schol.*, *21*, (77–9).

JANZ, H. W. (1940), 'Klinische und experimentelle Untersuchungen über Konstitution and Krampfbereitschaft bei Epileptikern', *Arch. Psychiat. Nerven*, *112*, (136–220).

JENKINS, R. and GLICKMAN, S. (1946), 'Common Syndromes in Child Psychiatry', *Am. J. Orthopsychiat.*, *16*, (244–61).

JENKINS, R. L. (1966), 'Psychiatric Syndromes in Children and Their Relation to Family Background', *Am. J. Orthopsychiat.*, *36*, (450–7).

JENSEN, R.A. (1947), 'Importance of the Emotional Factor in the Convulsive Disorders of Children', *Am. J. Psychiat.*, *104*, (126–31).

JEWKES, J. S. (1961), *The Genesis of the British National Health Service*, Oxford: Blackwell.

JONAS, A. D. (1967), 'The Emergence of Epileptic Equivalents in the Area of Tranquilizers', *Int. J. Neuropsychiat.*, *3*, (40–5).

JONES, J. (1965), 'Employment of Epileptics', *Lancet*, ii, (486–9).

JUS, A. and JUS, K. (1963), 'Experimental and Theoretical Electroclinical Evaluation of Some Memory Disturbances', *Neurol. Neurochir. Psychiat. Pol.*, *13*, (895–900).

JUUL-JENSEN, E. (1964), 'Epilepsy—a Clinical and Social Analysis', *Acta Neurol. Scand. Suppl.*, *5*, (40).

KALLMANN, F. and SANDER, G. (1948), 'The Genetics of Epilepsy', *in* Hoch, P. and Knight, R. (eds.), *Epilepsy*, London: Heinemann.

KAUFMAN, I. (1962), 'Crimes of Violence and Delinquency in Schizophrenic Children,' *J. Am. Acad. Child Psychiat.*, *1*, (269–83).

KAYE, I. (1951), 'What are the Evidences of Social and Psychological Maladjustment revealed in a Study of Seventeen Children Who have Idiopathic Petit Mal Epilepsy?', *J. Child Psychiat.*, *20*, (115–60).

KEATING, L. (1960), 'A Review of the Literature on the Relationship of Epilepsy and Intelligence in School-children', *J., Ment. Sci.*, *106*, (1042–59).

KEATING, L. (1962), 'Epilepsy and Behaviour Disorder in Schoolchildren', *J. Ment. Sci.*, *107*, (161–80).

KEITH, H. (1963), *Convulsive Disorders in Children*, London: Churchill.

KELLAWAY, P., CRAWLEY, J. and KAGAWA, N. (1959), 'A Specific E.E.G. Correlate of Convulsive Equivalent Disorders in Children', *J. Pediat.*, *55*, (582–92).

KELMAN, H. (1965), 'The Effect of a Brain-damaged Child on the Family', *in* Birch, H. (ed.), *Brain Damage in Children*, London: Ballière.

KENNARD, M. (1953), The Electroencephalograph in Psychological Disorders', *Psychsom. Med.*, *15*, (95–115).

KENNEDY, C. and RAMIREZ, L. (1965), 'Brain Damage as a Cause of Behaviour Disorder in Children', *in* Birch, H. (ed.), *Brain Damage in Children: Biological and Social Aspects*, London: Ballière.

KIMURA, D. (1964), 'Cognitive Deficit related to Seizure Pattern in Centrecephatic Epilepsy', *J. Neurol. Neurosurg. Psychiat.*, *27*, (291–5).

KISSEL, S. (1967), 'The Positive Spiral in Parent-child Relationships', *Mental Hygiene*, *51*, (21–6).

KLUCKHOHN, C. and MURRAY, H. (eds.) (1964), *Personality in Nature, Society and Culture*, New York: Knopf.

KOEGLER, R., COLBERT, E. and WALKER, R. (1961), 'Problems in the Correlation of Psychopathology with E.E.G. Abnormalities', *Amer. J. Psychiat.*, *117*, (822–4).

KORNRICH, M. (ed.) (1965), *Underachievement*, Springfield, Ill.: Thomas.

KRABBE, K. (1921), 'Myodonie-schizophrenie familiale', *Acta Med. Scand.*, *56*, (456–67).

KRAFFT-EBING, R. V. (1926), *Psychopathica Sexualis*, New York: Medical Art Agency.

KRAPF, E. (1928), 'Epilepsie und Schizophrenie', *Arch. Psychiat. Nervenkr.* *83*, (547–86).

KRYCH, Z., HURKALO, J., JACEQICZ, A., JANIK, J., KAPTURCZUK, R., OWCZARSKA, J., OWZARSKI, N. and WOJCICKI, A. (1965), 'Influence of Extra-clinical Factors on the Occurrence of Character Disorders in Children with Temporal-lobe Epilepsy', *Neurol. Neurochir. Psychiat. Pol.*, *15*, (863–8).

KUSHLICK, A. (1964), 'The Social Distribution of Mental Retardation', *Dev. Med. Chil. Neurol.*, *6*, (302–4).

LABOVITZ, S. (1967), 'Some Observations on Measurement and Statistics', *Social Forces*, *46*, (151–60).

LACEY, C. (1966), 'Some Sociological Concomitants of Academic Streaming in a Grammar School', *Brit. J. Sociol.*, *17*, (245–62).

Lancet (1953), 'The Epileptic Child', Annotation, ii, (387).

Lancet (1967): 'Services for Epileptics', Annotation, i, (259–60).

LANDOLT, H. (1955), 'Über Verstimmungen, Dammersustande und Schizophrene Zustandsbilder bei Epilepsie', *Schweitz. Arch. Neurol. Psychiat.*, *76*, (313–21).

LANDOLT, H. (1955), 'Über Verstimmungen, Dämmerzustände und schizophrene Zustandsbilder bei Epilepsie', *Schweitz. Arch. Neurol. Psychiat.*, *76*, (313–21).

LANDOLT, H. (1957), 'Die Bedeutung der Electrencephalographie für die Behandlung der Epilepsie', *Nervenarzt*, *28*, (170–6).

LANDOLT, H. (1958), 'Serial E.E.G Investigations during Psychotic Episodes in Epileptic Patients and during Schizophrenic Attacks', *in* de Haas (ed)., *Lectures on Epilepsy*, Amsterdam: Elsevier.

LAUFER, M. (1964), 'A Psycho-analytic Approach to Work with Adolescents', *J. Child Psychol. Psychiat.*, *5*, (217–29).

LAUFER, M. and DENHOFT, E. (1957), 'Hyperkinetic Behaviour Syndrome in Children', *Pediat.*, *50*, (463–74).

LAVITOLA, G. and VITZIOLI, D. (1955), 'Schizofrenia ed Epilepsia', *Osped. Psichiat.*, *23*, (168–70).

LEES, F. and LIVERSEDGE, L. (1962), 'The prognosis of Petit Mal and Minor Epilepsy', *Lancet*, i, (797–9).

LEFF, S. and LEFF, V. (1959), *The School Health Service*, London: Lewis.

LENNOX, W. G. (1942), 'Mental Defect in Epilepsy and the Influence of Heredity', *Am. J. Psychiat.*, *98*, (733–9).

LENNOX, W. G. and LENNOX, M. A. (1960), *Epilepsy and Related Disorders*, London: Churchill.

LEVINE, D. (1965), 'Some Key Problems in Simmel's Work', *in* Coser, L. (ed.), *Georg Simmel*, New Jersey: Prentice-Hall.

LEVY, L., FORBES, J. and PARIRENYATWA, T. (1964), 'Epilepsy in Africans', *Cent. African J. Med.*, *10*, 7 (cited in *Nature* 1964), *204*, (735).

LEVY, S. (1959), 'Post-encephalitic Behaviour Disorder—a Forgotten Entity: a Report of 100 Cases', *Am. J. Psychiat.*, *1–5*, (1,062–7).

LEVY, S. (1966), 'Hyperkinetic Syndrome in Pre-adolescence and Adolescence', *Devel. Med. Child Neurol.*, *8*, (626).

LEWIS, H. (1954), *Deprived Children (the Mersham Experiment): a Social and Clinical Study*, London: Oxford University Press.

LIBERSON, W. T. (1955), 'Emotional and Psychological Factors in Epilepsy: Physiological Background', *Amer. J. Psychiat.*, *112*, (91–106).

LISANSKY, E. S. (1948), 'Convulsive Disorder and Personality', *J. Ab. Soc. Psychol.*, *43*, (29–37).

LIVINGSTON, S. (1954), *The Diagnosis and Treatment of Convulsive Disorders in Children*, Oxford: Blackwell.

LIVINGSTON, S. (1963), *Living with Epileptic Seizures*, Illinois: Thomas.

LOTT, M. and JENKINS, R. (1953), 'Patterns of Maladjustment in Children', *J. Clin. Psychol.*, *9*, (16–19).

LOVELAND, N., SMITH, B. and FORSTER, F. (1957), 'Mental and Emotional Changes in Epileptic Patients on Continuous Anticonvulsant Medication', *Neurology*, *7*, (856–65).

LUCAS, A. R., RODIN, E. and SIMSON, C. (1965), 'Neurological Assessment of Children with Early School Problems', *Develop. Med. Child. Neurol.*, *7*, (145–56).

LUYSTERBORG, E. and SCHOLTE, H. (1965), 'A props d'un cas d'Epilepsie Psychique', *Acta Neurol. Belg.*, *65*, (134–41).

LYNN, R. (1955), 'Personality Factors in Reading Achievement', *Proc. Roy. Soc. Med.*, *48*, (996–7).

MCFIE, J. (1961), 'Intellectual Impairment in Children with Localized Post-infantile Cerebral Lesions', *J. Neurol. Neurosurg. Psychiat.*, *24*, (361–5).

McLAUGHLIN, R. and EYSENCK, H. (1967), 'Extraversion, Neuroticism and Paired-associates Learning', *J. Exp. Res. Personal*, *2*, (128–32).

MACRAE, D. (1954), 'Isolated Fear—a Temporal Lobe Aura', *Neurol. Minneap.*, *4*, (497–505).

MAGUIRE, U. (1966), 'The Effects of Anxiety on Learning, Task performance and Level of Aspiration in Secondary Modern School Children', *Brit. J. Ed. Psychol.*, *36*, (109–12).

MANNHEIM, H. (1966), *Comparative Criminology*, London: Routledge.

MASLAND, R. (1960), 'Classification of the Epilepsies', *Epilepsia*, *1*, (512–20).

MATTHEWS, C. and KLØVE, H. (1967), 'Differential Psychological Performances in Major Motor, Psychomotor and Mixed Seizure Classifications of Known and Unknown Etiology', *Epilepsia*, *8*, (117–28).

MAUDSLEY, H. (1873), *Responsibility in Mental Disease*, New York: Appleton.

MAURA RIBERO, R., ARMBRUST FIGVERIREDO, J. and MAURA RIBERO, V. (1964), 'Abdominal Epilepsy in Children', *Arch. Neuro-Psiquiat.* (*S. Paulo*), *22*, (44–50).

MCNEMAR, Q. (1955), *Psychological Statistics*, New York: Wiley.

MAXWELL, A. E. (1961), *Analysing Qualitative Data*, London: Methuen.

MAYER-GROSS, W., SLATER, E. and ROTH, N. (1955), *Clinical Psychiatry*, London: Cassell.

MAYMAN, M. and RAPAPORT, D. (1948), 'Diagnostic Testing in Convulsive Disorders', *in* Hoch, P. and Knight, R. (eds.), *Epilepsy*, London: Heinemann.

MERRITT, H. (1959), *A Textbook of Neurology*, London: Kimpton.

MEAD, G. (1956), *On Social Psychology*, University of Chicago Press.

MEADOW, K. (1969), 'Self Image, Family Climate, and Deafness', *Social Forces*, *47*, (428–38).

METRAKOS, J. and K. (1960), 'Genetics of Convulsive Disorders. I. Introduction, problems, methods and base lines', *Neurology*, *10*, (228–40).

METRAKOS, J. and K. (1963), 'Is Pregnancy Order a Factor in Epilepsy?', *J. Neurol. Neurosurg. Psychiat.*, *26*, (451–7).

MEYERS, R. and BRECHER, S. (1941), 'The So-called Epileptic Personality as investigated by the Kent-Rosanoff Test', *J. Ab. Soc. Psychol.*, *36*, (413–22).

MICHAEL, S. T. (1961), 'Neurotic Symptoms in an Urban Population', in *I. Congressus Psychiatricus Behemoslovenicus cum Participatione Internationali 1959*, eds. O. Janota and E. Wolf, Prague: State Printing House.

MILNER, B. (1954), 'Intellectual Function of the Temporal Lobes', *Psychol. Bull.*, *51*, (42–62).

MILSTEIN, V. and STEVENS, J. R. (1961), 'Verbal and Conditional Avoidance Learning during Abnormal E.E.G. Discharge', *J. Nerv. and Ment. Dis.*, *132*, i, (50–60).

MITCHELL, W., FALCONER, M. and HILL, D. (1954), 'Epilepsy with Fetishism relieved by Temporal Lobectomy', *Lancet*, ii, (626–30).

MONTAGU, A. (1964), *Life Before Birth*, New York: Longmans.

MORONEY, M. (1956), *Facts from Figures*, London: Penguin Books.

MORRIS, C. (1956), *Varieties of Human Value*, University of Chicago Press.

MOYA, G., JULIAN-RAMO, S. and GRANDAS, I. (1968), 'Spanish Public Opinion on the Subject of Epilepsy', *Rev. Sanid. Hig. Publ.*, *42*, (203–76).

MÜLLER, G. (1930), 'Anfalle bei schizophrenen Erkrankungen', *Allg. Z. Psychiat.*, *93*, (235–40).

MULLIGAN, D. G. (1964), 'Some Correlates of Maladjustment in a National Sample of Schoolchildren', Ph.D. thesis, University of London.

MURPHY, G. (1947), *Personality: A Biosocial Approach to Origins and Structure*, New York: Harper.

NAVRATIL, L. and STROTZKA, H. (1954), 'Die Kind Mutter-Relation bei Epileptischen Kindern', *Arch. f. Psychol.*, *4*, (36–53).

NEUMAN, C. J. and KRUG, O. (1964), 'Problems in Learning Arithmetic in Emotionally Disabled Children', *J. Amer.-Acad. Child Psychiat.*, *3*, (413–29).

NICHOLLS, J. V. (1962), 'The Retarded Reader', *Postgrad. Med.*, *31*, (66–71).

NORWOOD EAST, W. (1936), *Medical Aspects of Crime*, London: Churchill.

NOTKIN, J. (1928), 'Is there an Epileptic Personality Make-up?', *Arch. Neurol. Psychiat.*, *26*, (799–803).

NUFFIELD, E. (1961), 'Neuro-physiology and Behaviour Disorders in Epileptic Children', *J. Ment. Sci.*, *107*, (348–58).

OLESSEVICH, A. and PROTASSEVICH, L. (1936), 'Experiences in a Neuropsychiatric Clinic with the Occupational Therapy of Epilepsy and Mental Deficiency in Children', *Sovet. Pediats.*, *5*, (108).

OPPLER, W. (1933), 'Erbbiologische Nachkommenuntersuchungen bei Einem Fall von Huntingtonscher Chorea mit Schizophren gefaebter Psychose', *Zeitschr. Neurol. Psychiat.*, *144*, (769–83).

OSWIN, N. (1967), *Behaviour Problems amongst Children with Cerebral Palsy*, Bristol: John Wright.

OUNSTED, C. (1955), 'The Hyperkinetic Syndrome in Epileptic Children', *Lancet*, ii, (303).

OUNSTED, C. and SMITH, H. M. C. (1955), *The Psychology of the Patient and Relatives as a Factor in Successful Treatment: the Mental Welfare of Children after Tuberculosis Meningitis*, trans. NAPT 4th Commonwealth Tuberculosis Conference, June, (280–3).

OUNSTED, C., LINDSAY, J. and NORMAN, R. (1966), *Biological Factors in Temporal Lobe Epilepsy* (Clinics in Develop. Med.), London: Heinemann.

PAGE, J. (1947), *Abnormal Psychology*, New York: McGraw-Hill.

PAMPIGLIONE, G. (1955), 'The Recurrent Abdominal Syndrome in Children: Clinical and E.E.G. Observations in 52 Cases', paper read at the Institute of Neurology, London.

PANTELAKIS S. BOWER D. and JONES H. B. (1962), 'Convulsions and Television Viewing', *Brit. Med. J.*, ii, (633–8).

PARNELL, R. and SKOTTOWE, I. (1962), 'The Significance of Somatype and Other Signs of Psychiatric Prognosis and Treatment', *Proc. Roy. Soc. Med.*, *55*, (707–16).

PARSONS, O. and KEMP, D. (1960), 'Intellectual Functioning in Temporal Lobe Epilepsy', *J. Consult. Psychol.*, *24*, (408–14).

PARSONS, T. (1937), *The Structure of Social Action*, New York: Free Press of Glencoe.

PARSONS, T. (1964), *Social Structure and Personality*, New York: Free Press of Glencoe.

PARSONS, T. and SHILS, A. eds. (1951), *Toward a General Theory of Action*, New York: Harper & Row.

PASAMANICK, B. (1951), 'Anticonvulsant Drug Therapy of Behaviour Problem Children with Abnormal E.E.G.', *Arch. Neurol. Psychiat.*, *65*, (752–6).

PATTERSON, G. and BRODSKY, G. (1966), 'A Behaviour Modification Programme for a Child with Multiple Problem Behaviours', *J. Child. Psychol. Psychiat.*, *1*, (277–95).

PATTERSON, G. R., JONES, R., WHITTIER, J. and WRIGHT, M. (1965), 'A Behaviour Modification Technique for the Hyperactive Child', *Behav. Res. Ther.*, *2*, (217–26).

PENFIELD, W. and FLANIGAN, M. (1950), 'Surgical Therapy of Temporal Lobe Seizures', *Arch. Neurol. Psychiat.*, *64*, (491–500).

PENFIELD, W. and JASPER, H. (1954), *Epilepsy and the Functional Anatomy of the Human Brain*, Boston: Little, Brown.

PERSCH, R. (1938), 'Heredodegenerative Schizophrenia bei kombinierter Systemerkrankung', *Psychiat. Neurol. Wschr.*, (311–13).

PETERMAN, M. (1958), 'Behaviour in Epileptic Children', *J. Pediat.*, *42*, (758–69).

PINANSKI, J. (1947), 'The Vocational Problem of the Epileptic Child', *Nerv. Child.*, *6*, (105–14).

POND, D. (1952), 'Psychiatric Aspects of Epilepsy in Children', *J. Ment. Sci.*, *98*, (404–10).

POND, D. (1957), 'Psychiatric Aspects of Epilepsy', *J. Ind. Med. Prof.*, *31*, (1,441–51).

POND, D. (1961), 'Psychiatric Aspects of Epileptic and Brain-damaged Children', *Brit. Med. J.*, ii, (1,377–82, 1,454–9).

POND, D. (1963), 'Maturation, Epilepsy and Psychiatry', *Proc. Roy. Soc. Med.*, *56*, (710–13).

POND, D. (1965), 'Towards Better Treatment of Epileptics', *Guardian*, 11 May.

POND, D. (1965), 'The Neuropsychiatry of Childhood', *in* Howells, J. (ed.), *Modern Perspectives in Child Psychiatry*, Edinburgh: Oliver & Boyd.

POND, D. and BIDWELL, B. (1954), 'Management of Behaviour Disorders in Epileptic children', *Brit. Med. J.*, ii, (1,520).

POND, D. and BIDWELL, D. (1960), 'A Survey of Epilepsy in Fourteen General Practices: II. Social and Psychological Aspects', *Epilepsia*, *1*, (285–99).

POND, D., BIDWELL, B. and STEIN, L. (1960), 'A Survey of Epileptics in 14 General Practices: I. Demographic and Medical Data', *Psychiat. Neurol. Neurochir.*, *63*, (217–36).

POPPER, K. (1961), *The Poverty of Historicism*, London: Routledge.

POSER, C. and ZIEGLER, D. (1958), 'Clinical Significance of 14–6 per Second Positive Spike Complexes', *Neurology*, *8*, (903–12).

PRATT, R. (1965), 'Epilepsy and Schizophrenia', Sandoz Lecture, National Hospital, London, 3 November.

PRECHTL, H. and STEMMER, C. (1952), 'The Choreiform Syndrome in Children', *Dev. Med. Child. Neurol.*, *4*, (119–27).

PRICE, J. C. (1950), 'The Epileptic Child in School', *Ohio State Med. School*, *46*, (794–805).

PRICE, J. and PUTMAN, T. (1944), 'The Effect of Intrafamily Discord on the Prognosis of Epilepsy', *Am. J. Psychiat.*, *100*, (593–8).

PRITCHARD, D. (1963), *Education and the Handicapped*, London: Routledge.

PRITCHARD, M. (1963), 'Observation of Children in a Psychiatric In-patient Unit', *Brit. J. Psychiat.*, *109*, (572–8).

PUTNAM, T. J. and MERRITT, H. H. (1941), 'Dullness as an Epileptic Equivalent', *Arch. Neurol. Psychiat.*, *45*, (797–813).

QUAY, H., MORSE, W. and CURTER, R. (1966), 'Personality Patterns of Pupils in Special Classes for the Emotionally Disturbed', *Except. Child.*, *32*, (297–301).

RADCLIFFE, B. (1864), *Lectures on Epilepsy, Pain and Paralysis*, London: Churchill.

RECHTENWALD, (1920), 'Ueber Einer Familiaren Fortschrittenden Muskelschwund in Verbindung mit Schizophrener Verbloedung', *Zeitschr. Neurol. Psychiat.*, *53*, (203–14).

REES, W. L. and EYSENCK, H. J. (1945), 'A Factorial Study of Some Morphological and Psychological Aspects of Human Constitution', *J. Ment. Sci.*, *91*, (8–21).

REGISTRAR GENERAL (1961), *Classification of Occupations*, London: H.M.S.O.

REY, J., POND, D. and EVANS, C. (1949), 'Clinical and E.E.G. Studies of Temporal Lobe Function', *Proc. Roy. Soc. Med.*, *42*, (891–904).

REYNOLDS, E. H. (1967), 'Effects of Folic Acid on the Mental State and Fit-frequency of Drug-treated Epileptic Patients', *Lancet*, i, (1,086–9).

RICHARDSON, S. (1965), 'The Social Environment and Individual Functioning', *in* Birch, H. (ed.), *Brain Damage in Children: Biological and Social Aspects*, London Ballière.

RIMLAND, B. (1964), *Infantile Autism*, London: Methuen.

RIVER, J. P. de (1956), *The Sexual Criminal*, Springfield, Ill.: Charles C. Thomas.

ROBB, J. H. (1961), *Decentralization and the Citizen*, Oxford University Press.

ROBERTIELLO, R. (1953), 'Psychomotor Epilepsy in Children', *Dis. Nerv. Syst.*, *14*, (337–9).

ROBIN, A. and MALBRAIN, H. (1964), 'Abdominal Epilepsy in Children', *Acta. Neurol. Belg.*, *64*, (323–30).

ROBINS, L. (1966), *Deviant Children Grown Up*, Baltimore: Williams & Wilkins.

RODIN, E., LUCAS, A. and SIMPSON, C. (1963), 'A Study of Behavior Disorders in Children by Means of General Purpose Computers', *Proc. Conf. Data Acquisition in Processing in Biology and Medicine*, New York: Pergamon.

RODIN, E. and GONZALEZ, S. (1966), 'Heredity Components in Epileptic Patients', *J. Amer. Med. Assoc.*, *198*, (122–5).

RODIN, E., LYN, Y., GONZALEZ, S. and DENNERILL, R. D. (1964), 'The Application of Computer Techniques to Clinical Research in Convulsive Disorders', *I.E.E.E. Transactions on Biomedical Engineering*, January, (19–23).

ROGERS, M., LILIENFELD, A. and PASAMANICK, B. (1955), 'Prenatal and Paranatal Factors in the Development of Childhood Behaviour Disorders', *Acta Psychiat. Neurol. Scand., Suppl. 102.*

ROSE, A. (1962), *Human Behavior and Social Process—an Interactionist Approach*, Boston: Houghton Mifflin.

ROWS, R. and BOND, W. (1926), *Epilepsy: a Functional Mental Illness*, London: Lewis.

ROYO, D. and MARTIN, F. (1959), 'Standardised Psychometrical Tests applied to the Analysis of the Effects of Anti-convulsive Medication on the Intellectual Proficiency of Young Epileptics', *Epilepsia*, *1*, (189–207).

RUNCIMAN, W. G. (1963), *Social Science and Political Theory*, Cambridge University Press.

RUSHTON, J. (1966), 'The Relationship between Personality Characteristics and Scholastic Sucess in Eleven-year-old Children', *Brit. J. Ed. Psychol.*, *36*, (178–84).

RUSSELL, B. (1967), *The Autobiography of Bertrand Russell*, London: Allen & Unwin.

RUTTER, M. (1963), 'Some Current Research Issues in American Child Psychology', *Milbank Mem. Fund Quart.*, *41*, (339).

RUTTER, M. (1964), 'Intelligence and Childhood Psychiatric Disorder', *Brit. J. Soc. Clin. Psychol.*, *3*, (120–9).

RUTTER, M. (1965),'Classification and Categorization in Child Psychiatry', *J. Child. Psychol. Psychiat.*, *6*, (71–83).

RUTTER, M. (1967), 'A Children's Behaviour Questionnaire for Completion by Teachers: Preliminary Findings', *J. Child. Psychol. Psychiat.*, *8*, (1–11).

RUTTER, M., BIRCH, H., THOMAS, A. and CHESS, S. (1964), 'Temperamental Characteristic in Infancy and Later Development of Behavioural Disorders', *Brit. J. Psychiat.*, *110*, (651–61).

RUTTER, M., KORN, S. and BIRCH, H. (1963), 'Genetic and Environmental Factors in the Development of Primary Reaction Patterns', *Brit. J. Soc. Clin. Psychol.*, *2*, (161–73).

RUTTER, M. *et al.* (1966), 'Severe Reading Retardation: its Relationship to Maladjustment, Epilepsy and Neurological Disorders', paper given to Association for Special Education, London.

RYLE, A. and HAMILTON, M. (1962), 'Neurosis in Fifty Married Couples', *J. Ment. Sci.*, *108*, (265–73).

SANQUIST, J. and MORGAN, J. N. (1964), *The Detection of Interaction Effects*, Survey Research Centre: University of Michigan Monograph.

SARVIS, M. A. (1960), 'Psychiatric Implications of Temporal Lobe Damage', in Erssler, R. S., *et al.* (eds.), *Psychoanalytic Study of the Child*, Vol. 15, International Universities Press.

SCHAEFER, E. and BELL, R. (1959), 'Development of a Parental Attitude Research Instrument', *Child Devel.*, *29*, (339–61).

SCHORSCH, G. and HEDENSTROM, I. VON (1957), 'Die Schwenkungsbreite Hirnelektrischer Erregbarkeit in ihrer Beziehung zu Epileptischen Anfallen und Verstimmunszuständen', *Archiv. Psychiat. Nervenkr.*, *195*, (393–407).

SCHULZ, B. (1928), 'Beitrag zur Genealogie der Chorea Minor', *Zeitschr. Neurol. Psychiat.*, *117*, (288–314).

SCHUTTE, W. (1968), 'Epilepsy from the Patient's Point of View', *Nervenartz*, (296–301).

SCHWADE, B. and GEIGER, S. (1956), 'Abnormal E.E.G. Findings in Severe Behaviour Disorders', *Dis. Nerv. System.* *17*, (307–17).

SCHWEBEL, A. (1966), 'Aspects of Impulsivity on Performance of Verbal Tasks', *Amer. J. Orthopsychiat.*, *36*, (13–21).

SERAFETINIDES, G. (1965), 'Aggressiveness in Temporal Lobe Epileptics and Its Relation to Cerebral Dysfunction and Environmental Factors', *Epilepsia*, *6*, (33–42).

SETHNA, M. J. (1956), *Society and the Criminal*, Bombay: Leaders' Press.

SHAW, M. and CRUICKSHANK, W. (1957), 'The Rorschach Performance of Epileptic Children', *J. Consult. Psychol.*, *21*, (422–5).

SHELDON, W., STEVENS, S. and RUCKER, W. (1940), *The Varieties of Human Physique*, New York: Harper.

SIEGEL, S. (1956), *Nonparametric Statistics*, New York: McGraw-Hill.

SIEGEL, S. (1956), *Non-Parametric Statistics for the Behavioral Sciences*, New York: McGraw-Hill.

SIEGELMAN, M. (1965), 'Evaluation of Bronfenbrenner's Questionnaire for Children Concerning Parental Behaviour', *Child Develop.*, *36*, (163–74).

SIEGMUND, W. and PACHE, H. (1953), 'Die Roschachse Psychodiagnostik in ihrer Bedeutung die Prognose der Pyknolepsie', *Mschr. Kinderheilk.*, *101*, (191–2).

SKOTTOWE, I. (1965), 'Somatometry—a Second Look', *Brit. J. Psychiat. 111*, (4–9).
SLATER, E., BEARD, A. and GLITHERO, E. (1963), 'The Schizophrenia-like Psychoses of Epilepsy', *Brit. J. Psychiat.*, *109*, (95–150).
SMALL, J. HAYDEN, M. and SMALL, I. (1966), 'Further Psychiatric Investigations of Patients with Temporal- and Non-Temporal Lobe Epilepsy', *Am. J. Psychiat.*, *123*, (303–10).
SMALL, J., MILSTEIN, V. and STEVENS, J. (1962), 'Are Psychomotor Epileptics Different?', *Arch. Neurol.*, *7*, (187–94).
SOKAL, R. and SNEATH, P. (1963), *Principles of Numerical Taxonomy*, San Francisco: Freeman.
SOMERFELD-ZISKIND, E. and ZISKIND, E. (1940), 'Effect of Phenobarbital on the Mentality of Epileptic Patients', *Arch. Neurol. Psychiat.*, *43*, (70–9).
SPIRO, M. (1951), 'Culture and Personality—the Natural History of a False Dichotomy', *Psychiatry*, *14*, (19–48).
STAFFORD-CLARK, D. and TAYLOR, F. H. (1949), 'Clinical and Electroencephalographic Studies of Prisoners charged with Murder', *J. Neurol. Neurosurg. Psychiat.*, *12*, (325–30).
STARR, M. (1904), 'Is Epilepsy a Functional Disease?', *J. Nerv. Ment. Dis.*, *31*, (145–56).
STEIN, C. (1933), 'Hereditary Factors in Epilepsy: a Comparative Study of 1,100 Institutionalized Epileptics and 1,115 Non-epileptic Controls', *Amer. J. Psychiat.*, *89*, (989–1,037).
STEKEL, W. (1923), *Conditions of Nervous Anxiety and Their Treatment*, London: Kegan Paul.
STEKEL, W. (1933), *The Homosexual Neurosis*, Vol. II, New York; Physicians and Surgeons Book Co. (trans. J. V. Treslaar).
STEKEL, W. (1951), *Auto-eroticism*, London: Peter Nevill.
STEVENS, D., BOYDSTUN, J. DYKMAN, R., PETERS, J. and SINTON, D. (1967), 'Presumed Minimal Brain Dysfunction in Children', *Arch. Gen. Psychiat.*, *16*, (281–5).
STEVENS, J. (1966), 'Psychiatric Implications of Psychomotor Epilepsy', *Arch. Gen. Psychiat.*, *14*, (461–71).
STEVENS, S. (1957), 'On the Psychophysical Law', *Psychol.Rev.*, *64*, (153–81).
STEWART, M., PITTS, F., GRAIG, A. and OIEURUF, W. (1966), 'The Hyperactive Child Syndrome', *Am. J. Orthopsychiat.*, *36*, (861–7).
STONE, F. B. and RAWLEY, V. M. (1965), 'Children's Behaviour Problems and Parental Attitudes', *J. Genet. Psychol.*, *107*, (281–7).
STOTT, D. (1966), *Studies of Troublesome Children*, London: Tavistock.
STOTT, D. H. (1964), 'Sociological and Psychological Explanations of Delinquency', *Int. J. Soc. Psychiat.*, Congress Issue, ii, (35–43).
STRAUSS, A. and LEHTINEN, L. (1947), *Psychopathology and Education of the Brain Injured Child*, Vol. I, New York: Grune & Stratton.
STRAUSS, R. and KEPHART, N. (1955), *Psychopathology and Education of the Brain-Injured Child*, ii, New York: Grune & Stratton.
STUTTE, W. KLUGE, D. and DOBLER, A. (1962), 'Psychiatric Experience—Problems of the Inherent Psychic Activity of Ospolot', *Internat. Sympos. on Ospolot*, Vol. 4.
SULLIVAN, H. S. (1965), *The Fusion of Psychiatry and Social Science*, New York: Norton.
SYMONDS, C. (1955), 'Classification of the Epilepsies', *Brit. Med. J.*, i, (1,235–8).
SZASZ, T. (1966), 'Whither Psychiatry?', *Social Research*, (439–62).
TANNER, J. (1958), 'The Evaluation of Physical Growth and Development', in *Modern Trends in Pediatrics*, London: Butterworth.

TAPRA, F. (1965), 'Medication of Brain-Damaged Children', *Dis. Nerv. Syst.*, *26*, (490–5).

TATARENNO, N. (1930), 'Zur Frage der heredogenerativen Schizophrenie', *Monetschr. Psychiat.*, *77*, (364–71).

TELLENBACH, H. (1965), 'Epilepsie als Anfallsleiden und als Psychose über alternative Psychosen Prägung bei "forcierter Normalisierung" (Landolt) des E.E.G. Epileptischer', *Nervernarzt*, *36*, (190–202).

TEMKIN, O. (1945), *The Falling Sickness*, Johns Hopkins University.

TENNEY, J. W. and LENNOX, M. A. (1961), 'Children with Epilepsy', in Magary, J. F. and Eichorn, J. R. (eds.) *The Exceptional Child*, New York: Holt, Rinehart & Winston.

TEUBER, H. L. and RUDEL, R. G. (1962), 'Behaviour after Cerebral Lesions in Children and Adults', *Devel. Med. Child. Neurol.*, *4*, (3–20).

THODAY, J. M. (1965) in Meade, J., and Parkes, A. (eds.), *Biological Aspects of Social Problems*, Edinburgh: Oliver & Boyd.

THOM, D. and WALKER, G. (1922), 'Epilepsy in the Offspring of Epileptics', *Am. J. Psychiat.*, *1*, (613–27).

THOMAS, A. (1965), 'What shapes the Child?', *New Society*, 11 November, (13–16).

THOMAS, A., BIRCH, H., CHESS, S.,HERTZIG, M. and KORN, S. (1964), *Behavioural Individuality in Early Childhood*, University of London Press.

THURSTONE, L. (1947), *Multiple Factor Analysis*, Chicago: University of Chicago Press.

TIZARD, B. (1962), 'The Personality of Epileptics; a Discussion of the Evidence', *Psychol. Bull.*, *59*, (196–210).

TIZARD, B. and MARGERISON, J. (1963), 'The Relationship between Generalized Paroxysmal E.E.G. Discharges and Various Test Situations in Two Epileptic Patients', *J. Neurol. Neurosurg. Psychiat.*, *26*, (308–13).

TOMAN, J. E. P. (1962), 'Physiological Triggering Mechanisms in Childhood Epilepsy', *Amer. J. Orthopsychiat.*, *32*, (507–14).

TUCKER, W. and FORSTER, F. (1950), 'Petit Mal Epilepsy occurring in *Status*', *Arch. Neurol. Psychiat.*, *64*, (823–7).

TUCKMAN, E. (1963), 'Emotional Disturbance in 8 and 9-year-old Children with Disparity between Reading Age on Test and Non-verbal Intelligence Level', M.D. thesis, University of London.

TUKE, D. (1882), *History of the Insane in the British Isles*, London: Kegan Paul & Trench.

TUREEN, L. and WOOLSEY, R. (1964), 'Some Psychiatric Aspects of Convulsive Disorders', *Missouri Med.*, *61*, (91–8).

TURNER, W. A. (1927), 'Observations on Epilepsy', *J. Neurol. Psychiat.*, *7*, (193–207).

UNDERWOOD, E. (1955), *Report of the Committee on Maladjusted Children*, London: H.M.S.O.

VISLIE, H. and HENRIKSON, G. (1958), 'Psychic Disturbances in Epileptics', in De Haas, A. M. (ed.) *Lectures on Epilepsy*, Amsterdam: Elsevier.

WADA, T. and LENNOX, W. (1955), 'So-called "Temporal" Epilepsy', *Folia Psychiat. Neurol. Jap.*, *8*, (294–301).

WADE, N. (1969), 'The Hopi and the Hopewell: a Genetic Puzzle', *New Society*, 15 May, (745–6).

WAHLER, R., WINKEL, G., PETERSON, R. and MORRISON, D. (1965), 'Mothers as Behaviour Therapists for Their Own Children', *Behav. Res. Ther.*, *3*,(113–24).

WALKER, A. (1961), 'Murder or Epilepsy?', *J. Nerv. Ment. Dis.*, *133*, (430–7).

WALKER, A. (1967), 'Cultural Variants and Psychological Illness in West Indian and British Children', paper given to Institute of Race Relations Conference, London, 21 September.

WALKER, E. and KATZ, D. (1958), 'Brain-damaged Children: the Problem of Relations in the Family Group', *Calif. Med.*, *88*, (320–3).

WAPNER, I. THURSTON, D. C. and HOLOUACH, J. (1962), 'Phenobarbital: Its Effect on Learning in Epileptic Children', *J. Am. Med. Assoc.*, *182*, (937).

WATTS, C. (1962) 'Diseases of the Nervous System', in *Morbidity Statistics from General Practice*, Vol III, 53–66, London: General Register Office.

WEIDER, A. (1951), 'The Wechsler Intelligence Scale for Children and the Revised Stanford-Binet', *J. Consult. Psychol.*, *15*, (330–3).

WHILDIN, O. (1947), 'The Epileptic Child in the Public School', *Nerv. Child.*, *6*, (99–104).

WHIMBEY, A. E. and DENENBERG, V. H. (1966), 'Programming Life Histories: Creating Individual Differences by the Experimental Control of Early Experiences', *Multivariate Behav. Res.*, *1*, (279–86).

WHITLOCK, R. V. (1967), 'A Study of the Effects of Emotional Arousal on Learning', M. Phil. thesis, London.

WHITMORE, K. (1964), 'Epilepsy in Children', paper read to Association for Child Psychology. Psychiat. meeting, Royal Society of Medicine, 11 November.

WHITTY, C. (1956), 'The Diagnosis of Epilepsy', *J. Ind. Med. Prof.*, *3*, (1,268–80).

WIDROW, S. A. (1966), 'The Diagnosis of Minimal Brain Damage', *Med. Soc. N.J.*, *63*, (47–50).

WIERSMA, E. D. (1923), 'The Psychology of Epilepsy', *J. Ment. Sci.*, *69*, (482–97).

WILLIAMS, D. (1956), 'The Structure of Emotions reflected in Epileptic Experiences', *Brain*, *79*, (29–67).

WILLIAMS, D. (1963), 'The Psychiatry of the Epileptic', *Proc. Roy. Soc. Med.*, *56*, (701–10).

WILLIAMS, D. (1966), 'Temporal Lobe Epilepsy', *Brit. Med. J.*, i, (1,439–42).

WILSON, W., STEWART, L. and PARKER, J. (1960), 'A Study of the Socio-economic Effects of Epilepsy', *Epilepsia*, *1*, (300–15).

WILSON, W. P. and HARRIS, B. S. H. (1966), 'Psychiatric Problems in Children with Frontal Central and Temporal Lobe Epilepsy', *South. Med. J.*, *59*, (49–53).

WINSTON, E. and CHILMAN, C. (1964), 'Epilepsy, Some Social, Psychological, Educational, Economic and Legal Aspects', *Welfare in Review*, *2*, (1–9).

WODDIS, G. N. (1964), 'Clinical Psychiatry and Crime', *Brit. J. Criminol.*, *4*, (443–66).

WOLF, M. G. (1965), 'Effects of Emotional Disturbance in Childhood on Intelligence', *Am. J. Orthopsychiat.*, *35*, (906–8).

WOLFF, P. and HURWITZ, I. (1966), 'The Choreiform Syndrome', *Develop. Med. Child Neurol.*, *4*, (160–5).

WOOTTON, B. (1966), 'On the Criminological Treadmill', *Guardian*, 3 March.

WORLD HEALTH ORGANIZATION (1957), 'Juvenile Epilepsy—Report of a Study Group', *W.H.O. Techn. Rep. Ser.*, *130*.

WORTIS, H., BRAINE, M., CUTLER, R. and FREEDMAN, A. (1964), 'Deviant Behaviour in Two and a Half-year-old Premature Children', *Child Develop.*, *35*, (871–9).

YAWORSKY, W. and KEMP, J. (1966), 'A Study of Affects in an Emotionally Disturbed Child with a Convulsive Disorder', *Psychosomatics*, *7*, (315–17).

YATES, F. (1958), *The Design and Analysis of Factorial Experiments*, Harpenden: Commonwealth Agricultural Bureaux, Rothamsted Experimental Station.

YDE, A., LOHSE, E. and FAURBGE, A. (1941), 'On the Relation between Schizophrenia, Epilepsy and Induced Convulsions', *Acta Psychiat. Scand.*, *16*, (325–88).

ZIMMERMAN, F. T., BURGERMEISTER, B. B. and PUTMAN, T. J. (1951), 'Intellectual and Emotional Make-up of the Epileptic', *Arch. Neurol. Psychiat.*, *65*, (545–56).

ZWEIG, F. (1965), *The Quest for Fellowship*, London: Heinemann.

Author index

Subject index

For Product Safety Concerns and Information please contact our
EU representative GPSR@taylorandfrancis.com Taylor & Francis
Verlag GmbH, Kaufingerstraße 24, 80331 München, Germany